# THE ESSENTIAL GUIDE TO FOODS THAT HEAL

Suzannah Olivier is a qualified nutritional therapist and best-selling author. She acts as consultant to a number of companies including Multibionta and Organix. She writes regularly for national newspapers and many magazines and websites. She is the author of *Healthy Food for Happy Kids*, *Banish Bloating*, *Natural Hormone Balance*, *Allergy Solutions*, *The Detox Manual* and *The Breast Cancer Prevention and Recovery Diet* and several other books.

# THE ESSENTIAL GUIDE TO FOODS THAT HEAL

Suzannah Olivier

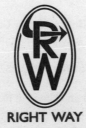

**RIGHT WAY**

Constable & Robinson Ltd
55–56 Russell Square
London WC1B 4HP
www.constable.robinson.com

Originally published in the UK under the title *Food Medicine*,
this edition published in the UK by Right Way,
an imprint of Constable & Robinson, 2012

A copy of the British Library Cataloguing in
Publication Data is available from the British Library

ISBN: 978-0-7160-2327-2

Printed and bound in the EU
1 3 5 7 9 10 8 6 4 2

# Contents

## Part 4: A–Z of Nutrients, Signs of Insufficiency and Food Sources  331

*I would like to thank Dr Margaret Rayman, Professor Joe Millward and Mrs Julie Paice who put together the nutritional medicine masters degree course at Surrey University to make the science, practice and art of nutrition available to those in the medical profession who are interested. In 2002, the Royal College of Physicians, in their publication* A Doctor's Responsibility, *said 'Doctors' knowledge of nutrition and its clinical relevance remains poor . . . Every doctor should recognize that proper nutritional care is fundamental to good clinical practice.' Medical schools have, to date, offered little training in nutrition other than in the most limited sense, but this is bound to change with the swell of interest in the subject from the general public, their physicians, and the input of dedicated and far-sighted people such as these.*

# Important Note

The advice in this book should not be used as an alternative to your doctor's advice. Patients on medication must not stop or reduce any prescribed drugs without consulting their medical advisors. In the first instance you are advised to seek correct diagnosis of any condition from your doctor and to discuss a treatment plan that includes nutritional elements if appropriate. It is important to take care with any changes and to use common sense. If a condition worsens, stop making the change and seek medical advice. By and large sensible nutritional intervention is usually extremely beneficial. This book aims to point out the disadvantages as well as the advantages, but concentrates on nutritional measures which are the best researched and the safest.

# Introduction

The last 15 years or so have seen an explosion of interest in how nutrition can prevent, stabilize, improve or even cure many conditions. Healthy eating messages have become the clarion-call of health professionals and government health departments. We are in a new era where the individual is advised to take responsibility for his or her own health. Nowadays, nobody would seriously dispute the advantages of incorporating the basic healthy eating messages into their lives to avoid the major killer and degenerative diseases – along with other lifestyle changes such as stopping smoking, remaining physically active, and moderating the use of alcohol.

The practice and art of nutrition goes back into the mists of time with every family, village and region having its favourite recipes and 'cures'. Going back to around 400 BC, Hippocrates, dubbed the father of medicine, penned the Hippocratic oath to which all doctors subscribe. He also said, famously: 'Let food be your medicine.' Even at the beginning of the twentieth century doctors were prescribing rest cures with fortifying tonics and specific foods for particular ailments: liver for its blood restoring properties (it is rich in iron), cod liver oil for joint problems (it provides anti-inflammatory fatty acids), and carrots to improve night vision (vitamin A, made from betacarotene in carrots, is vital for the health of the retina).

With the advent of more impressive medical interventions, however, health care became the province of the pharmacist. It seemed for a while that nutrition was relegated to the status of, at best, a feel-good approach or, at worst, the province of quacks and charlatans. The only areas of medicine to continue routinely to advocate excellent nutrition, for disease prevention and optimal health, have been in dentistry and obstetrics.

Adverse reactions to *prescribed* drugs cost the health services over £0.5 billion. The most common adverse reactions are to familiar over-the-counter pharmaceutical medicines such as aspirin (which can cause internal bleeding). It makes much more sense to improve health and to avoid the need for prescription drugs wherever possible. If you can lower cholesterol, lower blood pressure, reduce menopausal problems and get rid of pain or headaches with diet – why not do so? Finding the cause of the pain, or other health problem, instead of simply subduing it, is a guiding principle of nutritional therapy.

## Nutritional Medicine

Nutritional medicine works. Give the body what it needs for its biochemical processes and, for the most part, it fixes itself. It is a longer-term approach than simply masking symptoms with drugs. For instance, if you have frequent headaches, premenstrual problems or joint aches, simply to take painkillers is to subdue the messenger. Whatever is causing the particular problem will cause it to continue and possibly to manifest later in life as a more life-threatening condition.

Nutrition has a wealth of good strong scientific evidence behind it. All the answers are far from in, and anyone who would like to have the definitive answer on how, say, tomatoes or onions might influence health will have to wait a bit longer. But we are gaining valuable clues and insights. If you type the words 'human nutrition' into a medical research database you will get back over 140,000 references – and the evidence is growing exponentially.

Having said this, nutrition is still the poor cousin of research, mainly because not very much money can result from findings. The reason for mentioning the poor financing of nutrition research is to highlight the fact that we are still, to some degree, dependent on traditional use and observation. This is not necessarily to be sniffed at. Indeed the way that foods interact with body chemistry and the compounds isolated from foods and plants are often at the core of drug research.

The cutting edge of nutrition research is in the field of genetics. Nutritional research is taking yet another fascinating turn as the twenty-first century dawns. It is firmly placing the use of specific nutritional measures, virtually on a prescription basis for individuals, on a scientific footing. Common sense, and the old saying 'one man's meat is another's poison', tells us that not all dietary approaches suit everyone. It also tells us that different dietary changes yield results in some people but not in others. All is now becoming clear as we learn about the specifics of genetic research – a brand new but fantastically exciting direction for research. This is discussed further in Chapter 8.

## What Areas of Health can Nutrition Improve?

The logic of nutrition is immutable. Our bodies are turning over cells at a terrific rate – faster when we are younger, slower when we are older. The cells lining the digestive tract replace themselves every four days, the skin every six weeks and (most) bone every one to two years. This means that the body has a need for excellent raw materials. The quality of the food we eat determines the availability of raw materials. This means, literally, that from the moment that food quality improves so does our health and almost any condition linked to some aspect of poor quality of nutrition can be improved.

The ideal is to use nutrition as a preventive tool. By adopting healthy eating habits we can improve cardiovascular health, reduce cancer risk, forstall some eyesight problems and many other degenerative diseases. Most importantly, nutrition holds a vital place in creating a healthy child from healthy sperm and egg and healthy growth in the womb, thus setting the infant up with a 'reserve' of health to carry it through into adulthood. Nutritional measures will not be effective at righting very long-term damage such as macular degeneration (eye damage), dental decay or osteoarthritis, though it can help to prevent these in the first place and halt progression of these diseases. It is a testament to the power and effectiveness of nutritional intervention that the contents list of this book is as long as it is!

## Is Nutritional Therapy Safe?

Changing diet for the better is nearly always a safe option. For some people making abrupt changes can lead to transitory effects: withdrawal symptoms such as headaches when giving up coffee; digestive discomfort when eating more fibre; or even jaw-ache when eating more salads! But these are highly unlikely to be detrimental and taking a slower approach to changing habits will resolve short-term problems.

This book concentrates on foods you can use in everyday life to enhance your health and well-being and help to deal with specific ailments. Nutritional supplementation (vitamins and minerals) at sensible levels are generally safe and reported adverse reactions are but a fraction of the adverse reactions reported for medicinal drugs. Where supplements are mentioned it is only where there are such overwhelmingly positive results from research that to ignore them would not be sensible.

## Can Nutrition Really Make a Difference to My Health?

Yes. But it all depends on your initial health status, how much you are willing (or need) to change habits, and what your expectations are as to whether it is working or not. There is no point in trying something for a couple of days or a week and deciding it is not working if you really need to persevere for a month. Equally there is no point hammering away at a dietary change for six months if you should expect to see a change in three. Wherever possible, an expectation of the time period in which results should be seen is given.

This book concentrates on nutrition. This does not imply that nutrition is the sole answer to all health problems and genetics, medicine, stress management, hygiene, environmental exposure and exercise are all factors that play their part in health. But whatever the approach – be it taking a treatment prescribed by a doctor or an aromatherapy massage – a person's underlying nutritional status acts as scaffolding to underpin their health and plays its part in how responsive a person is to any given treatment.

# PART 1:

# FOOD POWER

# 1

# The Principles of a Healthy Diet

A balanced diet is the cornerstone of good health. While the main health messages have been received loud and clear by great numbers of people, there is great inertia in making the necessary changes. Why? In part it is to do with easy availability of snack and fast foods, in part because we all live busy lives, and in part because people have lost touch with basic cooking skills. But it is also linked to the fact that there is confusion about *how* to implement the guidelines.

On average, according to the National Diet and Nutrition Surveys in the UK, too much sugar and salt are eaten; we only eat three portions of the recommended five daily portions of fruits and vegetables; and fish intake is half of the recommended amount. Common nutritional deficiencies include magnesium, iron, Vitamin D and omega-3 fatty acids, amongst others.

In the following sections I simplify the healthy eating message into easy-to-follow principles. If it seems like a lot to deal with initially, there is no reason not to slowly introduce one measure at a time at a comfortable pace.

## Health on a Plate

One of the simplest ways of visualizing if a meal is healthy is mentally to divide it into thirds. One third should consist of wholegrain starches, one third of low-fat protein and one third of vegetables or fruits. This might seem obvious and easy with a main meal, but it is also helpful to go through the same exercise for snacks, as these can easily undermine a balanced diet. Snacking on high-fat biscuits, crisps or nuts all the time and not balancing this out with low-fat fruits and vegetables or some protein to help stabilize blood sugar, leads to lack of dietary balance. It also adds to the risk of piling on the pounds or suffering from persistent low energy.

*One-third proteins*: This group includes (preferably lean) meat, poultry, game, fish. Vegetarian sources of protein include eggs, beans, legumes, pulses, cheese, nuts and seeds. Yoghurt and milk have useful amounts of protein, though it is best to choose low or reduced fat versions and they also provide calcium. Calcium is also available from a varied diet which includes wholegrains (see below), nuts, seeds, vegetables and fruits. One of the best sources of calcium is canned fish that include bones, such as salmon and sardines.

*One-third starches*: Starches and sugars are carbohydrates. Complex carbohydrates are wholegrains such as wholemeal bread, brown rice, pasta, muesli, porridge oats, flapjacks and oatcakes. Complex carbohydrates have the advantage of releasing energy slowly into the bloodstream for a steady supply of energy. They also contain fibre, which is good for the digestive tract. White bread, white rice, many cereals, biscuits and pastry made with white flour, as well as sugar, are called refined carbohydrates because they have been processed to remove the outer husk of the grain. While there is little harm in having a small quantity of these, by making them the sole source of starches in the diet many people encounter health problems including low energy, mood swings, digestive discomfort and weight problems.

*One-third fruits and vegetables*: These are discussed in detail in the next section.

Adjustments to meals and snacks can easily be made by using this approach. Some examples are:

- If a ham (protein) and bread (starch) sandwich is being eaten for lunch, the addition of some tomatoes or an apple (fruit and veg) would balance the meal
- If two or three biscuits (starch) and a cup of tea make up a snack, a small handful of nuts (protein) and dried apricot (fruit) replacing one or two of the biscuits would balance the snack
- A breakfast of cereal (starch) would benefit from the addition of fruit salad (fruit) and yoghurt (protein) to balance the meal
- A bowl of pasta (starch) could incorporate tuna (protein) in the sauce and a large side salad (vegetables).

By broadly taking this approach at every meal and snack, a wider variety of nutrients are being consumed and the diet is balanced and therefore minimizing nutrient deficiencies, improving satiety (feeling of fullness), reducing intake of high-fat and sugary foods, reducing early hunger signals and cravings before the next meal and keeping moods stable. The idea is not to eat more food, but to replace some of the meal with a component which provides more nutritional balance to the overall meal.

**Fruit and vegetables**
Experts advise that we eat at least five portions of fruit and vegetables daily. This is the minimum amount. In reality most people eat around two to three portions daily. The total five portions should come to around 400 grams – or 80 grams per portion. It is easiest to picture each portion as roughly the amount you can hold in the palm of your hand. For children the portion size is roughly the amount they can hold in their cupped hand.

It is easy to achieve five portions, a portion is eaten with each of the three daily meals (breakfast, lunch and dinner) and a portion is eaten as a snack mid-morning and mid-afternoon. This could be:

- A glass of (preferably diluted) fruit juice (not squash) with breakfast, or chopped dried fruit on cereal
- A few carrot sticks mid-morning
- A couple of tomatoes with a lunchtime sandwich
- A banana mid-afternoon
- A portion of broccoli with the evening meal.

It is not difficult to do, but the habit must be established from early age and stuck to and you must never lose sight of the importance of this health measure. In fact, if all other health advice is ignored, it could be argued that this is probably the one most important measure to incorporate into daily life: the potassium that fruit and vegetables contain partly offset highish salt intakes; the antioxidants they provide are protective against a wide range of diseases; the fibre they contain is vital for bowel health; they are low calorie and satisfying, which means they offset high-fat foods; and the sugar they contain has a minimal impact on blood sugar.

A single portion of fruit and vegetables is any one of the following:

- A whole apple, banana, orange or similar-sized fruit. A couple of small fruit such as plums or half a larger fruit such as grapefruit. A handful of very small fruit such as strawberries or grapes
- A tablespoon of dried fruit
- A handful, or half a mugful, of vegetables or chopped vegetables

- A full mugful or small bowl of loosely packed salad or vegetable soup
- A wine glassful of fruit or vegetable juice (only counts once a day as it does not include the benefit of fibre)
- A half-mug of cooked pulses (beans, lentils, chickpeas, peas) once a day.

What does not count as a portion of fruit and vegetables:

- Potatoes which count as a starchy food
- Jam, or raisins in a chocolate bar, which provide insufficient fruit
- Squash, cordial or 'fruit drinks'.

Fresh, frozen, canned or dried fruits and vegetables count equally, though it is best to incorporate at least half fresh or frozen produce. Canned foods which are high in salt are not meant to carry the 'five-a-day' logo (such as canned pasta in tomato sauce) because the overall effect on health is detrimental. However, many manufacturers ignore this and label their foods accordingly. Additionally, a variety is meant to be eaten (in other words, eating five different types of fruit and vegetables rather than five apples each day). Therefore, manufacturers should not label, for instance, soups as 'provides two portions of the five recommended daily portions' – though, again, they often do this.

## Nutrient-dense foods

The quality of the foods we eat is also vitally important. Nutrient-dense foods provide lots of vitamins, minerals, healthy fats, good quality carbohydrates and proteins. By eating food as close to its original state as possible there is a greater chance of benefiting nutritionally. In practice this means eating wholegrains instead of refined grains, eating natural sources of sweetness such as bananas and dried fruit instead of too much refined sugar, and eating naturally fatty foods such as avocadoes and oily fish instead of commercially prepared fatty foods. The merit of this is that these foods are more satisfying and healthy.

Foods which are very sugary or heavily refined, such as many breakfast cereals, processed white bread and many (or most) fast and convenience foods increase our intake of sugar, salt and fat beyond the recommended guidelines. Because they do not provide sufficient vitamins and minerals, these foods also increase the risk of poor nutritional status and susceptibility to disease. This means preparing more food from scratch. It does not mean forgoing 'treats' or outings to the fish and chip shop all the time, but it does mean limiting these in favour of better quality food. Ultimately the quality of the food we eat determines the quality of our health.

Examples of better quality food choices could include:

- Porridge or muesli instead of sugary cereals
- Brown rice instead of white rice dishes
- Grilled fish and baked vegetables instead of fish and chips
- A vegetarian pulse/bean chilli stuffed in baked potato instead of a visit to the burger bar
- An oat flapjack instead of a bar of toffee chocolate
- A fruit-based pudding such as banana mashed with yoghurt instead of an artificial whipped mousse.

One of the ways in which the average diet could be dramatically improved is by altering the types of fats eaten. The effects of fats on health is discussed in Chapter 2 in more detail. In essence we eat too many saturated, hydrogenated and trans-fats and not enough polyunsaturated fats. Making these simple changes can help to redress the balance:

- Eating one meal a week based on white fish (not fried or battered fish). Fish is a good source of low fat protein
- Eating one meal a week based on oily fish such as mackerel, sardines, sprats, tuna or salmon. These are sources of valuable omega-3 fatty acids
- Eating two meals a week based on pulses and beans, such as baked beans, lentils, kidney beans in a chilli, or chickpeas.

By making these simple changes and replacing meat or convenience foods with healthier options, the balance of fatty acids is changed. Fibre from pulses and beans, more wholegrains, more fruits and vegetables all help to improve digestive health. These foods are also very rich sources of vitamins and minerals.

Finally, salt and sugar are used by the food industry to disguise the presence of increased levels of fat, and other low-quality ingredients. By reducing a dependency on fast and processed foods, we can reduce salt and sugar intake. For advice on reducing salt intake, see Appendix II, page 357. To reduce dependency on sugary foods, see Appendix I, page 349.

## Snacks, drinks, desserts and take-aways

Snacks, drinks and take-aways are often the pitfall in a healthy eating regime. The trick is to make them good quality. By maintaining a steady blood sugar, the need to snack is reduced. However, poor snack and drink choices, the habit of snacking and stress can all conspire to upset the best intentions. Instead of choosing high-sugar, high-salt and high-fat snacks or high-sugar or heavily caffeinated drinks, there are better options which will help to keep you within healthy eating guidelines. Some suggestions include:

### Snacks

- A small handful of unsalted nuts with dried fruit
- A banana and a small plain yoghurt
- A couple of oatcakes with nut butter spread
- A couple of cubes of dark chocolate and a few strawberries
- Some carrot sticks and hummus or guacamole (avocado) dip
- A bran muffin and an apple
- A rye cracker topped with cucumber and sliced egg
- Strips of ham wrapped around four or five pitted prunes
- Sunflower seeds and cherry tomatoes.

### Drinks

- Iced fruit tea
- Tomato or vegetable juice
- Smoothie
- Diluted fruit juice
- A mini can of tonic water
- Carbonated apple juice
- Dandelion coffee (available from health food shops).

### Desserts

Get into the habit of eating fruit for dessert. To ring the changes have stewed fruit with yoghurt or some dried fruit. If a small treat is needed, then some plain chocolate can be very satisfying. Higher sugar and fat desserts are fine from time to time, but avoid making them a regular feature. Take every opportunity to serve these with some fruit on the side to reduce the portion size and increase fruit and vegetable intake. If baking, take every opportunity to include fruit in the recipe.

### Take-aways

Look for the more simply cooked dishes with the least amount of frying and heavy or creamy sauces.

- In an Indian restaurant: Tandoori grilled chicken, chick pea or lentil curry, vegetable dishes and plain naan. Avoid deep fried options such as samosas
- In a Chinese restaurant: Stir-fried seafood, broccoli and other vegetables and sweetcorn soup. Avoid deep fried options such as spring rolls
- In a Burger bar: Flame-grilled chicken, salad with very little dressing and a modest (the smallest) bag of fries. Avoid super-sizing
- In a Kebab bar: Chicken or lamb meat chunks or hummus with salad in pitta pocket. Avoid the shawarma kebab
- In an Italian restaurant: Minestroni soup, a modest portion of pasta served with grilled meat or fish and/or a large salad
- In a Pizza restaurant: Choose thin crust. Order half the cheese, double the tomato and extra toppings and a large side salad. The best toppings are vegetable or seafood, while salami and sausage are best avoided.

# 2

# Healthy Fats

Fats have had a bad press over the last 30 years and there continues to be a lot of focus on low-fat diets. But fats are not all bad. In fact they have important health roles in the human body, and essential fatty acids are needed for almost every aspect of human health. The most important factor to consider about the fats we consume is they should be of the right quality. Fatty acids from foods have a number of uses in the body. As well as being used for energy, they are incorporated into cell membranes, making them vital for the functioning of most cells. They are also used to make hormones, are essential for nervous tissue and for regulating inflammation.

Signs of a deficiency in healthy fatty acids include: dry skin; dry eyes; dry listless hair; depression and mood disorders; hyperactivity and learning disorders in children; most inflammatory diseases such as arthritis, inflammatory bowel, eczema and asthma; and hormone imbalances such as PMS.

In addition to righting the conditions mentioned above, essential fatty acids can have other less visible benefits. They help to prevent cardiovascular disease, ensure fertility, improve immune function, protect against some cancers and guard against the negative effects of diabetes.

This chapter may seem a little like a biochemistry lesson, but for certain conditions it is important to understand just how critical the role healthy fats have to play in human health. If you want to skip the technical information, go to the advice on the balance of fatty acids and on incorporating healthy fats into the diet, from p. 24 at the end of this chapter.

## General roles of fats

- All fats, saturated and polyunsaturated (more on this later), are needed for absorbing the fat soluble vitamins A, D, E and K
- Dietary fats provide *physiological* fats, which give us 'padding'. Not everybody thinks of this as an advantage. However this padding, in normal amounts, provides warmth, a reservoir of energy, is necessary for female fertility and protection for our internal organs
- Fat in food makes it more palatable and literally helps it go down. Some cuisines are lower overall in fat, such as traditional Japanese or Chinese cooking (not necessarily true of Chinese take-aways, which are tailored for Western tastes), so using the minimum of fats to achieve palatability is a sensible goal – information on this can be found in cooking methods on page 97.

## The vital roles of healthy fats

Certain fatty acids have important *structural* roles and these fats, from the omega-3 and omega-6 families, are vital for health:

- They make up a significant part of the outer layer of virtually all cells (called the phospholipids membrane). This is important for organ function, digestive and skin health
- They provide insulation for and are incorporated into the structure of all nerve cells, including in the brain. This has important ramifications for eye health, mood, hyperactivity, learning and behaviour disorders
- They have important 'signalling' functions which regulate the way that cells speak to each other – this has profound

effects on the inflammatory process (see page 30), and thus on immune health, which is involved in many human diseases such as allergies and arthritis

- A particular fatty acid, EPA, has an impact on blood viscosity (stickiness) and therefore on cardiovascular health
- Two of the fatty acids, vital for all the above roles, are called *essential* fatty acids (EFAs). They are essential to human health in the same way that vitamins are. They cannot be manufactured in the body (the exception being in breast milk, as the human infant is totally dependent on this source of nourishment) and without them deficiency diseases develop. The omega-6 EFA is linoleic acid and the omega-3 EFA is alpha-linolenic acid. All the other members of these two families are not strictly essential, as they can be made in the human body from these two EFAs, but they are sometimes called 'conditionally essential'. This means that sometimes the body doesn't make them very efficiently, usually when certain health conditions such as allergies prevail, as we age or in infancy. Obtaining these other fatty acids from the diet therefore becomes more important. Some of the conditionally essential fatty acids, which we will discuss below, include GLA, DHA and EPA – these abbreviations may be familiar to you already.

## Fatty acid 'families'

To understand the roles of these important fatty acids it helps to explain a little bit about fats in general. All fats and oils are chains made up of carbon links with hydrogen atoms attached to them. The terms saturated and polyunsaturated refer to whether the carbon links are 'full up' with hydrogen or not. There are three main groups of fats:

- *Saturated*: Mainly found in meat, milk, cheese and butter. The Western diet typically provides a bit too much of these types of fats. Those carbon chains that are 'saturated' with hydrogen are called saturated fats. The carbon chains tend to be shorter – between four and 18 links in the chain (there are a couple which are longer). Hydrogenated fats, artificially made to make cheap margarine and used in most commercial baked goods, can also be thought of as saturated fats, but are probably more damaging (more on this later).

- *Mono-unsaturated*: Mainly found in olive oil and also called omega-9. Mono-unsaturated fats have one (mono) hydrogen attachment missing (called a double bond). Mono-unsaturates are familiar because of the Mediterranean diet. Olive oil is linked to many health benefits, especially heart health. While not being 'biologically active', omega-9 fats may have benefits simply by displacing saturated fats in the diet (if you are dipping your bread in olive oil you are not spreading butter on it). Virgin olive oil also contains antioxidants from its dark green colour.

- *Poly-unsaturated*: Those fatty acids with carbon chains that have spaces which are missing links to hydrogen (double bonds), and are therefore not 'saturated' with hydrogen, are called polyunsaturated. (When fats are hydrogenated or rehydrogenated, the manufacturers are artificially adding back in hydrogen to saturate the chain.) These chains are a bit longer, with at least 18 links. It is the very length of these chains that physically permits more double bonds (hydrogen-free links), thus giving more diverse biochemical uses in the body. The fatty acids can be subdivided into two main groups – omega-6 and omega-3 – and each group has its own essential fatty acid. They are called '*essential* fatty acids' because we are unable to make them for ourselves and must get them from our diet.

Omega-6 is found mainly in cooking oils, grains, seeds and nuts. While particular members of the omega-6 group of fatty acids are valuable for health, modern diets tend to be much too high in this family of fats because of the amounts of cooking oils and oils used in food processing and convenience foods. The omega-6 essential fatty acid is called linoleic acid. This is made by the body into GLA (gamma-linolenic acid) which many people buy in evening primrose and borage (also called starflower) capsules. GLA has important anti-inflammatory actions which makes it helpful for regulating some conditions such as PMS, allergies and skin conditions.

Omega-3 is found in small quantities in a few nuts and seeds, their oils and soya. Particularly active types of omega-3s, called EPA and DHA, are found in high quantities in oily fish. The omega-3 essential fatty acid is called alpha-linolenic acid (which is the one we are able to convert in our bodies to the 'fish-oil-type' fats EPA and DHA). The health qualities of fish oils come from the fact that they are very unsaturated – in other words, they have lots of double bonds without hydrogen on the chain. They have 20–22 links in the chain, which allows them to have more unsaturated spaces. The degree of unsaturation makes them very flexible and highly biologically active. The body can make these 20–22-link, highly unsaturated fats from shorter 18-link fatty acids, but is sometimes inefficient at doing this. By eating oily fish you benefit from all the work the fish has already done in converting the fats in its diet derived from plankton and smaller marine animals, and your body then does not need to make this conversion.

In particular there are three types of fatty acids which are of such benefit to us and which are in fish oils:

- EPA (eicosapentanoic acid), which has significant anti-inflammatory effects and helps to reduce blood 'stickiness'. Also important for brain neurochemical signalling

- DHA (decosahexanoic acid), which is important for nerve and brain health. DHA makes up a significant proportion of the fatty acids that are incorporated into the structure of the brain (which is itself 60 per cent lipid – fatty structures called phospholipids)
- AA (arachidonic acid), contributes to eye health and also makes up a significant amount of the brain lipid structure.

Arachidonic acid (AA) is a vital component of brain and phospholipids structure (see above point). However, an excess in the diet, which usually comes from too much red meat and dairy – especially when not balanced out by omega-3 fish oils – has the effect of increasing inflammation. You will see many references throughout this book to reducing sources of AA in the diet, but this does not preclude its importance for nervous tissue health.

## Antagonists to healthy fats

The essential fatty acids (omega-6 linoleic acid and omega-3 alpha-linolenic acid) are converted, as already mentioned, into the active fatty acids GLA, EPA and DHA (and AA). To do this the carbon chains are made longer via elongase enzymes and made more unsaturated via desaturase enzymes. This makes them more biologically flexible and useful. In some people, mainly those with atopic allergies such as eczema and asthma, infants and the elderly, the desaturase enzymes do not work efficiently. Adding to this, the omega-6 and omega-3 'families' compete for the same enzymes, meaning that if there is more omega-6 in the diet than omega-3 (which there is) then the competitive element means even less efficiency of the desaturase enzymes. To further complicate the situation, quite a lot of things interfere with successful desaturase function, including smoking, caffeine, alcohol, saturated fats and hydrogenated fats – so a lifestyle that features these will further compromise the ability to make the useful compounds GLA, EPA and DHA. This is why it is important to adjust the total 'background diet' to improve the situation.

## Trans-fats and hydrogenated fats

Trans-fats and hydrogenated oils are making the health headlines these days and we are now advised to avoid them where possible.

Trans-fats are fatty acids which have altered chemical structures and so they are not recognized by the body and actually interfere with the correct functioning of healthy fatty acids. To envisage this, imagine the wrong key (trans-fat) being inserted into a lock (cell membrane) – it stops the correct key (essential fatty acid) fitting in and jams up the lock mechanism (cell function).

Trans-fats occur naturally in beef, lamb and milk. The problem is that they are also made artificially in food manufacturing during the process of making hydrogenated fats. They therefore find their way into all sorts of everyday foods: cereal bars, muffins, pies, pastries, crisps, chips, biscuits, frozen desserts and confectionery. The body can deal with relatively small quantities, but probably not so well when people choose to eat processed foods all day or use lots of cheap margarine. Current estimates for UK trans-fat intakes are as much as 1.2 per cent of daily energy – which is more than the average omega-3 intake which, conversely, is deficient in the diet.

Vegetable oils have been used for several decades in cooking oils and in food manufacturing. In the 1970s and

1980s, this was believed to be better for us, as they are derived from, and are sources of, unsaturated fatty acids. Since the 1990s, however, related health problems have become evident.

The problem with oils, from a food manufacturing point of view, is that they are liquid at room temperature and also go rancid pretty quickly. To overcome this they are made solid by hydrogenation. This involves bubbling hydrogen through the oils to change the chemical structure, which makes them solid like lard and extends shelf-life (which for a food manufacturer increases the economic viability of a product). We now know that the human body doesn't know what to do with large quantities of hydrogenated trans-fats and they have been blamed for contributing to a number of diseases, including heart disease, raised cholesterol levels, allergies, nervous disorders and cancer.

To reduce the use of hydrogenation, food manufacturers are turning to new processes called interestification and fractionation, but no-one knows if these will be any better in the long run. While some countries have banned hydrogenated fats or insisted on quantity declarations on food labels, in the UK there are no such requirements.

## Omega-6 and Omega-3 Balance

This is probably one of the most crucial concepts to take on board. Human evolution happened at a time when food availability was entirely different. In particular there was a vast difference in the balance of fatty acids that were consumed. Our ancestors ate diets that consisted of about equal quantities of omega-6 to omega-3, a ratio of 1:1. This is probably why omega-3s have such an important role in human physiology. At that time the meat that was eaten was free ranging, eggs came from free-ranging birds, coastal communities had free access to fish and, vitally, more leaves were eaten (rich sources of omega-3) while very few grains were eaten (rich sources of omega-6).

With the advent of agriculture, the feeding of livestock on grains, the reduction in fish eating and latterly the wide availability of convenience foods which feature grain and seed oils, the ratio of these two fatty acids in the diet has swung dramatically in favour of omega-6 and reduced the amount of omega-3. The ratio has gone from 1:1 to up to 15 or 20:1 omega-6 to omega-3. Human health is struggling as a result and clear links have been found to a wide variety of mental and physical conditions as a result of this change.

## Dietary Changes to Improve Fatty acid intakes

To sum up the above, in terms that most people prefer to think of them (ie: 'good' and 'bad'):

| TYPE OF FAT | SOURCES | ADVICE |
|---|---|---|
| Saturated fats | meat, butter, cheese, full fat or semi-skimmed milk | OK in moderation but reduce wherever possible |
| Hydrogenated trans-fats | convenience foods, take-aways, baked goods, crisps and sweets | Bad for health, but hard to totally avoid – reduce intake dramatically |
| Mono-unsaturated fats | olive oil | Good in moderation, still provide a lot of calories |
| Omega-6 | seeds, nuts, grains and their oils | Healthy sources such as seeds, nuts and |

| TYPE OF FAT | SOURCES | ADVICE |
| --- | --- | --- |
| | | cold-pressed oils which are not heated, to be encouraged. Aim for a dramatic reduction in unhealthy sources such as heavily processed cooking oils, convenience foods and take-aways |
| Omega-3 | oily fish, game, enriched eggs, walnuts, pumpkin seeds, flax oil, canola (rape seed) oil | To be emphasised much more in the diet wherever possible |

Remember:

- Eat foods cooked from fresh ingredients as often as possible
- Increase sources of healthy fatty acids from oily fish, nuts, seeds and cold-pressed oils
- Eat oily fish at least once a week, or if related health conditions are evident then twice or three times a week
- Eat a pulse-based meal twice a week to reduce dependency on saturated fats from meat
- Use olive oil or canola (rape seed) oil for cooking instead of corn oil, which is very high in omega-6
- Use flax, walnut or pumpkin seed oil for salad dressings (if necessary use half and half with olive oil for taste)
- Instead of butter, use other means of moistening bread, such as hummus, salsa, nut butters, mashed avocado or banana

- Most fatty, and especially crispy foods such as crisps, biscuits, cakes and crackers, use hydrogenated fats because they create the crisp texture
- Check margarine packets for the 'no hydrogenated or partially hydrogenated fats' declaration
- The cheaper the cake or chocolate, and the longer the shelf-life of any product that contains fat, the more trans-fats it will contain
- Deep-fried foods from take-aways include large quantities of omega-6 and trans-fats.

# 3

# Immune Health and Inflammation

The immune system is our defence against external 'invaders' such as bacteria, viruses, parasites, cancerous cells and irritants such as allergy-causing substances. It differentiates between 'friend' – when it does not attack – and 'foe' – when it does. Intimately linked to any involvement of the immune system is the process of inflammation. Inflammation is a natural and beneficial healing response which helps to bring immune compounds to the area that needs healing, and acts as 'nature's bandage' by creating swelling and pain to stop us from doing something that might further damage the area. In the normal course of events, when the inflammation dies down and the immune system has done its job, everything returns to normal and we get on with our lives. But when the inflammatory response is out of control and causing additional damage to body tissues, then it becomes a major contributor to many diseases both immediately visible (such as joint swelling and asthma attacks) and invisible (such as cardiovascular and digestive tract diseases). Nutritional status has a profound effect on immune health and the inflammatory response.

## Immune Health and Diet

Nutritionally speaking the food we eat has a three-fold importance in relation to immune health:

1. *To not antagonize the immune system.*

The most clear-cut case of this is in people with serious food allergies – around 1–2 per cent of the population. If you have a peanut allergy you must avoid this food in order not to provoke a potentially life-threatening overreaction of the immune system. Another similar clear-cut case is that of coeliac disease (not an allergy), in which the digestive tract atrophies when gluten (a protein found in some grains) is eaten. In this case the inflammation that results in the digestive tract is a major factor. Food intolerances and other adverse food reactions and their impact on overall health in general, and immune health and the inflammatory response in particular, are a more grey area.

2. *To provide the building blocks needed for the body to maintain a healthy, balanced immune response.*

Just as with any other body tissues, immune cells are manufactured from available resources. Some nutrients, for instance zinc and vitamin C, are essential for this process and deficiencies lead to impairment of immune responses.

3. *To relieve the immune system of some of its duties.*

This is where antioxidants and other phytochemicals come in. By being available to quench free-radical oxidation activity, and by interfering with disease processes, they reduce the impact on the immune system and also ensure that resources are better channelled into maintaining equilibrium. Consequently, one of the most important knock-on effects of eating sufficient fruits and vegetables daily is improved immune health; this can include improved wound healing, less severe asthma attacks, lowered risk of some cancers and other symptom improvements.

## Inflammation

Inflammation is at the core of a wide variety of human diseases. When it is out of control – when a person is in a 'hyperinflammatory state' – all sorts of things start to go wrong. Arthritis is a good example. Inflammation is also involved in a wide variety of health problems including inflammation of the digestive tract, ulcers and wounds that won't heal easily anywhere on the body, all allergies, many aspects of pre-menstrual syndrome, and possibly even in brain diseases such as dementia and Alzheimer's. Inflammation is also involved with heart disease: C-reactive protein is a biochemical measure of inflammation which is consistently elevated in those with cardiovascular conditions.

## Fatty acids and inflammation

Fatty acids form part of the phospholipids structure of cells and the type of fatty acids that lodge in this cell layer is intimately linked to the fats in our diet. A sample of fat tissue analysed in a laboratory will give a very clear indication of the types of fats that person habitually eats. These fatty acids regulate the chemical messengers sent out from those cells. These include prostaglandins and leukotrienes, which are involved in promoting or reducing inflammation. They are vital for all immune responses. All immune responses involve inflammation. Excess inflammation – when someone is in a hyperinflammatory state – is common. Low level, acute or chronic inflammation are linked to many diseases and thus the fatty acid balance in the diet plays a major role in many health conditions. Saturated, hydrogenated fats and an excess of refined oils which provide high amounts of omega-6 (convenience foods, corn cooking oil and fast-foods) will enhance and increase inflammation. Conversely, omega-3 (mainly from oily fish) and unrefined sources of omega-6 (such as nuts and seeds) will help to dampen inflammation. In these circumstances it is even more important to follow the advice in Chapter 2 on improving the balance of fatty acids in the diet.

## The Digestive System and Immune Health

Along with the skin, the digestive tract forms our interface with the outside world. It protects us against assault from bacteria, viruses, toxic compounds, parasites and undigested proteins. In the course of this work it makes a number of immunoglobulins, immune compounds, which protect the body. Because of these functions, the digestive tract can be thought of as our largest immune organ. It responds to irritants with a full range of immune responses, including inflammation, which is a major factor in bloating and bowel diseases. The ability of the gut to heal itself subsequently is intimately linked to what is pushed along the tract – in other words the food we eat. Bowel bacteria play a vital part in immune health and this is discussed in Chapter 4.

## Antioxidants

Antioxidants are important because they counter the effects of oxidation damage. Oxidation has been linked in one way or the other to over 80 human diseases by causing tissue damage. This is similar to the effects of oxygen on iron (causing rust) or on rubber (causing it to become brittle and disintegrate). Similarly, when an apple is cut in half and starts to go brown, it is due to the effects of oxygen on the flesh.

If you squeeze a lemon, rich in the antioxidant vitamin C, on to the apple flesh, it protects the apple against discolouration.

The outer visible sign of oxidation damage, which is just as easy to understand, is the effect of the sun on skin, producing a tan in the short term but coarser more 'leathery' skin from free-radical damage in the long term. Another example is cataract formation, when the lens of the eye clouds over as a result of free-radical induced 'cross linking' of proteins. Some of the many diseases that are progressed by oxidation damage include age-related damage to the rear of the eye, any disease involving inflammation (which is itself a major trigger of free radicals), some aspects of cardiovascular disease, Alzheimer's disease, allergies such as asthma and some cancers. Diabetes is a major promoter of free radical damage.

Free radicals cause oxidation damage by creating molecular imbalance as they career out of control and 'rob' tissues of electrons. Antioxidants 'quench' free radicals by absorbing free-radical electrons and thus preserving body tissues. The best-known antioxidants are the essential vitamins A, C and E and the essential mineral selenium. However, there are many other compounds in fruits and vegetables – such as carotenes and anthocyanins – which have antioxidant activity, though they have not been defined as having essential vitamin status (vitamins are partially defined by known deficiency diseases which result from their absence). The truth is that there are so many of these compounds, and they interact in such complicated ways, that the broad-brush recommendation to eat at least five portions of fruits and vegetables daily is the best approach.

Two improvements to this recommendation would be helpful if they were more widely understood by all of us:

- To eat from as wide a variety of fruits and vegetables as possible – thus ensuring exposure to different antioxidant chemicals

- Five portions is a minimum suggestion, not a maximum to aim for. Indeed, evidence is emerging that the more fruits and vegetables eaten the better the effect on, for example, bone or cardiovascular health. See Chapter 1: The Principles of a Healthy Diet, page 11, for portion sizes.

## Phytochemicals (Plant chemicals)

We are all familiar with the exhortation to eat a minimum of five portions of fruits and vegetables daily. But why? Apart from providing nourishment mainly in the form of carbohydrates, minerals, vitamins, fibre and water, fruits and vegetables are our source of antioxidants and a range of phytochemicals. In addition to antioxidants, plant foods are rich in a wide variety of chemicals which can either be toxic or beneficial (at normal intake levels). There are thousands of such compounds and it is only recently that we have begun fully to appreciate their importance.

Toxic compounds are well documented and we can either avoid a plant, or cook or peel it to remove compounds. To take some familiar examples, green shoots in potatoes or uncooked kidney beans are highly toxic. Other compounds such as tannins in wine or tea can have a significant inhibiting effect on some nutrients, though they are generally not considered harmful as the foods they come with have other benefits – it is a question of balance.

Beneficial compounds are just as potent – antioxidants, flavonoids, and possibly enzymes and plant hormones. Some of these are:

- The compounds which give plants their colour – mainly antioxidants – such as the carotenes and anthocyanins mentioned above

- Isothiocyanates in vegetables such as broccoli and Brussels sprouts, which give these vegetables their bitter taste, encourage apoptosis (cell death) in cancerous cells
- Compounds in citrus fruit which have a stimulating or dampening effect on the P450 detoxification enzymes of the liver
- Enzymes in very enzyme-rich fruits such as pineapples and papaya, which have a digestive enhancing effect
- Soya foods which have a sufficiently strong hormonal effect possibly to protect against menopausal and other female hormone-related problems.

# 4

# Bacterial Balance

We have more bacteria microbes in our guts than we have cells in our body, and we are only just understanding the importance of these to our health. We give bacteria a home, warmth and food in our guts, and in turn the 'good' bacteria provide us with several important health advantages:

- They make significant amounts of some B-vitamins (needed for energy and nerve health) and vitamin K (needed for blood clotting and bone health)
- They protect us from pathogenic 'bad' bacteria including food poisoning
- They produce an important food for digestive tract cells, called butyric acid, which provides 80 per cent of energy needs directly to the gut
- When the good bacteria are present in sufficient quantities they crowd out pathogenic bacteria. This stops the bad bacteria from producing toxins which damage the gut wall, a condition called increased gut permeability, more commonly known as 'leaky gut'
- They are involved in final stage digestion of starches and milk sugars
- They keep the bowel slightly acidic, which is believed to be necessary to protect against bowel cancer.

Bowel bacteria replicate themselves very quickly – in fact half of the weight of our stools consists of bacteria. However, the gut is a highly competitive arena, with around 400 different types of bacteria battling it out to maintain their foothold. Depending on diet, antibiotic use and the general health of the host (person), different species of bacteria find the circumstances favourable to flourish in. Consequently the dietary and lifestyle choices we make can affect the health of the gut, and this has knock-on consequences for many aspects of our general health.

Conditions that can be improved by ensuring a healthy bacterial gut population include:

- *Just about all aspects of digestive, gut and bowel health*: this is easy to imagine, as the bacteria are in close contact with the gut
- *Immune health*: healthy bacteria promote a tightly 'sealed' gut wall and protect against the adverse immune consequences of bad bacteria (see below)
- *Protection against allergies*: children with poor gut bacteria profiles are more likely to develop allergies and supplementation with beneficial bacteria may have a role in prevention of allergies
- *Skin health*: if the bowels are not working properly, then the body seeks to eliminate toxins elsewhere. The skin is the largest organ of elimination and spots and eczema are often related to poor bowel bacteria health
- *Mood*: toxins that enter the bloodstream as the result of a 'leaky' gut can directly affect the brain, resulting in poor mood
- *Energy levels*: Healthy bacteria produce sufficient energy from which the body and brain can directly benefit.

## The Infant and gut bacteria

Babies have sterile guts just before they are born. As babies pass through the birth canal, they are 'inoculated' with their first bacteria, which mirrors maternal bacteria within ten minutes. When they start to breast-feed, this process is continued until by the age of two, they have gut bacteria that are similar to an adult's. When babies are born by Caesarean section and when they are bottle-fed, the bacteria species in their gut in the first two years are quite different. This is probably linked to an increased risk of infantile diarrhoea and allergies later in life. Breast-fed infants have much lower risks of gut, respiratory and urinary tract infections compared to formula-fed babies. Recent improvements in formula milk, which can now incorporate prebiotics (see below) seems to be closing the gap in the make up of infants' gut bacteria. The manufacturers of formula milks are seeking to replicate the prebiotic content of human breast milk, which has around 130 different oligosaccharides (prebiotics) that are barely present in cows' milk.

## Ageing and gut bacteria

As we age we become more prone to digestive and gut problems. There are fewer beneficial bacterial species in the gut as we age, probably reflecting a lifetime of assault on the digestive tract from diet and other factors. Beneficial gut bacteria have important roles to play in stopping and reversing many of these age-related gut problems. Inflammatory bowel disease, ulcerative colitis and Crohn's disease have all been shown to be helped by improving beneficial bowel bacteria health. This can also lead to improvements in the time it takes the contents of the gut to go through it (reducing problems with constipation), often a problem as we age.

## Immunity, allergies and gut bacteria

Many people do not realize that the digestive tract is the largest immune organ in the body. It presents the greatest surface area which is exposed to allergenic substances, toxins and micro-organisms and so has a vital role in protecting against 'invaders' and ill health.

Healthy bowel bacteria enhance immune health in several ways. When beneficial bacteria are present in sufficient quantities (and so crowding out 'bad' bacteria) the digestive tract is not being aggravated by the toxins from 'bad' bacteria. A 'leaky' gut which can result from bad, pathogenic, bacteria leads to the immune system being challenged by toxins and incompletely digested food particles. By feeding the gut wall directly with 80 per cent of its energy needs (with butyric acid) beneficial bacteria enable the gut to repair itself and stay healthy. They actively produce antibiotic substances which have been shown to deter the ulcer bacterium *Helicobacter pylori* and food poisoning such as *E. coli*. Supplementation with beneficial bacteria can even reduce 'travellers' diarrhoea. Finally, allergies are less common in children with healthy bowel bacteria, probably because of enhanced immune health.

## Antibiotics and gut bacteria

Antibiotics wipe out bacterial colonies indiscriminately and this includes the beneficial bacteria in the gut. This is one of the reasons why a main symptom associated with antibiotic use is diarrhoea (particularly in children). But bacteria grow back very quickly. One short course of antibiotics is unlikely to have long-term consequences for bowel bacterial balance if the diet is healthy and features plenty of fibre, but two or more courses, or a very strong single course, of antibiotics can wipe out enough beneficial bacteria to have consequences for long-term health. In these circumstances it becomes particularly important to replenish bowel bacteria (see below).

## Improving gut bacteria balance

A healthy balance of bowel bacteria depends on several things, but mostly on a healthy diet. If a healthy diet has not been the case for a while, or if a person has particular health problems, there is often a case for supplementing probiotic bacteria as well as prebiotics (the food, or growth medium, for healthy gut bacteria).

- *Breast-feeding*: This is the best way to establish healthy gut bacteria in the infant. Many mothers only breast-feed for six to 12 weeks, but continuing breast feeding until six months is the best option
- *Formula feeding*: If a parent chooses formula for their baby, it is important to ensure that it is one that includes pre-biotics. These encourage the growth of healthy bacteria in the infant's gut
- *Dietary fibre*: This is most important and acts as food and therefore as a growth medium for beneficial gut bacteria. Following the advice in Appendix III, page 363 on fibre intake and sources of fibre is vital. To avoid problems with bloating, increase fibre in the diet very slowly until the desired amount is achieved. Do not be put off this change by adverse symptoms – just cut back and begin from a lower starting point. Favouring soluble fibre from oats, fruits, vegetables and pulses, instead of insoluble fibre from wheat bran is best – wheat bran is often irritating for the gut. Cooking beans and pulses very well (and draining off

the soaking and cooking water several times) can help, and canned beans are much less likely to cause adverse symptoms. A fibre supplement such as psyllium husks or ground linseeds may be very helpful

- *Negative dietary factors*: Dietary factors that discourage healthy bowel bacteria and which encourage 'bad' bacteria are: high levels of sugar in the diet (from sweets, soft drinks, sugary cereals, etc.), and excess alcohol (beer seems to be a particular problem). (See also the advice in Candida, page 146.)
- *Yoghurt*: The food which has been used throughout millennia to promote healthy digestion via its effect on gut bacteria is yoghurt. Choose live 'bio' yoghurt rather than sweetened fruit enhanced brands (which have little beneficial bacteria left) and eat it daily
- *Probiotic supplements*: These are widely available. If experiencing any relevant health problems, such as gut problems, immune health problems, allergies, skin problems, or lack of energy, taking a beneficial probiotic bacteria supplement can be very advantageous. It is safe to take these daily over the long term. Make sure the supplement is from a reputable manufacturer and that it is stored correctly to ensure viability of the bacteria it contains (many supplements need to be kept in the fridge, but new technology is offering freeze-dried supplements). Talk to your health food shop about good brands. Supplements should include both lactobacillus and bifidobacteria. Several different types of bacteria-enhanced health drinks are now available which are convenient and are likely to be of benefit when consumed regularly (they are sugary, which is necessary as the bacteria thrive on the sugars, but if overly sensitive to sugar then it may be best to take a pill or powder supplement)
- *Prebiotics*: Bacteria thrive on particular types of food and supplements called prebiotics are now available

which provide these. The most common is FOS (fructo-oligosaccharides). FOS is found naturally in fruits and vegetables. It can be bought as a sweet-tasting powder which makes an excellent substitute for sugar on cereals and in cold drinks – it is not good heated and can only be used up to 50 per cent in baking recipes to replace sugar. FOS should be used in moderation, up to a tablespoon or two daily, to avoid bloating. Inulin is another prebiotic used in supplements, which is found in large amounts in Jerusalem artichokes

- *Synbiotics*: This is the term used for supplements which include both probiotics and prebiotics. This new generation of supplements are probably the most effective
- *Antibiotics*: By supporting immune health (using the various means outlined in this book) overuse of antibiotics can be minimized, reserving their use for when really needed. After a course of antibiotics it is particularly relevant to take probiotic supplements. One which is formulated for this event is a seven-day intensive course called 'Replete' by Biocare.

# 5

# Food and Mood

The brain is a part of the body. Yet in conventional medicine mood disorders and the physical disorders of the body (and brain) are divided into two separate areas of treatment. We have 'head doctors': psychiatrists, psychoanalysts, psychologists, behavioural scientists, educational psychologists; and we have 'body doctors': general practitioners, surgeons, physiotherapists. But we increasingly understand that body and mind must work together and that treatment of the chemistry of the body (with good food, lifestyle habits and sometimes supplements) will affect the chemistry of the brain and thus mood.

The idea that food can affect mood is only just gaining currency, though it seems glaringly obvious to nutritionists. Food that enters the body goes to make the constituent parts of the brain, is turned into the neurochemical messengers that make the brain operate and provides the energy for the brain to function. The brain uses 20 per cent of our energy despite being only around 2 per cent of body weight. The energy available from glucose in the blood affects mood and the ability to concentrate throughout the day. Fifty to 60 per cent of the brain weight is made up of lipids (fats) and the balance of fats in the diet seems to have profound implications for rates of depression, behavioural disorders, postnatal depression and even suicide. Hormone imbalance in women, which can lead to pre-menstrual syndrome with accompanying mood swings and depression, can be affected by dietary intake.

The Food and Mood Project, run in conjunction with the mental health charity MIND, found that many people with mental health problems use diet to help their condition. The most popular strategies were to restrict sugar, saturated fat intake, eat more oily fish and to eat more fruits and vegetables – mostly these are the guidelines for a healthy diet. Dietary changes to help specific conditions are dealt with in the A–Z section of this book.

## Blood sugar

The brain is fairly picky about the fuel it uses and it mostly needs glucose to operate (there are a couple of alternatives, but these are not favoured). Consequently the level of glucose in the blood is kept constant, as far as possible, to feed the brain. A drop in blood sugar, such as occurs in those with blood sugar balance problems and in the morning after the night-time fast, leads to hunger and fatigue. It also leads to low mood. This feels very unpleasant and so in a bid to raise blood sugar quickly (to pep ourselves up, in other words) we are attracted to sugary snacks and drinks. This works in the very short term, but in the long term perpetuates the problem by worsening blood sugar swings. The solution is to eat complex (wholegrain) carbohydrates and proteins for more lasting energy supplies to fuel the brain.

## Brain lipids

As already mentioned above, the structure of the brain is largely dependent on fats in the diet and lipids make up a major part of the phospholipids structure of the brain. A large part of the brain consists of DHA and AA in a ratio of

2:1 (see Chapter 2: Healthy Fats for an explanation of these). These fatty acids, and EPA, are found in oily fish. The body of research that is confirming the importance of dietary sources of the fatty acids DHA, AA and EPA to resolve mood problems is becoming quite impressive. While DHA is needed for the structure of the brain, it seems that EPA is needed to help normal signalling in the brain.

## Brain chemicals

Another way in which dietary sugar affects mood is when we use sugar to appease feelings of low mood. This is very similar to self-medicating with alcohol, cigarettes and recreational drugs. It is true that these have other mechanisms by which they work to alter brain chemistry, but sugar shares a common effect on dopamine pathways in the brain with these other substances. Carbohydrates also have an effect on serotonin. Serotonin is an important mood brain chemical which is familiar to anyone who takes SSRI medication (such as Prozac); SSRI stands for selective serotonin reuptake inhibitors. It is not known how carbohydrates exert this effect – it used to be thought that they aided the passage of an amino acid (protein building block), tryptophan, into the brain to be used to make serotonin, but this is now known not to be the case. (Tryptophan is turned into serotonin via 5HTP, but not with the aid of carbohydrates, it now appears.) Nevertheless, while we do not yet know how this works it is undoubtedly the case that carbohydrates have a profound effect on mood and probably on serotonin. The solution is to follow the advice regarding the Glycaemic Index in Appendix I, page 350.

## Micronutrients

Vitamins and minerals are also important for brain function and mood. The most important are probably the B-vitamin group, and these are often thought of as mood vitamins. In fact they are needed for many facets of nerve health and for energy production, as well as influencing hormone health (which can have a knock-on effect on mood). There is good evidence for the role that zinc has to play in brain health and mood and behavioural disorders. Magnesium is another important nutrient, involved in 300 different enzyme processes, including nerve health and energy metabolism. A by-product of eating foods low on the Glycaemic Index (see points above) is that these foods are also rich in these nutrients and so benefit brain and mood health by supplying the necessary vitamins and minerals for optimal mood.

## Hormones

Mood swings can also be linked to hormonal imbalance. Anyone with suspected underactive or overactive thyroid conditions should ask their doctor to check their thyroid hormone levels. Specific dietary advice may also be of benefit (see pages 304 and 306). PMS used to be called PMT – pre-menstrual tension – because women often suffer mood swings in the week or two before menstruation. This is often resolved with changes in diet, though about two or three menstrual cycles need to pass to assess the success of a regime. It is best to tackle several aspects at the same time if you have severe mood problems and addressing blood sugar, food sensitivities, caffeine and nutritional deficiencies at the same time can be more effective than when trying one at a time.

When successful it is remarkably so, with women reporting that 'it is like a cloud lifting' and with many grateful partners agreeing. Menopausal mood problems can also be helped with diet and sometimes herbal supplements (see page 249). No woman should have to endure post-natal depression, which is especially cruel since it comes at a time when women expect to be happy (this, indeed, can add unrealistic pressures). Dietary advice for general depression is very relevant, though it is best acted upon before giving birth, which makes it difficult if a woman does not know if she is likely to be prone to the condition. Any woman who has had the problem previously can address it in later pregnancies.

## Food to feed the soul

Finally, food has a unique role to play in nurturing ourselves and our families. Unfortunately food is often used to abuse ourselves, particularly in those with eating disorders (which are very common). It is so important to switch the view of food from one of a 'prop', or to fill the gap or to medicate low moods, to one of nurturing and enjoyment. By enjoying shopping for food (possibly even growing food), preparing, sharing and enjoying food we can improve our mood. By the simple act of taking the time and trouble to select the best foods and choosing the foods that will promote health and a happy psyche, food can have a profound effect on mood.

# 6

# Changing Dietary Needs

Our nutritional needs are not static, but change throughout our lives depending on our age and the demands being placed upon our physical resources. This is recognized by government nutritional recommendations in the form of RDAs (recommended daily amounts) and RNIs (reference nutrient intakes). Examples are the increased need of menstruating women for iron, the increased need for vitamin D in the 65+ age group, and the increased calorie needs of late-pregnancy and of breast-feeding women.

There are other times when changing needs are more individual and not so obvious or quantifiable. For instance, when a child suffers from a long period of illness, this can affect growth rate and indeed may have been a significant reason why people used to be shorter when sanitation was not as good as it is nowadays. Another example is when a person undertakes intensive sports training – the professional athlete will be aware of the nutritional demands this places on the body, but the amateur – perhaps teenager – may not be so well informed, which can have a significant impact on health. Any time in a person's life of increased physical or mental stress may require a reassessment of nutritional needs.

## Pregnancy and breast feeding

During pregnancy and breast-feeding it is logical that the mother is growing and nurturing another person and that good quality building blocks are needed. To preserve her own health (because the developing infant will certainly draw on her reserves) the mother also needs excellent nutrition.

It is a mistake to think that a pregnant woman needs a lot more calories and 'eating for two' is no longer advised. In fact she only needs an extra 200 calories daily in the last three months of the pregnancy, when the baby is putting on weight and therefore increasing calorie needs. In real terms 200 calories only amounts to an extra couple of slices of bread daily, or a yoghurt and a couple of pieces of fruit. Breast-feeding requires an extra 500 calories daily as the infant is putting on weight at a tremendous rate at that stage. Five hundred calories translates into an extra sandwich and a bowl of soup.

Though the mother does not need many more calories (and no extra calories in the first six months), what she does need is superb nutrient-dense foods which are sources of all the vitamins and minerals she and the baby need. Therefore the food choices she makes on a daily basis will make a difference to her health, the progress of the pregnancy and to the health of her child. Consequently, as an example, eating a small jacket potato with cottage cheese rather than a packet of crisps – which have the same calorie value – will be a better choice.

Certain nutrients are needed in greater quantities during pregnancy; these include folic acid, vitamin D, vitamin C and sometimes iron. The fatty acids a woman consumes can have profound effects on the long-term health of her child. There are also commonly consumed items which are not advised in pregnancy, as they can possibly have a negative impact. These include alcohol, excess coffee, liver (which has too much vitamin A) and foods which may be sources of bacterial contamination and can induce birth defects. Most medicines must be avoided during pregnancy (refer to your doctor for advice). Many compounds cross the placenta into the developing baby, which is why substances such as alcohol and caffeine affect the baby.

For more on the best food choices during pregnancy, see page 274.

## Infancy and childhood

Children need supercharged nutrition, but generally are not getting it. The reason they need high quality nutrition is that they are growing and 30 per cent of energy is being used for growth in the first year. In the first six months they double their birth weight and triple it by the end of the first year. In the first six months of life a baby only needs breast milk, and breast milk is continued during the weaning phase. Undoubtedly *breast is best* because it is perfectly formulated for the growing human infant. In order for breast milk to be optimally nourishing, the mother's diet needs to be nutrient-rich. Many women choose to opt for formula feeding and formulas have improved dramatically in recent years, aiming to mirror breast milk as closely as possible, though they can never be as good.

Children grow and develop at a terrific rate, and their brains are also developing and growing. The brain uses up 20 per cent of energy in an adult, but in a child it requires around 30 per cent of energy – this is for an organ which is only around 2 per cent of our overall weight. To sustain this growth and development children need the best quality food possible, but the reality is that they are often eating worse quality food than adults. In the last 30 years we have seen the advent of special foods marketed specifically for children. The astounding thing about these foods is that they are often cheaper and therefore use poor quality ingredients. It is common for children to eat their meals separately from their parents, which means that they eat different meals.

For instance, a parent might eat an evening meal of 'meat and two veg' while their children will eat, earlier in the evening, chicken nuggets and chips, perhaps with peas or baked beans. For dessert the parent might have some fruit while the child has a pot of 'kid's' pudding. This scenario is very, very common and crosses the social and financial divides. The result is that the parents are eating reasonably balanced meals with controlled amounts of salt and fat, while the children are eating pre-packaged foods; these have high amounts of low nutrient fillers and binders which can make upto 40 per cent of the product, with high salt, sugar and fat levels.

There is, generally, no problem with children's growth rate – children today are taller than previous generations as they are getting more than sufficient calories. However, they are also growing width-ways as a result of the poor nutritional quality of the foods they eat and one in five children is now classified as overweight or obese. Of great concern is that while they are getting sufficient calories, they are not getting the micronutrients – vitamins and minerals – that they need. Government nutrition surveys have identified several dietary deficiencies in children: vitamin A, vitamin C, vitamin D, copper, iodine, iron and zinc. Nutritional deficiencies such as these can compromise immune health, mental performance and energy levels.

## Changing needs as we age

We are enjoying longer life-spans than ever before, but the payback is that we need to say healthier for longer. It is inevitable that more should go wrong as we age – after all most things deteriorate over long periods of time. In much the same way as we need to build a house with good materials, and repaint and repair it over time to stop it decaying, we also need to take preventative action to ensure our long-term good health.

As we age, our calorie needs drop and body composition changes. Lean tissue reduces as a proportion of overall weight, to be replaced by fat tissue. This reduces calorie needs and if a downward shift in calories isn't made, then more body fat tissue accumulates. Of course increased physical activity, particularly resistance exercise, can reduce or stop this effect. But at the same time high quality nutrition is needed to prop up the general decline in body tissues: joint, organ, muscle and brain tissue. This makes it vital that high quality food is eaten. Digestive function is also often compromised as we age, with a general slowing down of digestive processes. This can further compromise optimum nutrition. The solution is to make sure that diet fits digestive capability. This starts with looking after our teeth and ends with ensuring healthy bowel bacteria (the balance of bowel bacteria changes as we age).

Most of the age-related diseases with which we are all familiar – arthritis, decreased mental acuity, digestive slow-down, bone health, eye health – have a nutritional component which makes it important that a person in their thirties or forties needs to think about their diet in relation to future health. Women also need to make changes as a result of going through the menopause. This is quite a radical shift as far as nutrition is concerned, because their health risk profile shifts from one that is typically female to one which, to some degree, begins to reflect traditional health problems experienced by men, including stroke and heart disease (though there remain gender differences in how these manifest).

## Nutrition during sports and exercise

Sport and exercise are excellent ways of staying fit and enhancing health. Government advice is that more of us should lead active lives featuring regular exercise. The reality is that we are considerably more sedentary than previous generations. This, in part, is to do with the availability of labour-saving devices, car usage (which precludes walking or cycling), and increased TV watching and computer use. In these circumstances it is obvious that increasing activity levels to the minimum recommended amounts of half-an-hour daily of reasonably brisk walking is advantageous for cardiovascular health. Other cardiovascular activity options are swimming, team sports and racket games. Maintaining the strength of muscles by doing resistance exercise, such as rowing, weight training or push-ups, is also important. To improve bone density, impact or weight bearing exercise is recommended, such as the resistance exercise mentioned previously, skipping and using a mini-trampoline.

So, if some exercise and physical activity on a daily basis is good for us, then is it true that more must be even better? Yes and no. A more intense regime of physical activity, whether training for competitive sport, dance training or just incorporating more than the average amount of physical training into daily life, is undoubtedly health-enhancing overall, but also carries a nutritional price. To ensure that our health is not damaged by the effects of over-exercising, attention needs to be paid to the potential for damage. Obviously warming up and cooling down are important measures, but there are also nutritional considerations: oxidation damage to muscles, hydration, maintaining normal hormonal cycles and ensuring that iron-deficiency does not lead to exercise-induced tiredness all need to be taken into account. For more on exercise see page 193.

# 7

# How Nutritious is the Food We Eat?

You can get all you need from a balanced diet. How often have you heard this said? And is it true or not?

The first response to this statement is that few people really know what a balanced diet is. (For more information on this see Chapter 1.) But there are also questions raised by how our food is produced and what is added to it during processing, along with lifestyle habits that might interfere with nutritional balance.

## Refined Grains

We are missing a huge nutritional opportunity by generally preferring refined grains over wholegrains. The starchy centre of any grain, for instance white rice, or white flour used for bread and baked products, provides calories for energy but little else. Wholegrains retain the husk and the germ of the grain. By stripping away the outer husk of a grain we lose B-vitamins, magnesium, calcium, chromium, iron, zinc and other micronutrients, as well as fibre. The germ provides essential fatty acids. In recognition of these deficiencies the law partially remedies the situation by insisting that white flour is fortified with iron, calcium and some B-vitamins, but this only goes part of the way to solving the problem and many other nutrients are missed out.

## Salt and Sugar

While a little sodium (found in salt) present naturally in foods is necessary for our bodies to function, a lot, such as in processed foods, is very bad. We consume, on average, nearly twice the recommended maximum of 5–7g of salt daily. Most of this comes from packaged food staples such as cornflakes and bread, and also from cheese, sausages, snacks, pre-prepared dishes and children's food. Lowering salt intakes is one of the key government health targets, as this could significantly lower blood-pressure in the population and so reduce cardiovascular disease risk – statistically the biggest killer. Aside from the health risks, and asking the question of whether our diet provides sufficient nutrients, salt is added for one major reason to processed foods: to disguise cheap, taste-less ingredients which are intrinsically low in nutrients. This is easy to visualize: imagine the taste of crisps without salt (greasy). The same is true of sugar: imagine the taste of a doughnut without sugar (greasy). A century ago we ate around 1kg of sugar annually per person, while now the figure is around 60kg. So salt and sugar are additives which in moder-ation bring out flavours in cooking, but in larger quantities are used to make cheap low-nutrient food taste better.

## Fatty Acid Composition

Our consumption of fish has dropped by 50 per cent in 60 years and this is having dramatic consequences for the intake of omega-3 fatty acids in the diet. Meat reared on grass or able to range freely has significantly higher proportions of omega-3 fatty acids (the 'fish oil family') and a lower propor-tion of saturated fatty acids. The same is true of eggs from chickens that are able to forage freely. This considerably healthier fatty acid profile mirrors the make-up that would have been found in our ancestors' diets throughout our evolution. The habit of grain feeding our livestock bulks the animals out – improving financial gain – but also dramatically alters fatty acid composition to favour saturated fatty acids which are linked to a variety of inflammatory disease states. The large quantity of omega-6 fatty acids in our diet, derived from cooking oils, margarine and processed foods also encourages inflammation by crowding omega-3 fatty acids out of our diets.

## Food Preparation and Cooking Methods

How we cook and prepare foods makes a difference to the nutritional contribution they make to our health. Cooking many foods actually makes nutrients more available for absorption. For instance, absorption of the carotenes (found in orange and red-coloured fruit and vegetables) is enhanced many times over by cooking or processing. Other foods just can't be eaten until they are cooked, such as beans and other pulses. However, overcooking food leads to a loss of the many vitamins which are heat sensitive. Additionally, boiling in water will lead to the loss of a significant amount of minerals (you can see this in the colour of the water, which we often then throw away). A loss of cooking skills has made this worse. Making stocks and soups and slow casseroles preserves these minerals, but these are often considered old-fashioned methods which don't fit with fast-paced modern lives. Eating too much cooked food, with little fresh, raw food in the diet will usually contribute to a loss of vitality. Enjoying fresh fruit and vegetables and their fresh juices is an excellent way to ensure beneficial nutrient intake. For more on food cooking methods, see page 97.

## Food Storage

Buying, and eating, fresh food is a foundation of a healthy diet. However, we tend to bulk buy these days, with 80 per cent of us making a weekly trip to the supermarket instead of buying fresh a few times a week. While this may seem convenient, leaving fresh produce for a week before eating it can dramatically increase vitamin-loss. A cabbage will lose half of its vitamin C (of which it is a rich source) in a short time and that is hastened by cutting and exposing to air. The produce you buy has often been sitting around in cold-store for a long time – it takes an average of six weeks for fruit to reach the customer's plate after it has been picked, and an apple can spend up to a year in cold store. The answer to this is to buy as locally and as seasonally as possible, from suppliers that you know (reducing 'food miles' is also good for the environment). If this is not possible, leave 'protected' foods to be eaten last – those with skins such as oranges or winter squashes will last longest. If convenience is important, frozen vegetables often have more nutrients because they have been picked and frozen almost immediately to preserve freshness and so nutrient loss is minimized.

## Food Additives

Many food additives, especially flavourings and colourings, are used to enhance the appeal of commercially prepared foods without adding any nutritional benefit. If this was all there was to the situation it would possibly not be an issue. However, frequently it is these additives which are disguising low-cost, low-nutrient, filler ingredients which are added to bulk out foods. These fillers include water, maltodextrine (a hydrolized – or partially broken down – starch), starch, fats and mechanically extruded meats. By packing up to 40 per cent bulking and filling agents manufacturers lower their costs dramatically but also lower the nutritional value of the food eaten. Additionally some of these food additives, particularly colourings and some preservatives, are suspected of causing health problems such as behavioural problems, asthma and skin rashes, especially in children (probably because foods targeted at them feature these additives widely).

## Nutrient Antagonism

Many aspects of diet and lifestyle interfere with the optimal absorption of vitamins and minerals from our foods. For instance a cup of tea or coffee immediately after a meal can reduce the uptake of minerals dramatically. Tea will reduce iron uptake by half and coffee will lower uptake of magnesium and B-vitamins. This information could be important if you are, for example, anaemic or inexplicably lacking in energy. It could be a better choice to drink a herbal tea which enhances digestion, such as mint tea, and save tea and coffee for mid-morning or mid-afternoon when drunk away from food. Similarly alcohol severely interferes with and depletes B-vitamins, and many common drugs interfere with nutrient uptake and metabolism. Sugar causes a net loss of the mineral chromium (which is needed for blood sugar regulation and insulin metabolism).

## Changing Nutrient Levels

There is a growing awareness that the odds are stacked against a person today getting as much nutritional benefit from their diet as someone 50-60 years ago, or even 4000 years ago (presuming that lack of food supply is not an issue). It has been estimated from comparisons of UK and USA nutrition tables that we get up to 50 per cent fewer vitamins and minerals from many common foods than 50 years ago. (There may be differences in the way foods were tested, but this is unlikely to result in such wide differences across the board.) There is concern that the nutrient levels provided from soil which is over exploited due to intensive farming methods is a core problem. The most stark example of how soil nutrient levels can affect human health is the drop in selenium level intakes in the last ten to 20 years. Wheat was the UK's main source of selenium, but after joining the EU imports from selenium-rich North America were reduced in favour of European wheat. This has resulted in an estimated 50 per cent drop in selenium intake, so that the average person may be deficient. Acid rain has probably also made this worse, since the acidity causes plants to increase uptake of silicon rather than selenium in from the soil.

## Plant Breeds

Modern tastes are for sweeter foods than were previously available. To this end the modern apple has up to 20 per cent more sugar in it than earlier common varieties. There is also concern that we might breed out the bitter taste of some vegetables such as broccoli, cabbage and Brussels sprouts to make them more popular. The problem with this is that the health promoting compounds are precisely those chemicals responsible for their slightly bitter taste.

The other major change that has happened to our food supply concerns choice. While it seems that we have greater choice because foods are available from around the world, the actual number of plant breeds used for common produce, as diverse as wheat, bananas and apples, has narrowed: a century ago, 200 or more varieties of apple were widely available, while now around ten varieties are favoured and grown to the detriment of others.

## The Benefits of Organic

People buy organic food for all sorts of reasons: environmental issues; in reaction to food scares; to minimize chemical intakes in the diet; and sometimes from a belief that organic foods are more nutritious. Organic food was the norm before World War II – a time before the advent of the thousands of artificial chemicals we now use. Certainly an organic diet reduces exposure to artificial chemicals, and additionally there has never yet been a case of BSE in organic cattle herds. Organic foods have higher nutrients and minerals, for example vitamin C, omega-3 fatty acids and Vitamin E in milk, and also higher levels of a compound called salycilic acid. It is unknown if there is an overall nutritional benefit to eating organic food; however, it is strongly suspected that the artificial chemicals used have hormone disrupting effects and it is likely that any cocktail effect of using several compounds together will be worse on the bodies of small children than for adults.

## Functional Foods

The addition of nutrients to foods is not a new idea, and food fortification has been a common practice with iron, calcium and some B-vitamins being added to white flour used for baking and bread production and the addition of vitamin A to margarine. But these have all been added to make up for what is lost in the processing of food. A new, commercially driven form of fortification is now available – these foods are variously called functional foods, neutraceuticals and designer foods. They have ingredients added, which would not normally appear in the recipe, specifically for enhancing the health promoting qualities of the product. In nature many foods naturally provide health enhancing effects and these are outlined in Part 2, A–Z of Superfoods. For example oats naturally lower cholesterol, oily fish naturally thin blood, broccoli has cancer fighting compounds, soya has hormone modulating effects and yoghurt contains bacteria which is beneficial for bowel health.

The functional foods now available would probably not be necessary if everyone ate a healthy diet which incorporated these foods, but in the same way that the vitamin and mineral supplement market has become popular because people want to optimize their health in the face of a fast-food culture, so functional foods are finding a niche. Examples of available foods include orange juice enriched with calcium, eggs enhanced with omega-3 fatty acids (by changing the diet of the laying chickens), cholesterol lowering foods which contain statins and stanols, and foods and drinks enhanced with pre- and probiotics (healthy bowel bacteria).

## Then and Now

Our bodies and brains – our physiology – have not changed significantly in the last 10,000 years, but our diets have. One aim of improving our background diet is to get much closer to the balance of nutrients that our paleolithic ancestors evolved to live on. By getting closer to this we give our bodies the best possible chance of righting any health problems. This is how the make-up of our diets has changed (on average):

|  | Then | Now |
|---|---|---|
| Protein % | 33 | 15 |
| Carbohydrate % | 46 | 45 |
| Fat % | 21 | 38 |
| Polyunsaturated fat/ saturated fat ratio | 1.4:1 | 0.4:1 |
| Omega-6/omega–3 fatty acid ratio | 1:1 | 10–20:1 |
| Fibre (grams) | 100 | 22 |
| Folic acid (micrograms) | 357 | 265 |
| Vitamin C (milligrams) | 440 | 74 |

It may be unfeasible for many people to redress the balance to the point where their diet reflects the exact balance of our ancestors: for instance very few people will reach the fibre levels of our hunter-gatherer ancestors who ate large quantities of roughage from roots, seeds, vegetable leaves and fruits. However, wherever possible the health guidelines suggested in this book will take this reference point into consideration, particularly in relation to the balance of fatty acids in the diet.

# 8

# Genetics – The New Frontier

Genetics hits the news daily with 'big-news', almost science-fiction, items such as the eradication of genetic diseases, the potential to grow new tissues and cloning. But of more practical everyday use for the average person is that genetic research is also telling us how our individual genetic profiles interact with our environment. This is likely to prove to be of real value for those who wish to alter and improve the course of their life-long health by changing their lifestyle and habits, the food they eat and, possibly, the supplements they take.

## Changes in Food Supply

We have evolved over millions of years, and our genetically identical ancestors were roaming the continents 10,000 years ago after the last ice age retreated. At about this time in our history a major shift took place in our food supply. As people settled into fixed communities and abandoned their nomadic lifestyles, farming became a possibility. At this time we generally ceased to be totally dependent on being hunter-gatherers, with the food that we gathered, scavenged or killed being the only food that we ate. The ability to grow grains evolved and the penning of animals became an option, with all the advantages of a fixed and abundant food supply.

This system obviously had a lot of advantages but also heralded a major change in the types of foods we ate. Grains such as wheat, corn and rice (depending on which continent people were on), became a mainstay of the diet, and for the first time dairy products from penned animals were introduced into everyday diet. These energy-dense foods also allowed us more time to evolve other aspects of society as we had more time on our hands. (A clear sign that our ability to physically adapt has not kept pace with the changes in diet is the number of lactose-intolerant people – those who can't digest the milk sugar lactase – who amount to around 70 per cent of the world population. These people are unable to digest fully milk because 10,000 years is just not enough time to adapt.)

In the twentieth century, our food supply changed even more radically. Food was able to be shipped in vast quantities across the world, new methods of food preservation were invented, refrigeration made a very important contribution to food storage and the reduction of food poisoning, and of course the supermarkets – which now supply 80 per cent of households – made their mark. Foods have become available year round, and convenience and low prices have become the most important criteria in a majority of households. But yet again there are downsides and the constant pressure of low prices and easy availability has driven the nutritional quality of much of the food we eat downwards and this is driving our health into a similar abyss.

## Changes in Disease Patterns

Over this time we have seen a change in the types of diseases to which we succumb. In earlier centuries, average, and maximum, life spans were much shorter. In our hunter-gatherer days we only lived to about our forties, long before any age-related diseases could set in (apart from arthritis from the heavy work of day-to-day living). The greatest impact on life span over the nineteenth and twentieth centuries came from improved sanitation, antibiotic use to limit the impact of bacterial-born disease, and anti- and post-natal care to improve child and maternal mortality statistics. While a good food supply would make the difference between good and poor health, it was not a major driving force on life span compared to these other interventions.

Now we are all living longer, however, we are experiencing a different set of problems that are intimately bound up with nutrition. The type of diseases to which we are subject are mostly degenerative diseases, many of which do not kill but just make life miserable, for example arthritis, Alzheimer's and depression. Allergies are also a major problem and have gone from a very low incidence to affecting over a quarter of the population. The killer diseases, cancer and heart disease, to which we are at least in part subject to precisely because we *are* living longer, also have major nutritional components.

## Genetics and the Environment

The point about this history lesson is that our genes have not changed markedly in recent millennia. What has changed is the environment in which we find ourselves. But we now know that there is a genetic component to many – perhaps most – diseases. Most interesting, though, is the fact that our genetic make-up interacts with our environment. Genes are not set in stone but respond to environmental factors and diet – this is called 'gene regulation'. The environmental factors to which our genes respond include: diet, smoking, alcohol intake, the exercise we take, stress levels, age of first having children, number of children we have, sun exposure, radiation exposure, toxic chemical exposure and many other factors. Not only do nutrients – and other environmental factors – change 'gene expression' (how a gene behaves) but genes also affect how we use nutrients and whether our needs are typical compared to other people's, or different.

How environmental factors affect us depends on our individual genetics. Someone with one genetic profile may be more likely to develop heart disease, another will be more likely to develop Alzheimer's and another will develop arthritis. Yet others, the lucky few, will defy all gloomy health predictions, smoking and drinking themselves into a very late and healthy grave because they are genetically programmed to do so. But most of us can't count on this!

At the moment this emerging genetic information has limited practical use on a day-to-day basis, other than intelligent guess work. A person who has had several members of their family succumb to a particular health problem – perhaps who is prone to being overweight, or prone to allergies, or prone to memory loss with advancing age, or prone to breast cancer – will have reasonable clues that this is an area of their health that they need to attend to. In very few cases, such as testing for the BRCA1 and BRCA2 breast cancer genes, are we able to find out definitively what our genetic risk factors are. This science is undoubtedly going to be applied to other health conditions in the not too distant future. It is not science fiction to imagine that we will be told in early years what our genetic health risk profile is and to be given dietary, nutritional supplement and drug prescription advice to optimize our health.

## Practical Steps

At the moment what we can do is to test for and make lifestyle changes to alter certain 'biochemical markers' of nutritional and genetic interactions. Whilst the genes are not being tested for, the biochemical changes that result from these gene/environment interactions are. For instance, people prone to high cholesterol, high blood pressure or high homocysteine can change their diet, and possibly take supplements and drugs to alter their risk profile. This is going to become much more common with other conditions.

We are finding out that certain groups of people are probably not metabolizing some nutrients as well as they should do, because of their genetics, and so supplementation is a possible way forward as they will not get sufficient of the required nutrient from their diets. Examples are:

- Women who have already had a child with a neural tube defect who need extra high levels of folic acid
- People from allergic families (atopic families) who do not metabolize the essential fatty acids properly due to a genetic inefficiency of the enzyme delta-6-desaturase, and who can benefit from supplementation of fatty acids such as from fish oils
- Around 25 per cent of the population seem to be prone to high homocysteine levels, with implications for heart disease, pre-eclampsia in pregnancy and senile dementia, and for whom a B-vitamin supplement with folic acid, B2, B6 and B12 may be the difference between disease and health
- Yet others may have higher than average genetic requirements for the important antioxidant mineral selenium which could ultimately help to protect them from developing cancer
- Those who are genetically programmed to produce a particular type of a protein called haptoglobin, which helps return free haemoglobin to the liver, are likely to benefit in cardiovascular risk profile when taking antioxidant

supplements. Others may have no benefit, while others may worsen.

- Genetics may dictate whether someone with asthma benefits, or has worse symptoms, from taking fish oils.

The point is that the science of nutrition is becoming more targeted. Watch this space!

# PART 2:

# A–Z OF SUPERFOODS

## Superfoods

For many years individual foods have been known to have particular therapeutic effects. This is increasingly being recognized with, for instance, specific health claims now permitted for oats, walnuts and soya-based foods in the US. Having said this, it is important not to overdo any one food just because it is supposed to be good for a condition you are wishing to improve. Eat it regularly, but remember to vary your diet and keep a balanced approach – by and large it is the entire diet which counts towards optimal health.

## Apples

These common fruit are particularly rich in quercitin, an antioxidant flavonoid which is highly supportive of the lungs. Apples also have high levels of a soluble fibre, pectin, which promotes bowel health. However, modern varieties such as Braeburn and Fuji are bred to have a much higher sugar content than older varieties such as Cox's Orange Pippin and Granny Smiths. This means that they are increasingly detrimental to teeth – therefore ideally you should eat them with meals.

*Useful for: Lung, bowel/digestive health*

## Apricots

Dried apricots are low on the Glycaemic Index (see page 350), making them ideal for snacking when compared to more sugary dried fruit such as raisins and dates. The betacarotene they contain is highly supportive of eyes, mucus membranes and general immunity. All dried fruit is an excellent source of iron.

*Useful for: Lung health, antioxidant protection, blood sugar control*

## Artichoke, globe

Research indicates that this vegetable has a strong bile stimulating and liver cleansing effect. It is eaten to relieve bloating, indigestion and the effects of alcohol.

*Useful for: Liver*

## Artichoke, Jerusalem

This root vegetable is particularly high in an invaluable compound called inulin. Unfortunately, this is also what gives the vegetable its 'windy' reputation. Inulin is a non-digestible fibre which acts as a prebiotic (promoting the growth of healthy bowel bacteria).

*Useful for: Bowels*

## Asparagus

Used as a traditional remedy for kidney problems, asparagus contains an alkaloid, asparagines, which while it stimulates the kidneys, turns urine dark and gives it a distinctive smell. This is an indication that its diuretic actions are working. Choose green asparagus for more of a nutritional punch than white asparagus can deliver.

*Useful for: Kidneys*

## Avocado

Spurned by many for its high calories, avocados are an excellent way to satisfy the urge to eat some fat without resorting to saturated fats. Mashing onto bread instead of butter to 'moisten' a sandwich is a good example. High in vitamin E, which works with vitamin C, avocados are excellent for the skin.

*Useful for: Skin health*

## Banana

This favourite fruit is convenient for a quick snack. To reduce the impact on blood sugar choose slightly less ripe fruit, but to increase digestibility choose riper fruit. Being high in potassium, bananas benefit nerve (and so brain) health and the kidneys. Bananas are effective in reducing fat and sugar levels in the diet, as they can be chopped into cereals, used in baking and mashed into sandwiches.

*Useful for: Brain, kidney health*

## Barley

This grain is much underused, but is very adaptable to many dishes as a replacement for rice or when used in stews. Barley is rich in fibre, calcium, iron, magnesium and potassium. It is very low on the Glycaemic Index (see page 350), giving it a stabilizing effect on blood sugar and making it an ideal substitute for grains such as wheat and rice. This makes it valuable for diabetics. Barley water is a time-honoured herbal remedy for kidney, intestinal and bowel disorders.

*Useful for: Blood sugar control, kidney, digestive health*

## Beer

A modest intake of traditionally brewed beer is a good way to ensure B-vitamin levels. B-vitamins are essential for all aspects of energy production, for nerve health and for stress hormone production. Beer is also a good source of silicon, an important mineral for skin, hair and nails, as well as for bones. One pint contains around 11mg of silicon.

*Useful for: Brain function, energy*

## Beetroot

An extremely rich source of betacarotene which converts to vitamin A, vital for the health of the retina. Also traditionally used to alleviate anaemia (iron deficiency).

*Useful for: Eyes, skin, possibly anaemia*

## Berries

Red/purple berries such as strawberries, raspberries, blackberries, blackcurrants and others are rich in anthocyanins, which give them their colouring. These have potent antioxidant properties. Strawberries and blackcurrants are also particularly rich sources of vitamin C. Bilberries (blueberries) help to improve vision. Blueberries are one of the richest sources of antioxidants known. Cranberries and blueberries have particular properties which stop adhesion of pathogenic bacteria in the urinary tract, making them potent allies against cystitis. Vitamin C and the flavonoids that berries contain keep blood vessels and capillaries strong.

*Useful for: Skin, protecting against infections, heart disease, cystitis, stomach ulcers, anti-cancer*

## Bitter and peppery vegetables

The bitter compounds in many vegetables are what make them therapeutically useful. For instance, the slightly bitter taste of broccoli gives it its anti-cancer effect from those compounds that are biologically active. Watercress is a member of the mustard family, as are radishes, which make them both ideal for catarrhal conditions. Radishes are also useful for kidney health. All the bitter and peppery vegetables and salad ingredients tend to have a positive effect on the liver by promoting detoxification processes and stimulating bile production.

*Useful for: Liver, kidneys, catarrhal conditions*

## Buckwheat

Also known as kasha when cooked, buckwheat is not actually wheat. It is a rich source of the flavanoid rutin, which aids vascular health. Being free of gluten, it has many uses for those who are intolerant to wheat. It can be cooked like rice, made into a porridge and the flour cooked as pancakes (blinis).

*Useful for: Blood sugar balance, gluten intolerance*

## Cherries

Like all the dark red, blue and purple berries, cherries are excellent sources of antioxidant anthocyanins. Cherries are so high in salicylates that 20 cherries have been found to have analgesic properties similar to aspirin. Two hundred grams daily (a lot!) is protective against build-up of compounds that cause gout.

*Useful for: Antioxidant protection, pain relief*

## Chocolate, dark

Chocolate has a bad name mainly because it typically is made with a high amount of sugar and is also fatty. However, dark, high-cocoa content (60–70 per cent cocoa solids) chocolate is almost a health food – as long as it is eaten in moderation. Cocoa is high in antioxidants; because milk inhibits their absorption, dark, rather than milk, chocolate is preferable. Chocolate is high in a saturated fat, stearic acid. This converts into oleic acid in the body, a mono-unsaturated fat of the kind found in olive oil, which is linked to health benefits. There are mixed reports about the advantages of this fat profile. On the one hand, chocolate does not raise the damaging LDL cholesterol levels, which is a good thing as far as heart disease is concerned. However, it seems that the good HDL cholesterol is suppressed. On the other hand, the antioxidant compounds in chocolate help to protect from heart disease. Chocolate docs not particularly encourage dental caries, as the cocoa butter coats teeth and protects them from harmful bacteria. Dark chocolate is a very good source of magnesium and iron. A little goes a long way, which is just as well because dark chocolate is also a strong source of caffeine. Theobromine in chocolate is more effective than codeine medication for soothing a cough.

*Useful for: Antioxidant protection, tooth health*

## Citrus

All citrus fruit is high in vitamin C. The pith also contains the important flavonoids rutin and hesperidin, which complement the actions of vitamin C and strengthens blood vessels. This makes them important for wound healing and vascular health. Vitamin C is also needed to make collagen in skin and for energy production (the energy cycle is called the citric acid cycle, after vitamin C). The rind of (preferably unwaxed) lemons is valuable for the compound limonene, which aids liver P450 enzyme detoxification pathways (see page 239). Grapefruit juice should be avoided when taking some medication (see chapter 8 for more on this).

*Useful for: Immune health, skin elasticity, wound healing, energy, cardiovascular health*

## Cress and other sprouts

The young sprouted plant, whether the more familiar cress or alfalfa, or the less familiar sprouted beans or seeds such as mung, chickpea or sunflower (although these are not widely available some health food shops have them, or sprout them at home) are unique power-houses of nutrition. At the point when the plant has just sprouted, it is benefiting from the stored nutrition in the seed and has just started to trap energy from sunlight, giving it its green colouring; this makes sprouts richer as a nutritious food than at any other time in the plants' growing cycle.

*Useful for: Anti-cancer, nutritional deficiency*

## Cruciferous vegetables

This family of vegetables, also known as brassicas, includes broccoli, cabbage, Brussels sprouts, cauliflower, cress, horse-radish, radish, kale, bok choy, swede (rutabaga) and turnip. They are known to have important anti-cancer properties. The slightly bitter taste of these vegetables comes from a chemical they contain called singrin. This is converted on cooking or eating into allyl-isothiocyanate (AITC), which encourages apoptosis (cell death) in cancer cells. Broccoli, cabbage, Brussels sprouts and cauliflower are also all extremely good sources of vitamin C.

*Useful for: Anti-cancer*

## Fish

Oily fish provides the fatty acids DHA and EPA. These are essential for brain and nervous tissue development and health, cell membrane structure and production of anti-inflammatory compounds. EPA also reduces blood platelet 'stickiness' and clumping. White fish such as cod, haddock and plaice are not significant sources of these oils, but are still beneficial as they are very low fat sources of protein. Fish are also important sources of iodine, vital for thyroid health, and selenium, needed for over 14 critical enzyme processes including antioxidant and thyroid hormones and for sperm motility.

*Useful for: Brain health, behavioural problems, cardiovascular health, learning, anti-inflammatory, thyroid, fertility, pregnancy*

## Fruit, tropical

Fruits such as pineapple, papaya and kiwi have high levels of enzymes that can benefit the digestive system. In particular bromelain and papain digest proteins, which means that they have a role in cleaning up dead tissue in the digestive tract and helping to reduce ulceration. Papain, from papaya, also seems to have a positive effect on bowel flora. There is some evidence that these enzymes can have a positive effect on reducing blood clotting.

*Useful for: Digestion, ulceration*

## Game

Meat from game such as deer, pheasant and partridge has advantages over reared meat. Like reared meat, these meats are high in iron and zinc, but they are also very lean. Because of the animals' wild lifestyle, they are not fed fattening forage foods and so their fat profiles have very little saturated fats and good amounts of omega-3 fats (the type also found in oily fish). At certain times of the year in rural communities, game is relatively inexpensive.

*Useful for: Low fat*

## Grapes

Dark grapes contain anthodyanins and resveratrol. White and dark grapes contain ellagic acid and also pterostilbene. All these combined serve to improve many aspects of heart disease risk including blood lipid levels and blood pressure.

*Useful for: Heart disease, high blood pressure*

## Green, leafy vegetables

Vegetables such as cabbage, kale, spinach and Brussels sprouts get their green colour from chlorophyll, which is extremely rich in magnesium. This mineral is needed for over 300 functions in the body, including nerve health, a healthy heart, the stress reaction, for bone structure, and to reduce migraines and PMS. These vegetables are also rich in folic acid, essential for cell reproduction and the formation of nerve insulation. Finally, they are also particularly rich in vitamin K for healthy bones and for blood clotting.

*Useful for: Nerve health, cardiovascular disease, healthy pregnancy, anti-cancer, stress, migraines, PMS, bone health*

## Honey

Honey is not much better than sugar as a source of sweetness. However, raw, unpasteurized, honey cultivated locally may have a use in an 'inoculating' effect against hay fever in any given region. Manuka honey, which comes from New Zealand, has potent antibacterial properties, known from fairly extensive research, which makes it very useful in the treatment of internal and external ulcers, and is particularly helpful against *Helicobacter pylori*.

*Useful for: Hay fever, ulcers*

## Linseeds

Also known as flax seeds, these tiny seeds are high in compounds called lignans. When swollen with liquid (either from pre-soaking, being added to yoghurt or milk in breakfast cereal, or when mixed with digestive juices in the digestive tract) they produce a mucilaginous gel-like fibre which enhances bowel movements dramatically. This coats and protects the digestive mucosa, bulks out and softens stools, making them easy to pass. The phytochemicals from linseeds are acted on by bowel flora to improve oestrogen profiles, making them an ally in managing breast cancer. Linseeds are best cracked (in a coffee grinder) or soaked before adding to dishes. People with diverticulitis should not take linseeds unless they have been milled to a powder, as the small seeds can lodge in the diverticuli. It is important to drink sufficient water, or other liquid, when taking linseeds.

*Useful for: Bowel health, breast cancer*

## Liver

Along with other offal, liver has gone out of fashion. Yet because the liver is the storage organ for many vitamins and minerals it is also a particularly rich source of these nutrients. A small portion of liver once every two or three weeks would probably be equivalent to taking a vitamin and mineral supplement daily. However, as the liver is also the processing area in the body for toxins and pollutants, eating organic liver is probably the best option. Women who are planning a pregnancy or who are pregnant are advised to avoid liver and liver products such as pâtés because of high levels of vitamin A, which could damage a foetus.

*Useful for: Nutritional deficiencies, anaemia*

## Meat, lean

For lean meat cut away all visible fat, and drain off fat when cooking (for instance, mince or stews). Alternatively choose naturally very lean game meat such as pheasant or venison. Meat provides the most absorbable form of iron. Including some protein, such as meat, with meals and snacks helps to dampen the glycaemic effects of carbohydrates (see page 350) and so helps to keep blood sugar control within a healthy range. Meat is also one of the richest sources of zinc, needed for building all body tissues, hormones and brain chemicals. Vegetarians need not be deficient in iron and zinc, as the same nutrients are found in cheese, eggs, beans, pulses, nuts and seeds.

*Useful for: Anaemia, Blood sugar balance, building tissues and hormones*

## Mushrooms, Oriental

Cultivated mushrooms are the ones that are most frequently eaten in the UK. However, other countries have traditions of mushroom hunting and of using wild mushrooms medicinally. Oriental and wild mushrooms are increasingly available in supermarkets and speciality food shops. Maitake and coriolus are used interchangeably for their effects on boosting white blood cell counts. Coriolus may be slightly preferred, as it seems to have a more sustained effect, and it is helpful for treating ME (chronic fatigue). Reishi, also called the longevity mushroom, is effective in controlling allergies such as asthma and hay fever, as it lowers histamine levels. Ganoderma is another mushroom that is used for allergies. Both are useful for lowering cholesterol levels, and they are well tolerated when used in the long term. All the medicinal mushrooms have applications for improving blood sugar control in diabetics, though reishi might be the best choice. Cordyceps is useful for the elderly and for people in a weakened state. It is safe over the long term.

*Useful for: Immunity, allergies*

## Nettles

The traditional use for this leafy vegetable is as an iron and nerve tonic. Nettle tea is also a favourite to help reduce hay fever symptoms. Nettles can be used to make soup (but pick young leaves, unsprayed with pesticides, and wear gloves).

*Useful for: Anaemia, hay fever*

## Nuts

Many people avoid nuts as they are high in fat and can seem disastrous for those on calorie controlled diets. However, the fats they contain are mainly omega-6, with some nuts featuring omega-3 and omega-9. This means that they are healthy sources of fats as long as you don't eat too many. All nuts also contain good amounts of the antioxidant vitamin E, which keeps oils from going rancid and also works in harmony with vitamin C. Different nuts have specific properties:

- Walnuts are known to reduce risk of heart disease
- Brazils are the richest source of selenium and two or three a day provide the required daily intake
- Peanuts (not nuts, but actually legumes) have a beneficial effect on cholesterol levels. Peanuts (and peanut butter) are also high in copper which protects against heart disease
- Chestnuts are particularly low in fat, making them ideal in weight-loss regimes.

*Useful for: Heart health, blood sugar control*

## Oats

Rich in soluble fibre, oats are excellent for enhancing bowel health and for reducing cholesterol levels. Whole oats are quite low on the Glycaemic Index making them useful for blood sugar control. They are also used traditionally by herbalists to induce sleepiness, which may account for the popularity of oat-based night-time drinks (though making your own is a better option than pre-made mixes, which are very high in sugar). Porridge, flapjacks, sweet or savoury crumble toppings and oatcakes are all ways to enjoy oats.

*Useful for: Bowel health, blood sugar control, cholesterol, wheat intolerance*

## Okra

The high mucin content of okra (also called bindi or ladies' fingers) makes it very soothing for the digestive tract mucus membrane and is ideal for those with ulceration.

*Useful for: Digestive tract ulceration*

## Onions

Along with apples, onions are one of our main sources of the important antioxidant quercitin, which is excellent for lung health. Other members of the onion family, shallots, leeks and spring onions, have similar properties and the sulphur compounds they contain are highly supportive of immune and liver health. For garlic, see Culinary Herbs and Spices page 94.

*Useful for: Immune protection, lung health, liver health*

## Orange-coloured fruits and vegetables

Carrots, apricots, pumpkins, cantaloupes and mango get their colouring from carotenoids. Betacarotene is converted in the body into vitamin A as it is needed, which is important for eye and skin health. Betacarotene is supportive of the mucus membranes which line the lungs and digestive tract, making it useful against allergies. Carotenoids also have antioxidant properties in their own right, which fight cancer. Special carotenoids are also found in dark green leafy vegetables such as spinach (see page 89).

*Useful for: Eyes, immunity, lung health, anti-cancer*

## Pear

Because of their unusually high pectin soluble fibre content, pears are excellent for encouraging bowel movements when you are constipated. Eating three or four in a day during a constipation crisis can work wonders!

*Useful for: Bowel health*

## Peppers

Peppers are higher in vitamin C than most other fruit and vegetables and the red/orange-coloured ones are also very high in betacarotene, so they are especially good for immune health. They are ideal as a sweet-tasting low-calorie snack, as crudités for dips and are sweet when baked.

*Useful for: Immune health*

## Prunes and Figs

On a scale of sources of antioxidants conducted by Tufts University, prunes came out at the top of the list. Both prunes and figs have a beneficial effect on bowel health, as they are very rich in gentle sources of fibre.

*Useful for: Bowel health*

## Pulses, beans, lentils

These are a good source of protein and can be substituted for meat in vegetarian meals. In earlier days they were often added to casserole dishes to 'stretch' the budget, as meat was expensive – in France it is still common to have lentils or flageolet beans as a meat accompaniment. This adds many nutritional benefits to a meal. As they are low-fat, they reduce the overall fat content of a meal. Being rich in soluble fibre they are excellent for bowel health and also help to lower cholesterol. They are also rich in the minerals iron and zinc. Finally, being low on the Glycaemic Index (GI), they are an ideal meal substitute for higher GI foods such as bread, rice or potatoes.

*Useful for: Blood sugar control, bowel health, cholesterol*

## Rice, wholegrain

Brown rice takes longer to cook than white rice, but it has health benefits that makes it worth this effort. Wholegrain brown rice retains all the nutrients, such as B-vitamins, chromium and calcium, which are lost when rice husks are discarded. Whole rice is also lower on the GI than white rice, making it a better option for blood sugar control. Finally, brown rice is a source of gamma-oryzanol (GO) which helps to heal the gut wall and maintain its integrity, especially when ulcerated, in gastritis and IBS (irritable bowel syndrome). GO acts on the autonomic nervous system to normalize gastric secretions.

*Useful for: Digestive health, cholesterol, wheat intolerance*

## Rye

Bread made from rye is dark, with a slightly sour and nutty taste, and is commonly eaten in Eastern Europe.

Rye crackers are more commonly eaten in the UK. Rye was also a staple in the UK until a few hundred years ago when it fell out of favour and wheat bread became more popular. Rye is also very often tolerated by people in whom wheat causes digestive upset (though not in the case of gluten sensitivity). It is very rich in fibre and minerals.

*Useful for: Wheat intolerance, female hormone balance*

## Seafood

All seafood, such as prawns, oysters, crab, mussels and lobster, are ideal low-fat foods (prawns have some cholesterol but this is not unhealthy for blood cholesterol levels – see Cholesterol page 149). Shellfish are an excellent way to vary the diet and provide rich sources of nutrients. Seafood is very rich in iodine for thyroid health, and selenium for immune health and in protecting against cancer. Oysters are the richest known source of zinc, and crab the best known source of copper. These two elements are needed for skin health and copper is needed for melanin pigment formation which protects against sun damage and protects the heart. Some shellfish also provide useful quantities of DHA, the beneficial omega-3 fatty acid important for nerve function and cardiovascular health.

*Useful for: Brain health, thyroid health, immunity, anti-cancer, low-fat*

## Sea vegetables

At one time seaweed was used as a fertilizer in coastal growing areas, but this has fallen into disuse. This is a shame because the nutrients in seaweed are really valuable for enriching the earth and thus the plant foods grown in it. Unfortunately seaweeds are not commonly eaten in Europe. They are fantastically rich sources of iodine, selenium, magnesium and other trace elements. The Japanese eat plenty of seaweed and their traditional diet, which is low-fat, high in fish and seaweed, has many benefits. Indeed their recent changes in diet to reflect Western diet have led to an increase in Western degenerative diseases. Lava-bread from Wales and samphire from East-Anglia are remaining vestiges of our sea-vegetable eating past. Seaweed sheets, for toasting and flaking as a crunchy topping, or seaweed granules for grinding (they have a salty and not a fishy taste) into savoury dishes are available from health food shops. Traditionally-made sushi uses seaweed as a wrapper. If you have thyroid deficiency you can benefit from seaweed (kelp), but you should check with your doctor as it can make it worse in some situations (see Thyroid, page 304). Being so high in nutrients, sea vegetables are ideal to help boost overall nutritional status. Some seaweeds can be high in salt, however.

*Useful for: Thyroid health, nutritional deficiencies*

## Seeds

Being 'potential plants' with stored nutrients, seeds share many of the benefits of nuts (see above) and cress and other sprouts (also see above). Seeds are powerhouses of nutrients and are rich in essential fatty acids as well as many minerals. This makes them ideal for a number of conditions linked to essential fatty acid deficiency, such as skin and immune health, and inflammation. Sunflower and pumpkin seeds are ideal as snacks instead of biscuits. Whole and toasted, chopped or ground they can be added to savoury and sweet dishes to add fibre, healthy fats and micronutrients. When eating watermelon try crunching some of the seeds as they are particularly blessed with potassium, which helps to reduce fluid retention and high blood pressure.

*Useful for: Essential fatty acid deficiency, skin health, allergies, immune health*

## Soya

There are several potentially health-promoting effects of soya. The isoflavones genistein and diadzein have mild oestrogenic effects which can help to balance hormonal shifts in women. Where oestrogen is deficient, these can top levels up and thus reduce symptoms of the menopause such as hot flushes and bone degeneration. Conversely, in the case of oestrogen-sensitive problems such as menstrual bloating or some breast cancers, these mild oestrogens have been shown to block oestrogen receptor sites on cell surfaces and thus stop the excessive effects of other body oestrogens. Soya proteins have also been found to reduce the risk of heart disease and improve bone health. Many people with dairy allergies or intolerances choose soya, though 25 per cent of those with a true milk protein allergy are also allergic to soya.

*Useful for: Anti-cancer, PMS, menopause, bone health, heart health, dairy allergies*

## Spinach

Two members of the carotene family, leutine and zeaxanthine, are found in spinach and other dark green leafy vegetables. The orange colour of these carotenoids is disguised by the dark green colour of the leaves. These two carotenoids have been found to be particularly relevant in reducing the incidence of age-related macular degeneration, the leading cause of blindness in the over-sixties. Spinach is a reasonable source of iron, but not more so than other green vegetables. It is not easily absorbed and its Popeye reputation is probably not really deserved.

*Useful for: Eye health, nerve health, immunity*

## Sweet potato, yam

These vegetables make an ideal substitute for potatoes in many dishes. As an excellent source of betacarotene which converts to vitamin A they help to protect eye health. As they are much lower on the Glycaemic Index (see page 350) than potatoes and many other starches they make a valuable contribution to controlling blood sugar levels. They are high in the antioxidant vitamin E.

*Useful for: Blood sugar control, eye health*

## Tea, black

As tea may be drunk several times daily it makes an important contribution to the daily intake of antioxidant flavonoids (though it does not count as a portion of fruit and veg!). Tea drinking has been linked to reduced risk of cardiovascular disease. However, it may be best to drink it between meals if you are anaemic, as the tannins in tea dramatically reduce the absorption of iron. Adding milk or lemon to tea reduces this negative effect to a degree.

*Useful for: Antioxidant protection*

## Tea, green

Green tea has about a quarter of the caffeine of black tea, making it more acceptable to those who are caffeine-sensitive. A compound isolated from green tea, epigallocatechin-3-galate (EGCG), has been studied extensively. It appears there are several anti-cancer mechanisms in green tea, as long as sufficient amounts are drunk: about 10 cups daily.

*Useful for: Anti-cancer*

## Tomatoes

These fruit are the richest source of the powerful singlet-oxygen scavenger, lycopene. Lycopene is found in very few other red fruit: watermelon, guava and pink grapefruit. Singlet oxygen is one of the most damaging species of free-radical generators. Lycopene is 'liberated' and made more available for absorption when tomatoes are cooked or processed, such as in cans of tomato, tomato paste or juice. Lycopene, from daily tomato intake, has been strongly linked to a reduced risk of prostate and breast cancers.

*Useful for: Prostate and breast cancer, antioxidant*

## Water

Women need about 2.7 litres of water daily and men around 3.7 litres. We excrete around 1.5 litres of water daily in our urine, sweat, breath and faeces. There is much controversy over whether we really need to drink water for optimal hydration or whether any liquid will do. Certainly it is true that we get a significant amount – around 20 per cent – of our water intake from food. It is also true that nobody is likely to keel over if they drink gallons of coffee and no water at all. However, whether these various drinks will permit the body to function at its best is open to debate. One indisputable fact is that we evolved drinking only water and it is arguable that this is what our bodies are adapted to. Plenty of people swear that making the simple switch to drinking 1.5–2 litres daily of water (from any source, tap, bottled or filtered) has resolved many health complaints from creaky joints to headaches to skin problems.

The people most at risk from dehydration are those who suffer diarrhoea or vomiting (both of these may require special rehydration treatment rather than just water if severe), those who are elderly and hospitalized, children who engage in very active sports and those who move rapidly from a cool climate to a hot climate. Children have been shown to improve their concentration at school by the simple measure of keeping their liquid intake – water – up, and while thirst may be a good signal for dehydration for most people, children in particular are likely to override this signal if they are distracted with other activities. Anyone who is constipated should ensure they drink more water.

*Useful for: Hydration, constipation, concentration, sports performance*

## Wine, red

Red wine is rich in a polyphenol called resveratrol, which is believed to protect against heart disease and may explain some of the French diet effect: they eat more saturated fat than the British but have less heart disease (however, they do have more alcohol-related problems). Wine has an advantage over other alcohol sources as it tends to be drunk with meals, slowing down the effect of the alcohol. However, red grape juice or cranberry juice will afford similar antioxidant protection as red wine, and the protective effects on the heart of moderate alcohol consumption may well be related to any alcohol and not just red wine.

*Useful for: Antioxidants, cardiovascular health*

## Yoghurt

The cultures which are still active in 'live' or 'bio' plain yoghurt have a beneficial effect on bowel bacteria. Yoghurt consumption has been linked to better functioning immune health, probably via its effects on bowel health. Yoghurt is often tolerated even by those with a lactose intolerance: the bacteria in yoghurt breaks down the milk sugars (lactose) giving it its characteristic slightly sour taste. The same bacteria also partly pre-digest the milk proteins, making them more digestible and producing B-vitamins.

*Useful for: Bowel health, immunity, allergies*

## Culinary Herbs and Spices

Many day-to-day herbs used in the kitchen have impressive therapeutic effects. Medicinal herbal remedies are sold over the counter, but many more are simply found in the kitchen.

### Basil

The most potent effect of this herb is as a sedative and a good dose of pesto sauce with pasta will ease sleep. It also has antibacterial properties. Basil is used to increase the flow of milk in breast feeding. Do not use medicinally (i.e., repeated high doses) in pregnancy.

### Cayenne

Just a pinch daily (one-eighth of a teaspoon) can promote digestive health. Cayenne is a potent stimulant of digestion and of digestive enzymes.

### Cinnamon

A tree bark, this spice has a positive effect on the digestive system, helping to counteract flatulence and diarrhoea. It has been shown to inhibit the growth of *E. coli* and *Staphylococcus aureus*. One gram a day of cinnamon significantly improves insulin sensitivity. It can be taken as a supplement or one gram (one-third of a teaspoon) can be added to food when cooking. *Cinnamon verum* and *cinnamon zilanicum* are the same spice and have the same effect.

### Cloves

Clove oil has been used for a long time to reduce dental pain by numbing the gum. Clove is a very effective antibacterial: a 1 per cent clove tincture is three or four times stronger in action than carbolic acid, which was used in the early days of surgery.

## Coriander

Also called cilantro. Coriander is used in ethnic cooking to impart a distinctive flavour, but it is also effective at fighting food bacteria such as salmonella. A decoction (tea) is very useful to help dispel trapped wind and flatulence and can be used for babies as gripe water.

## Cumin

A traditional Indian remedy for indigestion, which is one reason why it appears in many curry recipes.

## Garlic

Probably the most important health-promoting herb in the kitchen, garlic has potent anti-bacterial, anti-viral, anti-parasitic, anti-blood clotting and cholesterol-lowering effects. The compound alliin converts to the active compound allicin, with its characteristic smell, when garlic is cut or crushed and exposed to the air. A clove a day really will, for the most part, keep the doctor away.

## Ginger

Take as a tea by steeping fresh slices in boiling water, use in cooking, or enjoy as crystallized ginger (which is very delicious medicine). The main uses for ginger are as a potent anti-nausea remedy, to improve circulation, and in irritable bowel or diarrhoea where no inflammation (ulceration) exists. It helps to promote sweating for fever and so to reduce body temperature. Ginger also encourages secretion of gastric juices in the elderly. As an anti-inflammatory, ginger can help with pain management. Ginger is contra-indicated in kidney disease, however.

## Mint and peppermint

A herb with a long history of use to ease digestive upsets and also for travel sickness, the active compound in mint is menthol. The most effective therapeutic effect is to take a mint tea after meals to settle the stomach. The leaves can also be shredded and added to salads and sweet dishes. Peppermint oil (available as supplements) is healing for digestive tract ulcers.

## Parsley

Rich in calcium, potassium and silica, parsley is used most often in the UK as a garnish. This herb is undervalued, except for its well-known properties as a breath freshener which counteracts garlic. It makes an excellent addition to salad if you need a higher dose. It has antibacterial properties and anti-rheumatic effects. It is useful for prostate problems and for fluid retention. Used for healthy skin, hair and nails due to its silica content, parsley is contraindicated in kidney disease.

## Rosemary

The oil in rosemary, which is responsible for its strong scent, rosemary camphor, is the active compound and can be effective against headaches. It has a tonic effect as a mild antidepressant.

## Sage

The purple variety is slightly more active than the green. It is a potent aid against menopausal hot sweats when drunk as a tea. It has antiseptic and antifungal properties and can be used as a mouthwash. Sage should be taken in moderation by breast-feeding women, as it can limit milk flow.

## Thyme

With strong antibacterial, antiviral, antifungal and antiparasitic actions, thyme can be used as a tea. As a gargle it is useful for throat infections. Pregnant women should avoid large doses.

## Turmeric

This spice from the Indian sub-continent contains curcumin (see cumin) as its active compound. This has powerful effects, including antiinflammatory and anti-cancer effects and also seems to protect against Alzheimer's. Curcumin is said to work as well as the steroid drug cortisone in relieving acute inflammation.

# Healthy Food Preparation Methods

The way we prepare food can make a difference to how nutritious it is. A perfect example is fish. If baked or steamed with a little drizzle of olive oil, lemon and a little wine and garlic, it is still a low-fat protein-rich dish – as well as being delicious. On the other hand, take the same piece of fish, dunk it in batter and deep fry it (the batter acts like a sponge to soak up as much oil as possible) and the fish is transformed into a high-fat dish. This is OK as an occasional treat, possibly, but as a dietary main-stay likely to reap disastrous health rewards such as weight gain and a worse risk of heart disease. There is some concern about the effect of high temperatures on carbohydrate foods as this can cause compounds called acrylamides, which are carcinogenic. Acrylamides are found in crispy processed foods such as cream crackers and rye biscuits, as well as French fries. Acrylamides are also produced when cooking carbohydrates at home, but it is not known if high levels are a real problem or not.

## Baking

Because baking tends to concentrate flavours and to make the best of natural juices in the food, it means that a minimum of oil can be used.

## Grilling

This is useful if you are cooking a small amount of food. Brushing the food with oil minimizes the amount of fat used. Take care not to burn food as this produces carcinogenic compounds.

## Steaming

The best means of cooking food and retaining its nutrients, steaming is ideal for delicate foods such as fish. Make sure not to overcook food – vegetables should still have some 'bite'.

## Juicing

Freshly made juices, using a special juicer for hard produce such as carrots or apples, or a blender for soft fruit, is an ideal way of consuming a concentrated source of vitamins and minerals. Many people swear by the therapeutic effects of regularly drinking home-made juices. However, unless a juice has been made in a blender, it will be devoid of fibre and so should be drunk slowly to minimize the effect on blood sugar and will only count as one of the daily portions of fruits and vegetables.

## Raw or cooked food?

We undoubtedly evolved on a diet which features more raw foods than are typically eaten today. Chewing raw fruits, vegetables, salads, nuts and seeds is very satisfying as it involves lots of jaw power. Certainly you can achieve a certain vitality by including lots of fresh raw produce in the diet. However, it is probably not a good idea to concentrate solely on raw foods. It is likely that, during our evolution, cooking was the process which liberated nutrients and allowed us to develop larger brains. Some antioxidants, particularly the carotenes such as betacarotene and lycopene, are also made more available to the body by cooking and processing. As with most aspects of nutrition it is probably best to achieve a balance – at the very least aim to incorporate some raw food with each meal: a piece of fruit for breakfast, a couple of tomatoes at lunch and a salad or crudités with your evening meal.

## Using fats

Fat used in cooking makes food taste better. However, choosing the most healthy fats can make a significant difference to your overall health. For a full run-down on the different health effects of fats, see Chapter 2. In terms of cooking, remember that heat can change the chemical composition of various fats, rendering healthy fats less so. Therefore it is ideal to:

- Avoid heating fats to the point where they smoke – olive oil is a good cooking choice but not if it smokes as this creates harmful compounds
- The best cooking fat is saturated fat such as butter or coconut butter as they can't be 'denatured' by heat. Having said this, we need to moderate the amount of saturated fat in our diets, so use the tiniest amount
- To control the amount of fat used and to avoid cooking in fat, steam foods or bake them and then dress them at the last minute with a healthy oil
- When dressing salads, ideally choose oils which are high in omega-3 fats such as cold-pressed canola (rape), walnut, pumpkin and flax, or in omega-6, such as cold-pressed sunflower or safflower.

# PART 3:

# A–Z OF COMMON CONDITIONS AND DIETARY APPROACHES

## Acne

Acne affects 80 per cent of adolescents aged 12–18 years, but can strike at any age. Whilst mainly affecting the face it commonly also occurs on the shoulders, arms, back, chest or buttocks. The sebaceous glands in the hair follicles, being oversensitive to production of the hormone testosterone, increase sebum production, forming blackheads. Bacteria infects the blackheads, leading to inflammation. Adolescent acne usually clears over time but may leave scarring. In women the contraceptive pill can trigger acne, in which case a different pill prescription or form of contraception can be sought. Women with PCOS (polycystic ovary syndrome) produce excess testosterone, which can trigger acne (see page 271). Acne is probably not caused solely by diet but a poor diet can make symptoms worse (however if comments are made about diet not affecting acne at all, recall that the standard references are now nearly 30 years old and were poorly designed trials).

- *Antioxidants*: A diet featuring antioxidant rich fruits and vegetables is the cornerstone of dietary changes – seven to eight portions daily.
- *Omega-3s*: Fatty acids from oily fish may help – Inuit populations who consume high levels of omega-3s have no acne until they move to a Western diet. Omega-3s have a potent anti-inflammatory action and eating three portions a week, while reducing trans- and saturated fats could be effective over the long term.
- *Saturated fats*: A fatty diet is often mooted as a cause, though research does not yet back this up (even though – observationally – the worst cases of acne often seem to be in those who work in fast-food chains!). What is most likely to be responsible is the balance of fatty acids between those

that promote inflammation and those that damp inflammation down. Chocolate has long been considered to be a problem; however, research has not found a link. Now, though, it is recognized that the research was done in the days before the effects hydrogenated trans-fats have on health were understood. As a result, the research was flawed by using hydrogenated vegetable oils as 'controls' for the chocolate with no adjustments for background diet.

- *Trans-fats*: Hydrogenated trans-fatty acids found in processed foods such as pastry, crisps, biscuits, ice cream, confectionery and some margarines are implicated in acne because of their effect of increasing inflammation.
- *Zinc*: Deficiency is a possible link and studies have shown that those with acne have lower zinc levels. Zinc is needed for normal skin functioning. Seeds, nuts, oysters and lean meat are good sources of zinc. 30mg daily of zinc have been used in trials (but at this level it is sensible to also supplement 3mg of copper).
- *Selenium*: Around 200mcg daily can help acne, as selenium improves levels of an enzyme called glutathione-peroxidase, which is low in many people with acne. Around three to four Brazil nuts will provide this amount.
- *Vitamin A*: Needed for skin health, vitamin A may be inefficiently processed by those with acne due to sluggish liver function. Liver (the food) is an excellent source of vitamin A and a portion once every two or three weeks is sufficient. Vitamin A analogues, forms of retinoic acid, are prescribed by doctors to treat acne, but there are problems with toxicity from overuse. Avoid taking vitamin A supplements if on these medications. Vitamin A supplements and liver should also be avoided by women who may be pregnant.
- *Sugar*: A sugary diet will have adverse effects on bowel bacteria. Since both the bowels and the skin are major organs of elimination, if the bowel bacteria is upset the

skin will have to work harder at elimination and this will affect its functioning. Antibiotics, sometimes prescribed for acne, also can upset bacterial balance. For more on bowel bacteria, see page 138.

- *Other*: Iodine-rich foods such as kelp (seaweed) or kelp supplements might aggravate acne. Some medicines are also rich in iodine. Using diluted tea tree oil as an antibacterial wash can help. Sun exposure usually helps. Topical sulphur-based preparations are gentle and effective.

## Acne Rosacea

Acne rosacea affects about 1 per cent of the population, mainly women in the 30–50 age group. Whilst more common in women, it tends to be more severe in men. This is a chronic congestion of the 'flush' area of the face – the area that is activated when we blush. This leads to the formation of red papules and redness of the skin. It may be triggered and then dampen down initially, but eventually becomes a permanent redness and can be accompanied by enlargement of the nose from excessively enlarged sebaceous glands. The eyes can be affected with a type of conjunctivitis. Early medical treatment must be sought, as scarring can result if left untreated.

- *Food Triggers*: In the initial stages flushing can be brought on by alcohol, a spicy meal, hot drinks, sunlight (using sun block can help) and vigorous exercise.
- *Food sensitivities*: These may make it worse; prime suspects are caffeine, cheese, eggs, citrus, yeast extracts and wheat.
- *Citrus fruit*: If not adversely sensitive, citrus fruit may be beneficial as they are rich in vitamin C and rutin, which are involved in capillary repair and have anti-inflammatory actions.

- *Digestive aids*: Hydrochloric acid and pancreatic enzyme supplementation have been shown in five older trials to be effective. Such supplements are available from health food shops and can be taken with meals to improve digestion. Improving gut transit time, with fibre and probiotics, may be significant (see Digestive Health, page 181).
- *B-vitamins*: Supplementation featuring a moderately high dose of riboflavin (vitamin B2) was also included in some trials and showed effect.

## Addiction

The chemical aspect of addiction involves dealing with physical withdrawal from the substance – be it nicotine, alcohol, drugs or foods – with accompanying psychological and social consequences. Addictions of any description share a common feature, with 'highs' becoming harder and harder to achieve leading to increased use. It may seem obvious that nutritional advice is appropriate for food-based addictions; it is also relevant for other addictions on several fronts. Nutritional intervention is unlikely to be the sole answer to resolving a person's addiction problems, although it can certainly help. There is also a psychological benefit to helping oneself in this way. There are many organizations that help those with addictions and they are usually the best port of call as they have a wide experience of similar problems.

- *Quality of diet*: People who are addicted often ignore their health and simply do not eat properly, leading to nutritional deficiencies that can exacerbate the ill effects of their addiction.
- *Nutrient depletion*: Smoking, alcohol and drugs actively deplete certain nutrients, particularly B-vitamins, vitamin C and

zinc, meaning that people who consume these have a higher requirement than other people. As a minimum it is probably appropriate to take a multi-vitamin/mineral supplement.

- *Blood sugar regulation*: Dealing with withdrawal from addictive substances, and possibly from compulsive addictive behaviour, may be improved by helping to normalize blood sugar imbalance (and so reduce the overall effect of cravings and stress) and help in stabilizing brain chemistry. Blood sugar imbalance is a key feature of any addiction. This is partly the case because addiction involves stress hormones that raise blood sugar when adrenaline is activated by whatever substance is being abused (be it alcohol, cigarette, drug or cream cake). Sugar has a similar effect to opiates on dopamine neurochemical pathways in the brain. See Low Blood Sugar (Hypoglycaemia), page 136 for more on this.
- *Polyunsaturated fatty acids*: In one study, cocaine addicts were most likely to relapse anything up to a year after admission to an in-patient drug detox unit if their bodies were deficient in the n-6 and n-3 polyunsaturated fatty acids found in nuts, seeds, grains and oily fish.
- See also Smoking Cessation page 297 and Alcohol Excess page 109.

## Ageing

The fastest growing demographic age group is 65+ years. With longer life spans it is now important that we grow older healthily. Indeed, we tend to be much more active and not to have the limited horizons of earlier generations of 'seniors'. Ageing is associated with various health problems such as bone health, eyesight degeneration, heart disease, joint health, mental slow-down, poor dentition and varicose veins (each of these and other subjects are discussed in individual categories). While genetics and age can conspire to make these more likely, they are not necessarily a forgone conclusion. There is much that you can do to improve your chances of living a healthy long life. Staying active, employed, interested and mentally challenged is of tremendous value.

- *Body composition*: Changes in body composition from our forties onwards mean that, on average, a person loses 30 per cent of muscle mass by age 80, and this is replaced with fat. Hence the curse of creeping middle-age spread. In reality what this means is that metabolism slows down because fat burns less energy than muscle. Consequently, older people need fewer calories than younger people, but they still need as many vitamins and minerals. So foods chosen on a daily basis should be as nutrient-packed as possible. Older people should eat plenty of fruits and vegetables, lean meat, low-fat dairy products, complex carbohydrates and reduce dependency on processed salty, sugary and fatty foods.
- *Glycosylation*: The above mentioned basic eating approach also keeps blood sugar levels constant. It is called a low-GI diet (see Appendix I page 350) and is protective against many of the effects of ageing. Sugars interact with collagen, causing glycosylation (damage). This is visible in skin as the collagen cross-links, robbing it of its natural elasticity.
- *Sarcopenia*: This is age-related muscle wasting. High intensity resistance exercise such as weight lifting, but not aerobic exercise such as swimming or jogging, is highly effective at stopping muscle wasting. (If it seems inappropriate for elderly people to lift weights, there are many who do to provide the evidence for these trials – though it should not be attempted by those with osteoporosis or other conditions such as high blood pressure without appropriate

medical supervision.) Resistance of exercise also leads to a 15 per cent increase in energy needs, while aerobic exercise leads to compensatory decreases in activity and therefore energy intakes.

- *Dentition*: Poor dental health is a major inhibitor of healthy eating. Maintaining regular visits to the dentist to overcome dental problems is essential. If dentition is a problem – partial or total loss of teeth usually leads to a nutritionally depleted diet – it can be very helpful to work out a diet that is nutritious but easy to chew: for instance, creamed or grated carrots instead of raw, mince instead of steak.

- *Taste*: Loss of taste sensation can be a problem in later years (see page 303).

- *Vitamin D*: Intake is usually very low in the elderly, but this vitamin is important for bone health and balance. A supplement of 800ius daily is advised.

- *Omega-3s*: Commonly deficient in the general population, a range of symptoms manifest in the elderly after a lifetime of low intake. Conditions such as arthritis, cognitive impairment and decline and heart disease are all linked. Eating oily fish twice a week or taking supplements is beneficial.

- *Digestive health*: Achlorhydria and hypochlorhydria (non-existent or poor stomach acid production) is a problem in 20 per cent of elderly people. This impairs digestion, thus further reducing nutritional status. Hydrochloric acid supplements are available from health food shops (one is swallowed with each meal, but not chewed, and avoid with ulcers). Bowel bacteria is frequently imbalanced in the elderly who also suffer from many problems such as constipation as their digestive systems become more 'sluggish'. Two teaspoons of a fibre such as powdered linseeds or one teaspoon of psyllium husks can help, as can probiotics (see more on Digestive Health, page 181).

## Alcohol, Excessive Intake

A relaxing drink with friends, with a meal, or as an evening treat is a part of our culture. Many people drink daily without considering themselves to be alcoholics but still may be at greater risk of alcohol induced health problems than they realize. One or two drinks daily may be fine, but three or four is, generally speaking, not. Certainly anyone with a dependency needs to seek help. People have found success with counselling from approaches such as the 12-step programme, cognitive behaviour therapy, relaxation techniques, acupuncture and hypnosis. In recent years we have seen the emergence of the binge-drinking culture and young women, who have adopted 'male pattern behaviour', are particularly at risk.

- *What is a measure?*: The guidelines are that women should have no more than two to three units of alcohol per day and men no more than three to four units a day. One measure is either: one small 125ml glass of wine, one 25ml shot of a spirit, one-half pint of regular strength beer, one 50ml sherry, port or vermouth. Measures poured at home tend to be more generous than those measured out in a bar, but glasses of wine in bars are often larger than 125ml. A typical bottle of wine contains 9 units.
- *B-Vitamins*: Alcohol severely depletes B-vitamins, which are important for energy, brain function, mood, cardiovascular health and many other health factors. Eating a bowl of cereal fortified with B-vitamins before you go out if you think you are going to drink a lot is a good idea in order to replace lost nutrients, or eat some fortified cereal for breakfast the next day.
- *Hangover cures*: These have mixed results. A hangover happens when the body is unable to metabolize the amount

of alcohol drunk. Dehydration plays a large part in hang-over symptoms, so drinking water can certainly alleviate this. A breakfast containing protein can help to stabilize blood sugar. The traditional hangover cure of a raw egg is a bad idea as raw egg white contains avidin, which binds with biotin, a B-vitamin, and this can lead to deficiency if overdone. Artichokes have potent liver and bile supporting actions, which can help reduce the worst effects of alcohol. If eating lots of artichoke is not an option, supplements are available.

- *Isn't alcohol healthy?*: It is well publicized that alcohol intake protects against heart disease. But while a little is good, a lot is very bad. The most health benefits accrue between one to two units daily, but excess drinking (regular con-sumption of over three units for women or over four units for men) increases risk of heart disease, strokes and liver disease. And the studies only show benefit for men and for post-menopausal women. The antioxidants in wine may well have an effect in protecting against heart disease, but the same antioxidants can be found in non-alcoholic red grape juice and other red-coloured berry juices such as cranberry and blackcurrant. On the other hand, it may be that wine has no magical properties beyond the health effect of drinking moderate alcohol in general. The worst health profiles are in those who abstain completely, and in those who binge drink. It is not necessary to drink more than the recommended amounts but if the total is drunk in only one or two sessions a week (five or more measures at a go) then this has highly adverse effects on health. Even if less is drunk overall during these binges compared to very moderate but regular drinking, it still has an adverse effect. Drinking a small amount on a regular basis therefore seems to be the healthiest way forward. It has been theorized that evidence of benefit from low-level but consistent alcohol intake fits with the theory that early in our evolution alcohol would have naturally been consumed from fermenting fruits rotting on the ground.

- *Women and alcohol*: Women's bodies can't deal with alcohol as efficiently as men. This is for several reasons: a woman's liver is physically smaller than a man's, which means she has much less capacity; women tend to have much lower amounts of an alcohol-processing enzyme, alcohol-dehydrogenase; finally, alcohol interacts with oestrogen, amplifying its negative effects. This means that alcohol even in small amounts over one measure daily, increases breast cancer risk significantly in pre-menopausal women. Binge drinking in women is becoming a major social problem in the UK.

- *Pregnancy*: Women should not drink any alcohol at all in pregnancy. Alcohol crosses the placenta easily and in the first few months can act as a neurotoxin for the baby. In the last few months the baby is certainly more sensitive to alcohol than the mother, and clearance of alcohol from the baby's liver takes several times longer and so the baby is, effectively, tipsy for quite a long time. Heavy drinking can lead to foetal alcohol syndrome.

- *Race*: We have adapted over the millennia to drinking alcohol – it is believed that naturally fermenting fruit was the first 'tipple'. Indeed many animals seek these out. We also developed brewing as a means of sanitizing drinking water. Some cultures did not do this and in the East boiling water for tea is more common. A high proportion of Chinese people cannot metabolize alcohol and will get drunk quickly on just one drink.

- *Liver health*: This is damaged by alcohol. The liver takes about one hour to clear one measure of alcohol, so drinking a swift couple of double measures will overload the liver and will take it four hours to clear. Fatty liver degeneration and liver cirrhosis are the consequences of long-term excess alcohol intake. Milk thistle is a herb that has been used for a long time and has good evidence behind it for selectively helping to protect the liver and helping it to regenerate. It has liver-specific antioxidant effects.

- See also Addiction page 105.

## Allergies

One in three adults and one in four children in the UK are now affected by allergies. More than 1,000 people die annually from allergies, mainly asthma. The UK has a far greater incidence of allergies than almost any other country in the world. No one is quite sure why allergies are on the increase, but the assumption is that it has something to do with modern living. Possible theories include:

- Modern diets, heavily reliant on processed foods, may be weakening our immune systems. Low average fruit and vegetable intake will not provide sufficient antioxidants. Low fish intakes will provide insufficient omega-3 fatty acids, needed to suppress inflammation, while processed foods and margarine promote inflammation. Omega-3s may be particularly effective when introduced early in life (and while in the uterus).
- Lack of 'outdoor living' and being cooped up in cities is probably less healthy.
- The hygiene theory says that as we sanitize our environments our children's immune systems are less likely to be 'primed' by infections.
- Our houses are filling up with chemical residues as they are trapped in carpets and curtains, and are hermetically sealed in air-tight, centrally-heated houses.

- Our heavy use of antibiotics is not allowing our immune systems to be challenged and so to develop strength. They wipe out the beneficial bowel bacteria that help to protect against allergies.

For specific advice see: Food allergies page 202, Food intolerances page 205, Asthma page 122, Eczema page 186, Hay Fever page 212, Gut Bacteria page 138.

## Alzheimer's Disease

Half of all dementia cases involve Alzheimer's disease (AD) amounting to between 6 and 8 per cent of the 65+ age group. The first signs are often loss of memory and forgetfulness, which progresses to disorientation and sometimes paranoia. If concerned, a GP can refer a patient to a Memory Clinic. A definitive cause of AD has not been identified and it is probably multi-factoral, embracing genetic risk, dietary and lifestyle factors. The economic cost, in an ageing population, is huge and estimates outstrip combined cardiovascular disease and cancer statistics. Identifying early risk factors for AD, particularly mild, reversible, vitamin deficiencies in mid-life, could be highly cost-efficient and prevent much misery. There is a very real possibility that nutritional intervention implemented early enough can provide some protection against the age-related neuro-degeneration that leads to Alzheimer's. Anti-inflammatory drugs may have modifying effects.

- *B-vitamins and homocysteine*: Several recent studies have focused on the significant link between B-vitamin status, homocysteine, cognitive skills and AD. Evidence of folic acid, and vitamins B12, B6 and B2 supplementation lowering homocysteine is now an exciting development.

Neuronal tissue may be particularly susceptible to homo-cysteine damage, which seems to harm the hippocampus and amygdala in the brain. There is likely to be a strong genetic link to susceptibility to producing homocysteine in the presence of borderline folate and other B-vitamins. These vitamins are needed for detoxifying and recycling homocysteine. In one small study of nuns (nuns are useful to study as they live in identical circumstances, which elim-inate most variable factors) low serum folate correlated strongly to cerebral cortex atrophy in those with significant numbers of Alzheimer lesions. Most folate levels were within the 'normal' ranges, but these varied widely, sug-gesting that individual differences in uptake, metabolism or drug-nutrient interactions might be important.

- *Blood pressure and cholesterol*: Raised systolic blood pressure (the first of the two readings taken) and serum cholesterol are linked to AD and both are modifiable via dietary mea-sures. Indeed, the cholesterol-lowering Statin drugs may reduce AD incidence.
- *Malnourishment*: The elderly are often malnourished (not necessarily undernourished, which is insufficient calories, but malnourished, which is insufficient nutrient-rich foods). Possible contributing nutritional risk-factors to Alzheimer's include insufficient antioxidant protection. Antioxidant supplementation (particularly vitamin-E) may delay insti-tutionalization; and fatty acids, particularly omega-3, may exert an effect on nerve membranes. Food sources of antioxidants are all fruits and vegetables and the best sources of omega-3s are oily fish (see page 26 for more spe-cific sources). Fish consumption is linked to a reduced prevalence of AD in a seven-country European and North American study.
- *Metabolic syndrome*: This includes cardiovascular risks, which are common to AD.

- *Curcumin*: This is the active compound found in the spices turmeric and cumin. It has powerful antioxidant effects, which may explain its effect, seemingly, on reducing AD.

## Anaemia, Iron Deficiency

Iron deficiency anaemia (IDA) is the most common form of anaemia. Iron in haemoglobin, which carries oxygen around the body, gives blood its red colour. The main signs of IDA are fatigue and skin pallor, poor concentration and reduced resistance to infections, but also sometimes mouth ulcers, sore tongue, cracks at the side of the mouth, hair loss and poor appetite. Women of child-bearing age are at risk of IDA as a result of menstruation, pregnancy and lack of iron repletion. Around 4 per cent are anaemic and 10 per cent are borderline, while 1 per cent of men are anaemic. Babies who are exclusively breast fed for more than six months are at risk of IDA, as breast milk does not provide enough iron for the size of the baby beyond that time. Children who consume too much milk are also at risk, as milk is a poor source of iron and excess milk blunts appetites for other foods which could provide iron. In children IDA is a particular problem, as it has an irreversible impact on IQ levels. It is the most common worldwide deficiency disease in children. Your doctor will be able to run blood tests to determine if IDA is a problem for you.

- *Requirements*: Children, men and non-menstruating women need 6.7mg of iron daily, while menstruating women need 11.4mg daily. Women who bleed more heavily when they menstruate will need more than those who have light periods.
- *Lean meat*: This is the best source of iron (called haem-iron), which the body can absorb readily. The darker the meat the

more iron there is, therefore dark turkey and chicken leg meat is more iron-rich than light breast meat. Vegetarians who do not make appropriate adjustments to their diet may be at risk of IDA.

- *Plant sources of iron*: Cereals, beans, pulses, lentils, nuts, seeds, eggs, dried fruit and parsley.
- *Absorption helpers*: Plant sources of iron (called non-haem iron) are abundant but are not so readily absorbed. Consuming a source of vitamin C alongside a non-meat based meal will double iron-uptake. Suitable vitamin C sources are citrus juice, citrus fruit, cauliflower, cabbage, broccoli, Brussels sprouts, kiwi, strawberries, blackcurrant and other vitamin C rich fruit.
- *Absorption inhibitors*: Iron absorption is inhibited by two-thirds by a cup of tea, so it is best to drink tea separate from meals. Phytic acid in cereals reduces uptake, but then calcium improves uptake: iron-fortified breakfast cereal (usually served with milk) provides the major source of iron in the average person's diet.
- *Weight-loss diets*: Women who are on weight-loss diets are at risk, because they often do not consume enough iron.
- *Pregnancy*: Pregnancy related drops in iron are often related to increase in blood volume. It is no longer routine to supplement with iron unless overt IDA is found.
- *Internal bleeding*: This is a common cause of IDA, in those who do not tolerate aspirin or steroids, with Digestive tract ulceration (see page 307), Colitis (see page 157), Crohn's disease, undiagnosed coeliac disease or cancer.
- *Iron tonics*: Traditional tonics for restoring iron status are nettle tea, dandelion tea (or young, unsprayed, leaves used in salads) and cooked or raw beetroot. Ferrogreen and Spatone are gentle iron tonics available from chemists.
- *Iron supplements*: The iron generally prescribed, ferrous sulphate, is most likely to lead to the side-effect of constipa-

tion. Organic forms of iron such as iron ascorbate or iron malate are less likely to cause this reaction, and are more readily absorbed. It is not wise to take high-dose iron supplements unless properly diagnosed as anaemic, because high levels of free-iron have negative consequences as they cause oxidation. A small percentage of the population are affected by haemachromatosis, though they may not be diagnosed in the early stages. This is a genetic condition where the person accumulates iron in their body and this is very damaging to their livers and other organs. These people should not take iron-containing supplements.

- *Other anaemias*: Megoblastic anaemia is a different type of anaemia, where the red blood cells grow large and cannot divide; this relates to folic acid and vitamin B12 deficiencies. Pernicious anaemia is a type of megoblastic anaemia which results from B12 deficiency; this prevents folic acid from doing its job – usually corrected with B12 injections. Haemolytic anaemia, hypoplastic anaemia and apoplastic anaemia are all conditions which must be treated by a doctor. Sickle cell anaemia is an inherited condition. There is also a rare, genetically linked, type of anaemia called favism, which is triggered by cating fava (broad) beans because the individual lacks a particular type of digestive enzyme.

## Antibiotic Resistance

The antibacterial effect of penicillin was discovered by Alexander Fleming in 1929. Along with improved sanitation and obstetric care, antibiotics were responsible for the great improvement in mortality reduction seen during the early twentieth century. However, we have now learned that antibiotics are not a panacea. They are life-savers in the right situation, but the bacteria they are designed to eradicate are able to adapt very quickly. This means that many bacterial pathogens have become partially or very nearly wholly resistant to antibiotics. Hospitals have been plagued by the rise of the MRSA 'superbug' (methicillin-resistant *staphylococcus aureus*), which infects 100,000 patients and is fatal in 5,000 cases annually. This has been exacerbated by overuse of antibiotics in circumstances that do not fully warrant their use, and in their use in the food chain (they are given to animals as growth enhancers and for disease prevention, rather than cure). For this reason, guidelines are now in place to limit their use. It is also suspected that heavy-handed antibiotic use is contributing to the epidemic of allergies we are seeing. Your doctor will be aware of the problems of over-prescribing antibiotics and will take a view on the necessity of prescription in individual cases. However, there are many steps that individuals can also take.

- *Immune Health*: Prevention is better than cure. A strong immune system will be able to better overcome bacterial infection, reducing the risk of need for antibiotics. See Chapter 3 page 28.
- *Hospital stays*: If in hospital, make sure that anyone who examines, or even touches, you washes their hands thoroughly. The MRSA bacteria survive on taps, door handles and doctors' pens even after thorough cleaning of the environment. Spend as little time as possible in hospital – ask about day surgery for instance, or if a procedure can be carried out under local anaesthetic. Wash all over with an antibacterial soap in the week before admission to reduce bacterial contamination from your own skin through a wound.
- *Honey*: Manuka honey is a potent antibacterial agent, effective against MRSA even when used topically. It is not a

substitute for medical advice, but may be used as an adjunct (see Leg Ulcers page 309). Another topical antibacterial that is highly effective is tea tree oil.

- *Garlic*: A potent antibacterial, one clove a day per person in cooking is highly protective. Do not use garlic topically, as it burns.
- *Bowel bacteria*: Replenishing healthy bowel bacteria after, but not during, a course of antibiotics is wise. Taking a pre-biotic supplement in the weeks before admission to hospital (if possible) is also a good idea, to promote immune health. Choose a product with the probiotics acidophilus, bifidobacteria and with prebiotics such as FOS or inulin. If you need to take two or more courses of antibiotics, it becomes even more important to replenish bowel bacteria with a specific course of pro and prebiotics designed for this purpose, such as Replete from Biocare. Repeat courses are particularly implicated in the risk of candida infections, ME, inflammatory bowel disorders and repeat ear infections. For more, see Bowel Bacteria, page 138.
- *Bacterial production of vitamins*: Bowel bacteria produce significant amounts of vitamin K (important for blood clotting and for bone health) and B-vitamins, including biotin. Repeat antibiotics can wipe out enough bacterial colonies to induce deficiency. Vitamin K-rich foods are all leafy green vegetables such as cabbage, broccoli, kale, spinach and Brussels sprouts.
- *Smoking*: It is obviously desirable to stop in any event. But if you are going to be hospitalized, stop smoking for one week beforehand – this will improve wound healing. If you can't or won't stop, take 500mg of vitamin C daily to compensate.

## Arthritis

Arthritis means inflammation of the joints. There are several forms of arthritis, including spondylitis and gout, but the most common are osteoarthritis and rheumatoid arthritis (RA).

Osteoarthritis is a 'wear and tear' disease. It happens uni-laterally (in other words does not automatically affect joints on both sides of the body) and is often related to repetitive use of a joint – hence, for instance, nursemaid's knee and tennis elbow. It most commonly affects the hips and knees. The con-dition is caused by breakdown of the inter-joint cartilage that pads the joint: the bones literally rub together, causing inflam-mation and pain. The new thinking on osteoarthritis is that it is an active disease process in which the ability to heal damage is unbalanced.

RA is an autoimmune condition (where the immune system attacks the body), which leads to inflammation of the joints. The causes are unknown, but there are several dietary factors that can make a difference to the severity of the disease.

- *Oily fish*: Fish oils are the most potent nutritional anti-arthritic compounds. The omega-3 fatty acids have strong anti-inflammatory effects. Eating oily fish two or three times weekly has a therapeutic effect and on average arthritic people who eat the most oily fish use the least medication. Cod liver oil in trials has been shown to have the same anti-inflammatory effect of influencing the COX-2 (a cyclooxy-genase enzyme) pathways that COX-2 anti-inflammatory medication has. Cod liver oil (CLO) has about one-half the potency of fish oils (which come from muscle meat), although CLO has vitamin A and D, which may have an effect. If choosing CLO, ask for a high strength formulation, but you should check any other supplements you are taking to avoid taking in too much A and D.

- *Overweight*: Excess weight is a major contributor to osteoarthritis because it increases the pressure on joints, so if you are overweight, losing weight is an important goal.
- *Antioxidants*: A fruit- and vegetable-rich diet is vital for all forms of arthritis because antioxidants help to dampen down inflammation.
- *Vitamin D*: An observational study found that women with the highest vitamin D intakes from food had a 28 per cent less chance of developing RA and those taking supplements had a 34 per cent lower risk. While this sort of study can't establish cause and effect, it is an indicator of possible effect. Since women may be advised to take vitamin D for bone health (see Osteoporosis page 261) the knock-on effect may be of value.
- *Hydration*: Drinking plenty of liquids, particularly water, helps to maintain hydration in the joints.
- *Food intolerances*: Some people find that food intolerances, particularly wheat, dairy, tomatoes and citrus, exacerbate arthritic symptoms, particularly in rheumatoid arthritis. They do not directly cause arthritis, but may reduce the effectiveness of the individual's healing mechanism. One researcher said (talking about food intolerances), 'about 36 per cent of my patients who have manipulated their diet have done well and some have been able to stop taking drugs for several years.'
- *Supplements*: Sulphur, green-lipped muscle, bromelain and devil's claw are all supplements (or compounds) that have been found to be effective against arthritis. Glucosamine sulphate provides the building blocks that make up synovial fluid, which protects joints.
- *Helpful foods*: A traditional remedy for arthritis is to drink celery juice, a mild diuretic also high in organic sodium, which is said to counteract inorganic sodium chloride. Celery juice is best combined with something less potent

tasting, such as fresh apple or pear juice. Parsley has anti-rheumatic effects when eaten in reasonable quantities (it makes a good salad ingredient with other salad leaves).

- *Bone broth*: This is traditionally used to replenish bone nutrients. It is made with beef, lamb, chicken or fish bones, including the cartilage which is on the bones, and provides mucopolysaccharides. Try boiling them with vegetables and water for at least two hours, using something acidic such as two tablespoons of vinegar, lemon juice or white wine, to leach minerals out of the bones and use as a stock.
- *Vitamin B5*: Low levels of pantothenic acid (B5) have been noted in those with RA. Up to 2g daily of calcium pantothenate have been shown to reduce duration of morning stiffness and severity of pain.
- See also Pain Management, page 265.

## Asthma

Asthma is characterized by a narrowing of the airways, leading to breathlessness. It is a complex condition that is more likely to be 'controlled' than cured. A large genetic component influences who will suffer from this problem. However, it has been hugely on the increase in children in recent decades, which suggests that environmental aspects, including diet, have an important part to play.

Asthma can be terrifying and life threatening and for this reason it is important not to try to self-diagnose and self-treat. A GP's advice should always be sought. Airways can remain inflamed even between attacks and it is usually necessary to keep a preventive inhaler to hand to dampen this inflammation. As well as taking medical advice it is helpful to avoid triggers and adjust your diet. There are many well-known triggers that can set off an asthma attack including cigarette smoke, house dust mites, animal dander, pollens, moulds, household products, cosmetic products, perfumes, some aromatherapy oils, medicines such as aspirin and paracetamol and those with artificial colourings. Other triggers are atmospheric temperature changes, infections, the build up of chlorine gas in indoor pools, vigorous exercise and emotional stress.

Addressing some dietary concerns can be helpful in a number of ways. The overall aim is to reduce the threshold at which 'triggers' have their effect. Helping the body to control inflammation is one important goal and strengthening the mucus membranes of the respiratory tract is another.

- *Antioxidants*: Found in fruit and vegetables these are important for strengthening lung tissue and reducing inflammation and so lowering the number of asthma attacks. Quercitin, a plant flavonoid, found in abundance in onions and apples has been found to be particularly beneficial to lung health. Dark berries including cherries, blueberries, raspberries, blackberries and others are also lung specific. A useful aid is Sambucol, which is European Black Elderberry. Carrot juice is traditionally given for lung conditions, as betacarotene promotes mucus membrane health (mucus membranes line the lung bronchioles).
- *Fish oils*: Increasing oily fish consumption – as little as once or twice a week, but preferably three times – can significantly reduce asthma in some people but not for others; this may be due to genetic differences. If eating oily fish such as mackerel, sardines, tuna (fresh), salmon and pink trout is not manageable, then taking a daily fish oil supplement is an option. If symptoms worsen, as they can do in a minority of people, then cut back on fish oil intake.
- *Margarine*: Increased levels of asthma have been observed with increased margarine intake, though interestingly this

is more marked in boys. It may be linked to increased imbalance of omega-3-omega-6 fatty acids (see Chapter 2: Healthy Fats).

- *Food additives*: Benzoate preservatives (E210–219), sulphur-based food preservatives (E220–228) found in dried fruit, dehydrated vegetables (such as instant potato or packet soup), mushrooms, vinegar, grapes and grape juice are implicated. The artificial food colouring azo dyes, such as tartrazine, sunset yellow and ponceau 4R, are also suspected of triggering asthma.

- *Food sensitivities and allergies*: It is fairly common for asthma symptoms to improve when dairy and/or wheat (and sometimes all gluten grains, which are wheat, oats, rye and barley) are excluded. If this is the case, then sensible substitutions must be made, such as wholegrain rice and starchy vegetables such as potatoes, or calcium-rich foods and drinks if dairy is being avoided, to avoid deficiencies. For suitable substitutes for wheat and gluten grains see Coeliac Disease page 153 and for dairy substitutes see Lactose Intolerance and Dairy Allergy page 231.

- *Selenium*: Asthmatics have benefited from supplementation that supports the observations of lower asthma levels in those with higher dietary selenium intakes.

- *Herbs and spices*: Camomile tea is soothing, hemp nettle supports lung health, and compounds in liquorice root have a similar structure to cortisone and an anti-inflammatory action. The cortisone steroid effect of liquorice is more gentle than that of medication and does not suppress the immune system in the long run. You should seek the advice of a medical herbalist and should not stop prescribed medication. Garlic and onion contain allicin compounds, and mustard contains isothiocyanates, which help to dampen COX-induced inflammation.

- *Overweight*: Asthma may be linked to being overweight.

- *Vitamin C*: High dose supplements of 1000g (for adults, 50 per cent dose for children over age seven) half an hour before exercise can help to minimize the risk of exercise-induced asthma.
- *Salt*: High salt intakes have been linked to asthma in some studies, but not in others.
- *Green tea*: High in antioxidants, green tea drunk several times daily can be helpful to dampen down the frequency and severity of attacks (unless you are adversely sensitive to green tea).
- *Magnesium*: Severe acute asthma can respond to magnesium sulphate infusions given in hospital.

## Autism and Asperger's Syndrome

See Behavioural Disorders, page 127.

## Bad Breath (Halitosis)

Bad breath results from bacterial activity in the mouth. Oral hygiene is paramount – cleaning teeth twice daily, flossing between teeth and visiting the dentist and hygienist. Gentle tongue scraping using a special D-shaped tool (available from chemists) is also useful as this physically scrapes off a certain amount of bacteria from the surface of the tongue. In the absence of a tongue scraper a toothbrush can be used to clean the surface of the tongue. Toothbrushes should be changed regularly. Using an antibacterial mouthwash is also helpful although the alcohol content of many is too high: up to 27 per cent, which is twice as high as most wines. Alcohol dries the mucus membranes of the mouth and gums and feeds the bacteria, which worsens bacterial overgrowth. Alcohol-free mouthwashes are available from health food shops.

- *Deodorants*: Some people find that strong foods such as curry or garlic leave an unpleasant after taste. Parsley is a potent antidote to garlic and mint is an excellent mouth deodorizer.
- *Cloves*: Moderate use of a decoction of cloves steeped in boiling water (then cooled) is a useful mouthrinse as cloves have a strong antibacterial action. Other antibacterials include manuka oil, tea tree oil and eucalyptus oil used at 0.2 per cent concentrations.
- *Indigestion*: Those who suffer from indigestion many find that fumes float up from the stomach when they belch. For Indigestion see page 222.
- *Bowel bacteria*: As remote as it may sound, bowel health may be important to address in the case of halitosis. The compounds that cause smell in the mouth, the graphically named cadaverine and putricine together with indoles, are the same gases that are given off by bowel bacteria causing the bad smell of faeces. Improving bowel bacterial health can help in the long run (see Bowel Bacteria page 138).
- See also Dental Health page 169 and Oral Ulcers page 307.

## Balance

Feeling dizzy or unable to keep your balance can be distressing. There are many possible factors that can be checked for by your doctor: low blood pressure, postural hypotension, high blood pressure, inner ear infections, and anaemia being just some. There are some nutritional factors to consider as well.

- *Vitamin D*: In the elderly there is strong evidence to support supplementing 800ius of vitamin D, which has been shown to reduce the number of falls by 22 per cent due to an improvement in muscle function (falls in turn lead to bone breakages). In the winter in the Northern hemisphere, in particular, it is difficult to manufacture sufficient vitamin D from sun exposure. Ageing skin is also less efficient at making vitamin D compared to younger skin. Oily fish and cod liver oil are good sources of vitamin D.
- *Anaemia*: This may lead to fatigue and dizziness (see page 115).
- *Blood pressure*: Low or high blood pressure can lead to dizziness (see page 133).
- *Inner ear infections*: These can be worsened, in susceptible people, by food intolerances. In particular dairy products can increase mucus production and inflammation, and a high sugar diet can be linked to inner ear infections. Ear infections should always be checked by a doctor as permanent damage can result, but continuously prescribing antibiotics for a recurrent problem is obviously not finding the root cause. It is therefore well worth considering underlying dietary intolerances (see Otitis Media page 264).

## Behavioural Disorders

The missing link in the treatment of many behavioural disorders is the impact of nutrition on brain and neurological functioning. Nutritional measures are not always the sole answer to problems that may have genetic or environmental causal links – such as autism, bi-polar disorder (manic depression) or schizophrenia – or sociological causal links – such as disruptive behaviour or institutionalized offending. However, there is impressive evidence on the impact of improving the nutritional status of individuals caught up in these categories for whatever reason. It is important not to go down the route of self-treatment for any of these problems, but to seek out the help of those who specialize in their nutritional treatment – though at the moment these are few and far between. Access to information has improved dramatically via the Internet and so where possible helpful websites are included in Selected References and Resources at the end of this book.

Having said this, because the use of nutrition is so infrequent in standard treatment, anyone interested in this area is probably going to have to go down the route of investigating the possibilities themselves or with the help of a supportive GP. For ADHD (attention deficit hyperactivity disorder), where a number of cases can be treated extensively with nutritional measures if they are caught early enough, see page 220.

### Autism and Asperger's Syndrome

There are many theories about the cause of autism, none of which have a consensus of opinion. What *is* certain is that the incidence is on the increase – some would say as a result of better detection, but even this is not agreed upon. Asperger's syndrome is a milder version of autism and they are sometimes viewed as a continuum in the general spectrum of neurological problems that also includes ADHD, dyslexia and dyspraxia (see page 183). While boys are more likely than girls to be affected, it seems that girls are increasingly being affected. At the time of writing a plateau of incidence seems to be being reached. Nutritional intervention is not a 'cure' for autism and related problems, but is a means by which many individuals can be helped with an improvement in their symptoms.

- *Milk proteins*: A three-week experiment of casein removal from the diet to see if this improves symptoms. Casein is the main protein in milk and is a major source of allergy and intolerance. Milk, cheese, yoghurt and foods containing these must be avoided.

- *Gluten*: A three-month experiment with the removal from the diet of gluten to see if this improves symptoms. Gluten is the main protein in wheat, rye, oats and barley and is a major source of allergy and intolerance. In the case of both gluten and casein, the reasoning is that digestive tract integrity is impaired by these compounds and a 'leaky gut' allows through toxins into the bloodstream, which cross the blood brain barrier and affect brain function. The blood brain barrier normally keeps most substances away from the brain to protect it, but it is not 100 per cent effective.

- *Food diary*: Keeping a food diary to try to identify other foods to which the person could be sensitive (often frequently eaten foods), for example, corn, soya, tomatoes, beef, etc. This can be highly individual.

- *Yeast*: This may be a particular problem for these individuals (see Candida page 146).

- *Supplements and fish oils*: A general multi-vitamin and mineral supplement which provides 100 per cent of the RNI of most nutrients. A fatty acid supplement that provides good quantities of fish oils EPA and DHA, or a flax seed supplement for vegetarians, and an evening primrose oil or borage oil supplement, may be of benefit.

- *Sulphur pathways*: It is strongly suspected that these individuals are deficient in a particular detoxification 'pathway' in the liver called sulphation. A simple way to improve this is regularly bathing in a bath to which Epsom salts have been added: sulphur is absorbed in significant amounts across the skin.

- *Digestion*: There is also a case for taking digestive enzymes to improve the breakdown of food to reduce the likelihood of constituent parts causing toxic reactions.

## Schizophrenia and Bi-polar Disorder (manic depression)

It is essential not to attempt to treat these conditions by nutritional means alone and affected individuals must be under medical supervision. Antipsychotic and mood altering drugs are the usual methods of treatment. Some nutritional strategies are likely to help a significant number of people affected by these disorders.

- *Alcohol*: This will almost always worsen the conditions and must be avoided.
- *Supplementation*: Attention to healthy eating can be very poor (for some people this is fairly continual and for some there are 'good' and 'bad' episodes). At the same time, compliance with medication intake is often poor. It may be prudent, with the doctor's approval, to ensure there are no contraindications with medication, to take a multi-vitamin and mineral supplement to ensure the RNIs of the main nutrients are taken.
- *Omega-3 fatty acids*: There is good evidence that omega-3 fatty acids from fish oils can be important in the treatment of these conditions. There are reduced levels of these fatty acids in cell membranes, abnormal electroretinograms and other biochemical abnormalities that suggest insufficiency of these fatty acids. DHA has not been well studied in these conditions but EPA supplementation, at levels of around 2g daily, seems to be of value. Oily fish intake over time can help to build up levels in the cell membranes. Reducing intakes of fats that compete with EPA (and DHA) may also be advisable, the main ones being saturated fats and hydrogenated trans-fats.
- *Blood sugar regulation*: This is frequently a problem. Sugar can have a drug-like action on the brain. Eating more sources of complex carbohydrates and reducing sugar intake can

only be of value for most people. For more on this see Chapter 5: Food and Mood, and Appendix I Glycaemic Index, page 350.

### Antisocial Behaviour

There are many contributing factors to antisocial behaviour, but nutrition is rarely considered part of the problem. In fact it could well be of huge value for a number of those who are in the penal system, and it could provide adjunctive therapy to psychosocial support. Offenders often come into institutions after a lifetime of poor eating habits, alcohol and drug abuse. It is not a great leap of imagination to understand that a proportion of these will have nutritional deficiencies, which may compound the problem by affecting brain and nervous functioning. One advantage of studying people in prison is that they are subject to similar environmental and dietary influences. Very interesting work has been done giving inmates a simple proprietary nutritional vitamin, mineral and fatty acid supplement programme, versus a placebo, and monitoring their behaviour. The study was double-blind, placebo-controlled and found that, compared with placebos, the active group committed over one-quarter fewer offences. This led the researchers to conclude that antisocial behaviour in prisons could be modified with supplement use, with similar implications for those in the community with nutritionally-depleted diets. The trial has been praised for its rigorous methodology and has built on previous evidence from other studies.

See also ADHD page 220.

# Bloating

Bloating can mean different things to different people: distended stomachs, flatulence, water retention, thickened ankles or puffy eyes. Men and women can both experience bloating in its various forms, but for women the influence of hormones means that these symptoms can be worse before periods.

Digestive problems are usually the reason for non-specific bloating in most of its guises. Even hormonal related bloating can be resolved by focusing on the gut, because hormones are processed through the liver, which is affected in its turn by what is going on in the digestive tract. It is important to rule out diagnoses such as Crohn's disease or Coeliac disease. Acute problems with bloating should always be investigated by a doctor, as they could be a sign of blockage in the digestive tract.

- *Food sensitivities*: Finding out precisely what it is that leads to these uncomfortable and annoying symptoms can be an imprecise science. After finding a culprit and gaining relief, the problem may recur after a while – often because another food is now featuring more prominently in the diet and in turn is causing problems. The usual suspects, such as wheat products (bread, pasta and biscuits) or milk are most frequently found to be the cause of bloating. There are other likely culprits such as other grains (rye, oats, barley), soya-based foods, alcohol, coffee, potatoes and bananas. Unfortunately, the biggest hint that a food may be the cause is if the person eats it frequently and finds it hard to give up. For this reason, it is important to find convenient and nutritious substitutes. For instance, if you give up wheat for a while, you could eat dark rye bread, corn pasta, oatcakes, rye crackers, porridge, non-wheat breakfast cereals, rice and so on. Identifying suspect foods resolves around 50 per cent of bloating problems.
- *Food combining*: A further 25 per cent of people will respond to food combining. In the main, this takes the form of not

eating proteins (such as meat, fish, cheese and eggs) at the same time as starches (such as bread, rice or potatoes). In practice this means you can eat a meal based on, say, chicken with vegetables and salad, or a baked potato with vegetables and salad, but not chicken *and* potato. There is strong opposition to the principles of food combining (the idea that foods 'fight' in the digestive tract) amongst many nutritionists; however, it remains the case that a proportion of people find relief from bloating by this measure. See page 132 for more.

- *Yeast*: If these steps still don't work, a final 25 per cent of people will find that a diet to get the *candida albicans* yeast under control is likely to help them (see Candida, page 146).

- *Healing the digestive tract*: Identifying which eating plan is most likely to work is the most time consuming aspect, but not quite all there is to it. To ensure continued digestive health, which means the symptoms do not return and that intolerances are not created to new foods, it is well worth attending to repairing the gut wall. For this see Digestive and Bowel Health page 181.

- See also Fluid Retention page 201.

- See also Lactose Intolerance page 231.


## Blood Pressure, High (Hypertension)

High blood pressure (or hypertension) is a common problem and is linked to cardiovascular disease (heart attacks and strokes) as well as to eye, kidney and brain damage. When blood pressure is checked two numbers are provided (eg: 120/80). The first figure is the systolic and the second is the diastolic reading. Systolic is the point of maximum pressure when the heart has just pumped the blood through the arteries, while diastolic is the point of minimum pressure when the heart is momentarily at rest. A normal adult blood pressure reading is 120/80 mm/Hg with hypertension defined as greater than 140/90 mm/Hg. Major lifestyle contributors to high blood pressure are smoking and stress. Hardening and furring up of the arteries (arterio and atherosclerosis) occurs with increasing age and is exacerbated by smoking, excess alcohol intake, overweight and diabetes. Lack of exercise, high salt intake and raised blood fats contribute. If aged 35+, it is ideal to get your blood pressure checked every couple of years.

- *High salt intakes*: The idea that it is completely normal for blood pressure to increase with age is erroneous. Societies who eat less than 3g salt daily do not exhibit this effect (even with 'stressful' lifestyles) and populations such as Yi farmers in China moving from low-salt to high-salt diets exhibit changes in age-related hypertension. Salt-avoidance reaps relatively early hypertension-lowering rewards. We evolved on diets restricted in sodium, with added salt being introduced 5–10,000 years ago. Current UK/USA intakes are approximately 9–12g salt per day for adults. The kidneys are unable to excrete the levels of salt found in modern diets and so pressure in the arteries is raised. Current recommendations are a reduction from 9–12g to 5–7g salt per day. Current recommended targets are being questioned and recent USA daily sodium recommendations have dropped from 2.4g to 1.5g (equivalent to a drop from 6.0g to 3.8g salt). For more details see Appendix II page 357.
- *DASH Trial*: DASH (Dietary Approaches to Stop Hypertension) was a major study of diet and high blood pressure. The DASH-diet was based on high fruit and vegetable intakes (7–10 portions daily) and low-fat dairy

(fully, not semi-, skimmed milk), and reduced saturated fats and total fats, versus the SAD-diet (Standard American Diet). Over only 30 days the DASH-diet resulted in lowered blood pressures. The next phase of the trial – the DASH-sodium trial – subdivided these groups into high (3.3g), medium (2.4g) and low (1.5g) sodium (equivalent to 8.25g, 6g and 3.75g salt) and provided strong evidence that low salt diets reduced blood pressure in hypertensive people very significantly.

- *Potassium*: The mineral potassium directly antagonizes sodium from salt. Potassium is easily lost by the body, so keeping stores replenished on a daily basis is vital. All fruits and vegetables are high in potassium, one of the main reasons why the high fruit and vegetable intake on the DASH-trial is thought to have been relevant.
- *Overweight*: This increases problems with sodium excretion. About half of those who reduce sodium and lost 10lbs on average ceased the need for blood pressure lowering medication.
- *Calcium*: This is another mineral that is protective against high blood pressure and may be a part of the success of the DASH-trial's incorporation of low-fat dairy produce.
- *Alcohol avoidance*: In those with high blood pressure this can help to reduce hypertension. There is a dose-response relationship, which means that the more alcohol that is drunk the greater the effect on blood pressure.
- *Blood thinning*: One clove of garlic a day, and two portions of fish oils weekly are linked to improving blood thinning and therefore helping to normalize blood pressure.
- *Herbs to avoid*: Liquorice (the herbal root in supplements as well as liquorice sweets) should be avoided as it raises blood pressure significantly. Ginger and Ginkgo biloba should also be avoided when taking blood pressure lowering

medication, as they can increase the effects of the drugs (see Appendix IV, page 367 for more information).

- *Other helpful compounds*: Hawthorn is an effective herb. Vitamin C and CoQ10 have some evidence of helpful effects.

## Blood Pressure, Low (Hypotension)

Low blood pressure (or hypotension) is not a condition that is generally treated as a problem in the UK, unless symptoms such as dizziness cause real distress. Major stress can cause a sudden lowering of blood pressure in susceptible people, possibly as a part of the adrenal gland feedback mechanism (the adrenal glands produce stress hormones). Postural hypotension is common amongst the elderly, in those with ME and in pregnancy. The remedy is to get up from a lying position very slowly.

- *Salt*: The commonly prescribed solution to hypotension is to increase salt in the diet, to produce the opposite effect to that described in hypertension (above), but this may not be advisable in the long term.
- *Herbs*: The herb liquorice root can be very effective at raising, and thus normalizing, low blood pressure in cases of hypotension.

## Blood Sugar, Low (Hypoglycaemia)

The main fuel the body works with is glucose, which is delivered by the blood network to cells. The body needs to regulate blood glucose (commonly called blood sugar) very tightly so that a steady supply is trickled to cells and, most importantly, to the brain. If blood sugar levels are too high because sugary foods, or foods that have a sugary impact, are eaten the pancreas secretes insulin to stabilize blood sugar levels. Insulin clears the blood by storing glucose as fat. The reason it needs to do this is that high blood sugar levels cause cell and tissue damage. It is this damage which, in diabetes, causes blindness and peripheral circulation damage; this can lead to the need for lower limb amputation and heart disease. In the short-term, however, when insulin is called into play too often and with increasing impact, this leads to low blood sugar, as insulin is overcompensating and becoming trigger happy. It is a bit like a roller-coaster of sugary foods triggering too much insulin, which in turns lowers blood sugar too much, leading to low blood sugar symptoms. These symptoms are fatigue, light headedness, dizziness (as the brain is starved of sufficient fuel), and hunger pangs (particularly carbohydrate cravings). It is most common to assuage these symptoms by eating something quick and sugary – such as a biscuit, a chocolate or a slice of bread. This solves the short-term problem, but perpetuates the cycle and the problem in the long run.

- *Low Glycaemic Index (GI) foods*: Foods that release glucose slowly and steadily into the blood stream are preferred by the body to sugary foods, or foods which have a sugary effect such as white bread or rice. Slow-releasing carbohydrates are most often high in fibre. Carbohydrate foods have been quantified on a scale called the Glycaemic Index, which helps to quantify their effect on blood sugar. The foods are compared to glucose, which passes unchecked straight into the bloodstream and has been given a rating of 100. There are variations to where foods fit on the scale depending on how refined they are. Therefore whole porridge oats have a lowish score, but when the oats are milled finely they will have a higher GI score. This is because the finer particles are digested and absorbed more quickly, releasing sugar into the bloodstream.

- *Meal balance*: The GI score of foods is affected by the balance of other nutrients in the meal – fat and protein slow down the GI impact of carbohydrate foods. For a list of the GI scores of foods, see Appendix I, page 350.
- *Proteins*: Basing meals on a protein component, or at least including protein with each meal and snack helps to regulate blood sugar. When snacking this could mean a small handful of nuts, seeds, a tub of yoghurt, a hard-boiled egg, a matchbox-sized piece of cheese or some hummus on a cracker.
- *Coffee*: This does not have a rating; however, it does stimulate adrenaline, which in turn raises blood sugar.
- *Alcohol*: While alcohol has a GI rating of 0 in most cases (the exception being beer, though this still provides a moderate amount of carbohydrate) it can disturb blood sugar balance, as it interferes with the synthesis of glycogen (our glucose stores).
- See also Insulin Resistance page 227, Diabetes, page 176, and Low-carbohydrate Diets, page 323.

## Bowel Bacteria

Also called gut bacteria, gut flora and bowel flora. At birth, gut flora are inoculated into the sterile gut and from that time on we have an intimate and symbiotic (for the most part both host and bacteria benefit) relationship with the bacteria that colonize us. Advantageous human gut microflora compositions have many established health benefits. 'Beneficial' bacteria are responsible for vitamin B and K synthesis, producing compounds (called short-chain fatty acids) that act preferentially as food for the cells lining the bowel; acidification of the bowel, which protects against bowel cancer; controlling micro-organisms such as food poisoning bacteria via antibiotic compounds and competition; and enhancement of the protective barrier function of the gut. The vital importance of healthy bowel bacteria is covered in more detail in Chapter 4 page 35. Specific applications for improving bowel bacteria balance include: digestive health; bowel diseases such as inflammatory bowel disease; ulcerative colitis and Crohn's disease, which involve altered microflora and tissue damage; improving constipation; reducing diarrhoea; avoiding 'traveller's diarrhoea'; limiting the effect of antibiotic-induced diarrhoea; and enhancing immune function. Below are means by which a favourable balance of gut bacteria can be maintained.

- *Fibre*: Dietary fibre promotes healthy bowel bacteria. The most beneficial fibre comes from vegetables, fruits and beans/pulses/legumes. Oat fibre and other grain fibres are beneficial; however, for many people added wheat bran fibre is too aggressive for the digestive tract.
- *Make changes slowly*: Many people complain of excess wind when they switch to a higher fibre diet. In these circumstances it is advisable to make the changes slowly, increasing in steady increments over several weeks to permit the gut to adapt to increased fibre. Fibre specifically acts to increase bacterial fermentation in the gut – initially this may seem a problem, but it settles down eventually.
- *Sugars*: Sugars and refined carbohydrate (such as white bread and white rice), excess protein diets and alcohol adversely affect beneficial bacteria colonization.
- *Alcohol*: Excessive alcohol intake severely depletes healthy bacteria.
- *Antibiotics*: These drugs are non-selective and wipe out much of the bacterial colony in the gut. This re-establishes

itself very quickly but not always in an advantageous balance as 'unfriendly' bacteria get the upper hand. Repeat courses of antibiotics are more likely to cause longer-term problems and should really be followed by a course of pro- and prebiotics (see below).

- *Probiotics*: These are beneficial bacteria in foods and supplements. They are found naturally in foods such as fermented (live or 'bio') yoghurt and kefir. They are also added to yoghurt drinks and other foods. Probiotic supplements, such as acidophilus and bifidobacteria, are also available as supplements.
- *Prebiotics*: These are fibre compounds that specifically act to stimulate beneficial bowel bacteria. These compounds are found naturally in vegetables and fruits, but in quantities that would require us to be vegetarian or consume the quantities eaten by our close cousins, the great apes, to make a therapeutic difference. Common prebiotics are inulin and fructo-oligosaccharides (FOS) and they are added to increasing numbers of foods and drinks, as well as being available as supplements. They are sweet tasting and look like sugar, but have few calories as they are not digested and can make a pleasant addition to, for example, breakfast cereals or milk shakes.
- *Synbiotics*: This is the latest term which has been coined. These combine pro- and prebiotics for maximum benefit, and usually work much better than just probiotics on their own.

## Breast Tenderness, Lumpiness

Cyclical lumpiness and tenderness is common in women of menstruating age and relates to rising levels of oestrogen pre-menstrually. It can be very uncomfortable, in some cases requiring a bra to be worn in bed, not being able to bear being touched and affecting movement. It nearly always affects both breasts. Breast tenderness and lumpiness can be alleviated in a number of ways nutritionally. It is generally the case that at least two menstrual cycles need to pass before assessing the effectiveness of making dietary changes. Most lumps are non-malignant and can be cysts or fibroadenosis (fibrous tissue). All suspicious lumps in the breast and surrounding area (the collar bone, breast bone, armpits and the ribcage under the breast) must be checked by your doctor, particularly if irregularities occur in one breast/side only.

- *Caffeine*: High caffeine intake has been linked to breast tenderness and may be a particular problem for some women who are over-sensitive to caffeine. Caffeine is found in coffee, tea, chocolate (particularly dark chocolate), the herb guarana and some medications such as headache and pain medication.
- *Food intolerance*: A sensitivity to high levels of wheat in the diet can manifest in some women as increased breast swelling and tenderness pre-menstrually.
- *Soya*: This food is naturally rich in mild plant oestrogens that help to counteract the stronger effects of body oestrogens that rise pre-menstrually, causing breast tenderness.
- *Evening primrose oil (EPO)*: EPO is a source of the omega-6 GLA fatty acid, is licensed as a prescription item for breast tenderness and is routinely prescribed by doctors for the condition. However, the dosages used can be too low to achieve an effect in all cases. EPO has anti-inflammatory effects but when given against a background diet which is antagonistic to its effects, the impact can be only marginal. Excess saturated fats, hydrogenated fats, coffee and alcohol antagonize the metabolism of fatty acid and so need to be moderated to help the positive effects of supplementation.

. Very occasionally EPO will make the condition worse, probably because there is already an excess of omega-6s in the background diet. In this case eating more omega-3 fatty acids from oily fish is likely to be the answer.

- *Vitamin E*: As a supplement, vitamin E has been used successfully in many cases of breast tenderness at doses of around 800ius daily.
- *Herbs*: The herb Vitex agnus castus used over three months can result in a marked reduction in breast pain.

## Cancer Prevention

Cancer is actually a collection of around 35 different diseases. Most of them share a common beginning when healthy cells mutate into cancerous cells. When the body's immune system is functioning adequately these minute cancer cells are quickly killed off. However, when they manage to thrive, lay down their own blood supply network, produce a detectable tumour and go on to metastasize (spread) then cancer can be a killer as healthy tissue is eventually overwhelmed.

One of the most powerful ways in which nutrition can aid in this scenario is in prevention. It is recognized that at least 35 per cent – and perhaps as much as 70 per cent – of the causation of many cancers have a nutritional basis. Other factors are clearly involved in particular cancers: smoking is a major trigger, and radiation (sun, medical, industrial), genetic predisposition, industrial chemical hazards and even some viral infections can all lead to cancer.

Being aware of health changes, and visiting your doctor if you have any doubts, is one of the best diagnostic tools. Early detection for most cancers can make all the difference to successful treatment. Women should regularly examine their breasts, young men should check their testicles, older men should be aware of changes in urinary flow that might suggest prostate cancer. Unexplained headaches, rectal bleeding and any swelling, lump or inflammation should be reported to your doctor.

Whether or not nutrition can provide a 'cure' is a matter of huge debate and a large degree of scepticism. However, many people believe (myself included) that if you can keep the individual as healthy as possible, with their immune system in fighting shape, and able to deal with the assaults of medical treatment, then that person has the best possible chance of recovery.

In the meantime, what most experts who have studied cancer and nutrition do agree on is that some truly exciting and useful nutritional tools are available to avoid cancer in the first place. Some of the most widely accepted of these are:

- *Fruits and vegetables*: Five portions minimum daily are recommended for their protective effect against many diseases, including cancers. Some authorities, including the US, recommend higher amounts of seven or eight portions daily. Specific compounds have been identified that are protective, such as glucosinolates (found in cruciferous vegetables such as broccoli, Brussels sprouts, cauliflower and cabbage) and lycopene (a carotenoid found in tomatoes, which is highly protective against prostate and breast cancers). It was theorized for a long time that meat eaters had a worse cancer incidence compared to vegetarians because of red meat. However, it seems likely that vegetarians have more protection because of their high vegetable and fruit intakes. The message is that lean meat is not a risk factor, but fruit and vegetable intake is a protective factor.
- *Fibre intake*: Many studies have confirmed the benefits of high fibre intake, with a significantly lower risk of breast, prostate and colorectal cancers. Levels of 18g per day are

recommended in the UK and levels of 30–35g per day are recommended by the American Cancer Society.

- *Alcohol intake*: Two or more measures per day are negatively linked to breast cancer in pre-menopausal women (alcohol amplifies the effects of oestrogens). In post-menopausal women two units daily does not have adverse effects and may also protect the heart. Three units daily in men and women is associated with a higher risk of colorectal cancer.

- *Salt intake*: High salt intake increases the risk of stomach and oesophageal cancer.

- *Fish intake*: Protection against cancer from fish eating is probably linked to the omega-3 fatty acids in oily fish and possibly the low-fat content of white fish supplanting higher-fat meals centred on red meat. There are reduced risks of colorectal, prostate and breast cancers, as well as leukaemia, in those with the highest intakes of oily fish. Two to three portions weekly are recommended.

- *Selenium*: The risk of most cancers (but possibly not breast cancer) are reduced with adequate selenium intake. This mineral is involved in protective antioxidant systems. Typical daily intakes are half of the 60–75mcg that is recommended and 200mcg daily may be advantageous. For more see Part 4: A–Z of Nutrients page 331.

- *Soya*: This food is specifically rich in weak phytoestrogens which are thought to be protective against breast and prostate cancers. They protect by competing for oestrogen receptor sites against more powerful body, and possibly environmental, oestrogens that are linked to breast and prostate cancers. Around 50mg daily of soya phytoestrogens is believed to be the protective amount, and this can be obtained from about five weekly 100g portions of soya from foods such as tofu, soya yoghurt and soya milk.

- *Green tea*: This beverage is high in a compound called epigallocatechin-3-galate (EGCG), which is likely to work together with other compounds in the tea to be protective against a number of cancers. Around ten cups daily is probably needed.

- *Folic acid*: This B-vitamin is probably protective against breast and colorectal cancers.
- *Sunshine*: It is widely known that excess hot sun exposure can lead to melanoma skin cancer – for this reason it is important to stay out of the sun when at its hottest, to cover up with a shirt and hat and to use a barrier sun-screen. What is less widely known, but just as certain, is that sun exposure sufficient to produce vitamin D in the skin is protective against breast and prostate cancers. The middle course is thus to be recommended. Sun exposure early or very late in the day when the sun is milder, for a half-hour daily, and making sure that burning is not a risk, is likely to be beneficial overall.

These individual measures seem to have good science behind them. There are also many diets which concentrate on a more targeted 'curative' approach. Typical examples are diets that focus on drinking large quantities of freshly made vegetable and fruit juices, or exclude all dairy products, or a vegan approach. Each of these approaches have their proponents; however, you will always hear, when you question your medical advisors on the suitability of these, just to 'follow a balanced diet'. There is some truth in this and when devising diets it is important to ensure that all the major food groups are included (see Chapter 1: The Principles of a Healthy Diet) and certainly no diet should make you feel tired or malnourished – quite the opposite, you should feel revived and energetic on a diet that suits you individually.

See Menopausal Symptoms, page 246 for information on preventing breast cancer, and Prostate Health, page 282 for more on preventing prostate cancer.

# Candida

Candida is an opportunistic yeast, which is the culprit in thrush infections (vagina, mouth, anal area, skin), and which may get out of control in some susceptible people by invading the digestive tract. Bloating can be a dramatic symptom of a candida infestation. Overuse of antibiotics, regular alcohol intake and high sugar diets often predispose to candida. Candida is often implicated in ME (see page 244).

- *Foods to avoid*: An anti-candida diet focuses on eliminating all sources of sugar, all alcohol, refined grains and some very sweet fruits (including jams, dried fruit and juices which are very sweet), and yeast-based foods (such as bread baked with yeast, mushrooms, Quorn, Marmite), malted products (such as granary bread, malted drinks, some cereals – look at the labels), cheeses made with mould (and also stale mouldy food). The idea is to starve the candida of foods on which it thrives. If this seems difficult, the most important to avoid are sugar, alcohol, white bread, white rice and white flour products. These sugary compounds are known to activate yeasts (such as when making bread or wine).
- *Foods to enjoy*: On the other hand, you do not need to starve yourself and can freely eat soda bread, which is made without yeast, oat cakes, rye crispbreads, cottage and ricotta cheeses and fruits which are not overly sweet, such as green apples. Base meals on lean proteins, vegetables, wholegrains, less-sweet fruits and low-fat dairy products. Make pastry with wholemeal flour, use natural yoghurts, enjoy seeds and fresh nuts (make sure they are not old, as they can be mouldy).
- *Anti-candida foods*: Garlic has a strong anti-candida effect and one clove daily in food is advised. Propolis (sometimes called bee glue) has strong antibacterial and anti-candida

effects (not surprising, as it is used to protect bee larvae from outside invaders). Olive oil is also potently anti-candida, so making a garlic and olive oil salad dressing and using it regularly is ideal.

- *Bowel bacteria*: Improving bowel bacteria health is vital, as this is an important means by which the candida yeast can be kept in check (see page 138).
- *Food Intolerance*: If you have any food sensitivities (see page 205), it is important to deal with these as they can suppress the immune system's ability to deal with candida, which is an invasive yeast.

## Carpal Tunnel Syndrome

This condition results from compression of the nerves leading from the forearm to the hand and often is linked to inflammation of the 'tunnel' through which these nerves go. This leads to numbness and tingling and, when severe, to incapacitating discomfort as with repetitive strain injury. It can be a pregnancy-related symptom linked to fluid retention. Distal neuropathy (nerve tingling at the extremities), which seems similar, can be an early warning sign of diabetes (see page 176). Carpal tunnel often occurs at night or after carrying a heavy load. Your doctor may offer wrist splints, or in bad cases anti-inflammatory treatment. A surgical procedure called Carpal Tunnel Release relieves pressure on the median nerve. It is often successful but can take months for full recovery.

- *Overweight*: Lose excess weight – see page 315 for guidance.
- *Fluid retention*: If this is a problem, then following a low-salt, high fruit and vegetable diet (eight to ten portions daily) is the best course. Additionally, ensure an intake of two litres of water daily and avoid dehydrating coffee, excess strong tea (more than three cups daily), fizzy drinks such as colas

and alcohol. Diuretic herbs such as dandelion (use young unsprayed leaves in salad, make a tea, or take a supplement) and camomile (five to six cups tea daily) can help. See page 201 for more.

- *Evening primrose oil*: In diabetic neuropathy, treating the diabetes is the first concern. However, there is good evidence for evening primrose oil (EPO) supplementation. EPO is rich in a fatty acid, GLA, which is involved in nerve structure and inflammation. Interestingly, another more potent source of GLA, borage oil, does not seem to be effective against diabetic neuropathy (possibly because the GLA it contains has a slightly different chemical structure to that in EPO).
- *Vitamin B6*: B6 (pyridoxine) is another nutrient that has done well in trials, and even better when combined with magnesium.
- *Bromelain*: This is an enzyme found in pineapple, which has potent anti-inflammatory and pain-reduction effects. It is also available as a supplement.
- *Herbs*: Ginkgo biloba improves circulation to the extremities.

## Cataracts

There is excellent evidence on the effect of diet, smoking and sun exposure on cataract formation. The only problem is that cataracts take years to form and so any advice needs to be implemented no later than your thirties or forties to be of real benefit in stopping cataracts forming in your sixties.

Cataracts form when the proteins in the lens of the eye 'cross-link' to form a cloudy matrix. It is similar to the effect of the tanning process on animal skin to turn it into leather, or the process that turns egg protein from clear to white on cooking. This damage cannot be undone (other than by cataract surgery) so prevention is the best policy. Smoking and sun exposure are two major contributors, as they lead to free-radical damage.

- *Fruit and vegetables*: A diet rich in fruits and vegetables will provide the antioxidants needed to maintain eye health. Antioxidants directly disarm the damaging free radicals which cause the cross-linking in cataract formation. The carotenoids lutein and zeaxanthin are positively associated with reducing the incidence of cataracts by 22 per cent and they are found in spinach, other dark green leafy vegetables, orange and yellow vegetables and fruit such as carrots and cantaloupe melon.

- *Vitamin C*: Eye tissue contains about seven times higher concentrations of vitamin C than levels in the blood, which might suggest a need for it. Studies have concluded that long-term intake of vitamin C supplements, sometimes combined with vitamin E, reduces risk of cataracts. One study noted a 27 per cent reduction in cataract formation after five years' use; another found a 60 per cent reduction with long-term use (ten years) of vitamins C and E; yet another referred to a 70 per cent reduction in risk after ten years of taking vitamin C. 500mg–1g of vitamin C were used in the trials.

- *Diabetes*: This is a major risk factor for cataracts (see page 176 for more).

## Cholesterol, High

Cholesterol is almost universally thought of as a bad thing. But this fatty compound is actually the first stage in making a number of hormones including sex and stress hormones, vitamin D and bile acids, which aid digestion. These are very important functions. Having said this, unhealthy cholesterol levels are thought to be a risk factor for heart disease and strokes, though half of all heart attacks are in people with normal cholesterol levels, making this a contentious assumption. Cholesterol is most likely to be a risk factor for heart disease if it co-exists with other problems such as high blood pressure, family history of heart disease or smoking.

Many people have controlled their intake of dietary cholesterol ever since the egg-cholesterol scare of the 1970s when people were advised to cut out eggs because of their high cholesterol content. We now know that because cholesterol is such an important 'building block' in the body, the body will make as much as it needs. If you eat a lot, then the liver compensates somewhat and makes a bit less cholesterol, and if you don't eat enough the liver will make more. So limiting cholesterol in the diet only has a partial impact. What is more important is *how* the body makes cholesterol and the type of cholesterol it makes. And this can be intimately influenced by diet.

Cholesterol comes in two main forms: LDL (low-density lipoprotein) and HDL (high-density lipoprotein). Both have important roles in the body. LDL takes cholesterol around the body for use where needed, while HDL takes cholesterol back to the liver for re-processing. The amounts made of these two main types – and also other sub-divisions of these two, which fine-tune the system – are governed by how well the liver is working and the raw materials being supplied to it.

When having your cholesterol levels tested, the best test to look for is the ratio between HDL/LDL (the most useful measure) or HDL and total cholesterol:

Blood cholesterol levels

|  | Protective | Take action |
| --- | --- | --- |
| Total cholesterol/HDL | Less than 4.2:1 | More than 4.3:1 |
| LDL/HDL | Less than 2.5:1 | More than 2.5:1 |

Statins, which are prescribed as cholesterol-lowering medication and affect cholesterol metabolism in the liver, may not have much effect in women (even those who are prescribed Statins because they are not taking HRT). Statins are most likely to be of benefit in men who have already had a cardiac event. While Statins do indeed lower the risk of heart attack by one-quarter in healthy populations, with only a 4 per cent incidence this lowering to 3 per cent represents only 1 per cent of the population. Consequently dietary measures remain important.

- *Minimizing saturated fats*: Saturated fats 'shut down' the apparatus for making the healthier HDL-cholesterol. Saturated fats are found in meat, butter, cheese, cream and milk (apart from skimmed). They are also used extensively in food processing, so fast and convenience foods tend to have a lot of saturated fat. A low-saturated fat diet can reduce cholesterol levels by up to 14 per cent. Hydrogenated trans-fatty acids – found in margarines and, again, in convenience foods – have a negative effect similar to saturated fats.
- *New information about high protein diets*: Having said the above, one of the effects of high protein diets (which can also be fairly high in saturated fats) is that cholesterol levels are lowered (see page 324) in many people. This is new information, as the popularity of this way of eating is fairly new and early trials have only recently been conducted. This may suggest that it is the combination of saturated fat with refined carbohydrates that is the real problem, and we do know that sugar is a problem for heart disease (see Inflammation page 225). Indeed, in a review of studies where saturated and trans-fatty acids were replaced with carbohydrates, no benefit was found. However, if these problem fats were replaced with good quality unsaturated fatty acids from sources such as nuts, seeds, vegetables and

their (cold-pressed good quality) oils, improved cholesterol ratios were observed.

- *Walnuts*: Eaten daily, are beneficial for normalizing cholesterol levels.
- *Omega-3s*: Fish oils improve the ratio of HDL to LDL cholesterol.
- *Alcohol*: If liver health is not good, keeping alcohol to a minimum improves its ability to process cholesterol properly. With a seriously imbalanced cholesterol reading, it may be wise to avoid alcohol totally for three months to see if this has a beneficial effect. Conversely for those with healthy livers moderate alcohol consumption – one or two units daily – of wine or beer may help to improve HDL to LDL ratios.
- *Soluble fibre*: This has a cholesterol-lowering effect. In particular, oats – equivalent to two bowls of porridge or six oatcakes daily – and fruits are known to be of benefit. Pectin-rich fruits, such as grapefruit, apples and dried fruit are of particular benefit. Beans and pulses are also excellent sources of soluble fibre and a portion eaten four times a week is of benefit.
- *Antioxidants*: LDL cholesterol is particularly harmful when oxidized. Fruits and vegetables in the diet provide protection. A citrus juice called Sweetie juice has been shown to reduce cholesterol levels in patients given 100–200ml of juice after coronary bypass operations.
- *Garlic*: Taken regularly is beneficial. Trials using garlic powder showed a marked reduction in cholesterol levels.
- *Sterol and Stanol-ester cholesterol blocking foods*: Plant sterols and stanols are naturally found in some grain and plant foods and also in wood pulp. The average Western diet contains between 180 to 400mg/day of sterols; a traditional Asian diet contains 350–400mg/day; and a strict vegetarian diet contains 600–800mg/day. They are similar in structure to

cholesterol, but they are different enough not to be absorbed. They have a similar cholesterol lowering effect to statin medication, though the effect is achieved in a different manner (see point below). Two to three grams of sterols or stanols will reduce cholesterol by between 10–15 per cent. New foods with these cholesterol blocking factors are now available, such as Benecol (stanol-esters) and Flora Pro-activ (sterols) made as spreads, yoghurts and drinks. These are definitely of benefit in reducing cholesterol levels, but they are expensive. They can be used as an adjunct to statins drugs.

- *Sheep's milk*: There is limited evidence that switching to sheep's milk products (instead of cow's milk) lowers overall cholesterol, though it doesn't change the HDL/LDL ratio.
- *Exercise*: This can help to improve the ratio between HDL and LDL.
- *Statins and selenium*: Statins seem to interfere with selenium metabolism and as this is an important antioxidant, it may pay to eat a couple of extra Brazil nuts daily to compensate.

## Chronic Fatigue

See ME (Myalgic Encephalomyelitis), page 244.

## Coeliac Disease and Gluten Avoidance

Coeliac disease affects about one in 1,000 people. It is a complete intolerance to gluten, a protein found in certain grains. Gluten damages the wall of the small intestine; nutrients then can't be absorbed properly, resulting in malnutrition. Symptoms range from mild to severe and include digestive upsets, mouth ulcers, tiredness, breathlessness, anaemia, diar-rhoea and weight-loss. In children coeliac disease leads to 'failure to thrive'. Coeliac disease is diagnosed via blood tests and confirmed with a small tissue biopsy from the small intestine. As this is an invasive procedure, it is not carried out unless there are definite concerns. Coeliac disease is not the same as a food allergy (which results in hives, swelling or breathing difficulties) or a more generalized 'intolerance' to wheat or other grains (which can be unpleasant and involve various symptoms from bloating to headaches, but is rarely as serious a threat to health as Coeliac disease).

Coeliac disease is entirely different to wheat intolerance; however, the advice on appropriate substitutes that follows is of use to anyone aiming to avoid wheat and other gluten grains for whatever reason – coeliacs just need to be more precise about the nutritional changes.

- *Gluten grains must be avoided*: Wheat contains gluten and rye, barley and oats contain very similar proteins. Some coeli-acs can tolerate oats. Because these grains, and wheat in particular, are so common in staple and processed foods avoiding them involves careful attention. Tiny amounts of gluten can set off a full-blown reaction in a highly sensitive individual. Major sources of gluten are: bread, breakfast cereals and muesli, crackers (i.e.: oat, wheat or rye), pasta, pastry, biscuits, cakes, pies and puddings; in fact any food made with the flour of these grains. Manufactured and processed foods very commonly include flour or starch. These are used as thickeners, binders and fillers in all sorts of processed foods. Look out for the words 'flour' or 'starch' on labels, though if these are not included it is no guaran-tee that the food is gluten-free. Less obvious sources of gluten include: bulgar (wheat), couscous (usually wheat unless it specifies otherwise), spelt, sprouted wheat and tricale. It is very easy to trip up. For instance, an innocuous-looking chocolate could have gluten in it in small amounts. All sorts of foods contain gluten, especially those with sauces or 'composite' ingredients where full labelling is not required. Cross-contamination can also happen during food manufacture or storage.

- *Gluten-free foods can be eaten*: Meat, fish, eggs, cheese, milk, vegetables, fruit, nuts and seeds. The easiest way to plan meals is to offer a plain piece of fish or meat, without sauce (unless you are certain it has been only thickened with potato starch or cornflour), a non-gluten carbohydrate source such as potatoes, rice or special gluten-free bread or pasta, and vegetables. A gluten-free yoghurt or piece of fruit would be a suitable dessert.

- *Non-gluten grains and starches*: Many dishes can easily be made with other grains – for instance polenta cake or millet porridge. Grains that do not contain gluten are: corn (popcorn, polenta, cereals such as cornflakes, corn starch, corn bread, polenta cake, tacos, nachos – but check these don't include gluten-grains); rice (rice cakes, cereals such as Rice Krispies, pasta, Japanese rice crackers); quinoa (cooks like rice); millet (porridge, muesli); buckwheat (not wheat despite the name, used in pancakes and pasta); and kasha (toasted buckwheat). Other starchy foods which are gluten-free include: potato, sweet potato (yam), chestnut flour, sago, tapioca, gram (chickpea flour) and lentil flour (in popodums).

- *Gluten-free convenience foods*: There is a vast range of gluten-free packaged foods available from supermarkets, health food shops and large chemists. As they are labelled gluten-free, this eliminates the guess-work. While these foods tend to be more expensive, a diagnosed coeliac can get some of them on prescription from the doctor. Gluten-free foods include breads (usually made with rice flour and not hugely palatable), corn cakes (much better), mueslis, cereals, biscuits (which can be good but sugary), and pastas (made from various grains, they may have a different texture and cook slightly differently but work well).

## Cold Sores

A cold sore (*Herpes simplex*) is a viral infection. Four-fifths of people have antibodies to the virus, though most do not show clinical symptoms. The virus is normally acquired in childhood and kissing is the main means of infection (this should be avoided when an outbreak occurs). Cold sores tend to recur throughout life in susceptible people, usually when they are run down or feeling stressed (which it is wise to avoid as far as possible). Immunisation against flu has been shown to help people with recurrent herpes. *Herpes simplex* Type 1 causes cold sores, while Type 2 is the cause of genital herpes.

- *L-lysine*: This is an amino acid (protein building block) which reduces the frequency and severity of outbreaks and improves healing time. Taking a 300–1200mg L-lysine supplement when an outbreak is happening is a favoured treatment choice by many. L-lysine should not be taken long term, however, as it may increase cholesterol levels.
- *Arginine*: This is another amino acid, which works in opposition to L-lysine. While L-lysine is being taken the diet should be altered to reduce arginine as much as possible so that it doesn't conflict. Arginine is found in peanuts, chocolate, seeds and cereals.
- *Vitamin C bioflavonoids*: L-lysine works best with vitamin C with bioflavonoids (compounds which promote the action of vitamin C and are found, for example, in the pith of

oranges). Eating vitamin-C rich foods to give 100–200mg vitamin C daily – around three or four vitamin-C rich fruits daily – should help the L-lysine to work more effectively.

## Colitis and Crohn's Disease

Colitis is inflammation of the colon (the large intestine or large bowel). Gastro-enteritis due to food poisoning can be involved in acute cases. It is thought that ulcerative colitis may be caused by abnormal immune/allergic responses to bacteria or food. There is a strong familial tendency and it is also linked to Crohn's disease. Crohn's disease is chronic inflammation of the bowel. It may involve an overactive immune/allergic reaction, or bacterial, viral or parasitic infection – the causes are uncertain. Stools may be small, contain blood (this should always be checked by a doctor), pus-filled, and/or diarrhoea is present. Ulcers and fistula (pockets in the colon) develop. Many people with Crohn's disease are smokers and giving up can improve symptoms. It has been theorized that a possible cause of Crohn's disease is a bacterium found in milk which is not killed off during heat treatment (pasteurization) of milk and this possibility is still being investigated.

- *Fibre*: Harsh fibre, from sources such as wheatbread, cereals and pasta, should be avoided. Sources of soluble fibre such as fruits, cooked vegetables and lentils should be increased. Avoid bran, nuts, seeds and sweetcorn.
- *Food sensitivities*: These are probable irritants, but it may not be straightforward finding out which is the specific problem. In one study of Crohn's disease common culprits were corn, wheat, milk, yeast, egg, potato, rye, tea, coffee, apples, mushrooms, oats and chocolate. Many practising

nutritionists observe, anecdotally, that it is the foods eaten most commonly by an individual that are most likely to be suspect. Making sudden changes to the diet can worsen symptoms and slow removal and replacement may work better than suddenly altering the diet.

- *Malabsorption*: This is often a real problem. Malabsorption of vitamins and minerals can lead to a worsening of health as nutritional insufficiencies or even deficiencies lead to poor health. A general multi-vitamin and mineral supplement is advised, though this needs to be of top quality to improve absorption.

- *Fish oils*: Omega-3 fatty acids can help to repair the gut wall and have been shown to help two-thirds of those with Crohn's disease when taken over a year. Doses should be about 2g of EPA and 1g of DHA (the two main fatty acids found in fish oils). It is difficult to get this amount from the diet, but three portions of oily fish weekly can help; mackerel and sardines are particularly rich in omega-3s.

- *Bowel bacteria*: Probiotics are an essential treatment for both conditions. See page 138 for more on this. In a trial using very high-strength probiotics (giving 200 billion live organisms daily, much more than is found in typical supplements) almost complete reversal of ulcerative colitis was observed. The types of probiotics used may have differing degrees of success and this is currently being investigated by researchers. Prebiotics may have an adverse effect if used in too large quantities and these should be introduced extremely slowly.

- *Betacarotene-rich and vitamin A rich foods*: These help to repair the digestive tract. Liver (unless you are pregnant) once each week or two, and orange coloured vegetables and fruits on a regular basis help.

- See also Digestive Health page 181 and Anaemia page 115 (anaemia often results from internal bleeding).

# Concentration

A deterioration in the ability to concentrate can be frustrating. Concentration may be more important at some times than at others, for instance during exams or while doing difficult or dangerous work. There can be many reasons for loss of concentration such as boredom, distractions, weariness or establishing the habit of studying. Nutrition is not always the first consideration. However, there are a few nutritional issues that may contribute or help.

- *Dehydration*: This is a common reason for reduced concentration and studies have shown that children in schools who are given frequent water breaks are able to focus much better. In addition to drinking more water some drinks such as sugary drinks, alcohol, coffee and strong tea are dehydrating.
- *Caffeine*: This has been shown to aid concentration – but only in short spurts. It is a drug that aids alertness and so definitely has its place in emergency situations. However, drinking coffee regularly to aid concentration in the long term may be counterproductive as it can impair sleep patterns and tiredness may contribute to lack of concentration. Additionally caffeine-withdrawal headaches, often experienced at weekends when not near the office coffee pot, may not help.
- *Breakfast*: A nutritious start to the day is essential in order to be able to concentrate during the morning as it refuels the body and replaces energy reserves used up at night. Children and young adults are particularly noted for skipping breakfast, and in women this is often related to a desire to lose weight – which is erroneous. One-third of schoolchildren don't eat breakfast and one-quarter eat sweets and crisps for breakfast, which translates into lapses in concentration and poor performance. Glucose is essential fuel for

the brain, as it helps to make the neurotransmitter acetyl-choline, vital for concentration and memory. Those who eat breakfast work faster and have better memory recall than those who skip breakfast. In one study of nine to 16-year-olds, those who did not eat a proper breakfast performed mentally at the level of 70-year-olds. Breakfasts which include slow-releasing carbohydrates and a little protein are best for concentration and energy levels throughout the morning, so for example it would be better to eat beans on toast, or an egg and toast, than just toast on its own.

- *Iron*: Iron-deficiency anaemia can reduce oxygen supplies to the brain and so impair concentration. See page 115.
- *B-vitamins*: This group of vitamins is needed for optimal brain function. B-vitamin rich foods are fortified cereals, wholegrains, oatmeal, brewer's yeast, brown rice, legumes, liver, dark green leafy vegetables, egg yolks and yoghurt. Fish and meat are good sources of B6 and B12. The B-vitamin folic acid may have a particularly important role to play in age-related brain degeneration, particularly in reducing the risk of Alzheimer's.
- *Herbs*: Ginkgo biloba improves peripheral blood circulation and has a good reputation for improving concentration.
- *Omega-3s*: These fatty acids are important for overall brain health. Orange juice fortified with DHA is now available in some school vending machines and is marketed, with some possible justification, as a 'think drink'.

## Constipation

Some people may think it is normal to pass a motion only once or twice a week, but it isn't ideal and it is better to 'go' more frequently – the longer stools remain in the body the harder and less easy they become to pass. Chronic constipation is a debitating condition, which can be linked to several dietary factors. Prolonged stress can be involved as the stress response effectively shuts down the digestive system. If constipation alternates with loose bowel movements, it can be classed as IBS (see page 229). Constipation is more common in the elderly as their digestive system is working at a slower pace. Sitting on the toilet with an upturned bin under the feet to raise the level of the knees is extremely effective, as it changes the way the muscles of the colon work. Laxatives should be used as infrequently as possible because if the bowel becomes dependent on them, this makes it increasingly more difficult to respond to the 'call of nature'.

- *Low levels of fibre*: This is a leading cause. Fibre is needed to bulk out stools and to give the colon something to work on as it moves the stool along. However, adding bran to cereals is not usually the answer. Wheat bran is a form of 'roughage' which some people find quite irritating to the gut wall and it may cause other problems such as wind and bloating. Rice bran is a much better option. Soluble fibre found in fruits, vegetables, beans, lentils and oats is more gentle on the digestive tract and does a better job. Brown rice contains a substance called gamma-oryzanol as well as gentle fibre, which is very helpful for healthy bowel movements. Pears are exceptionally high in soluble fibre, making them ideal to resolve constipation gently. Figs and prunes are well-known remedies, three to eight per day being ideal. It is important to add bulky fibrous foods to the diet slowly to allow the digestive tract time to get used to them. Sudden changes can lead to discomfort and a worsening of symptoms, while slow changes can lead to a resolution.
- *Fibre supplements*: Soaked or cracked linseeds are an excellent solution to a short-term problem. Psyllium husks are

available from health food shops in powdered form (they are soaked in fruit juice or, less attractively, in water) and are ideal for resolving constipation. Extra water should always be drunk with fibre supplements.

- *Liquid levels*: The bowel extracts as much water from stools as possible and if you are dehydrated, insufficient liquid is left to keep the stools from becoming too hard. Breast-feeding is a common reason for constipation linked to low fluid levels, as fluid is being diverted to the breast milk. The solution is to drink more liquids, preferably water – at least two litres daily (or even three litres if breast-feeding).

- *Milk allergy or intolerance*: This is a common reason for con-stipation, especially in children. A simple exclusion period of two weeks will help to diagnose if this is a problem. Children should not avoid milk for longer than two weeks without taking great care to improve other calcium sources in the diet. Many dairy alternatives are now calcium enriched, however (see Lactose Intolerance, page 231).

- *Bowel bacteria*: These play a vital role in maintaining healthy bowel movements. They are involved in providing energy for healthy bowels and in improving peristalsis (gut movement). Bacteria constitute 50 per cent of the dry weight of stools. Eating live yoghurt daily or taking a probiotic supplement with bifidobacteria has been shown to help constipation. Prebiotics FOS (fructo-oligosaccharides) found in fruits and vegetables and inulin found in Jerusalem artichokes, help to encourage the growth of healthy bowel bacteria.

## Convalescence

Convalescence is a common sense part of recovery and allow-ing the body to recuperate before heading back into full activity can reduce the risk of becoming tired and ill again.

Bed-rest has to be balanced against inertia, however. Allowing time to heal and recover is important, but listen to your body and when you are ready, start moving again. This will enhance your sense of well-being and help you to keep a positive attitude. Prolonged bed-rest is not always the best thing, as it can lead to muscle wasting, sores, calcium loss from bones and increased thrombosis risk.

When it comes to surgery, not all surgical interventions are emergency procedures – indeed, most are planned well in advance. It makes sense to be as healthy as possible prior to planned surgery because surgery, whilst often necessary, has many side-effects. These include tissue damage, depressing the immune system and disturbing gut function from the surgical cutting, the anaesthetic and from the use of medication. The role of pre-surgical 'immunonutrition' is becoming better understood. In essence the person who is best nourished before, during and after hospitalization has reduced infection rates and reduced length of hospital stay. Apart from being malnourished as a complication of illness, 30 per cent of those admitted to hospital are malnourished. Hospital food can be fairly inadequate and the elderly in particular can be at risk as they may not even get fed if they are unable to feed themselves (this sounds astounding but happens frequently). Studies have shown that restricted diets (say enteral feeding, low protein, or low fat) lack several nutrients. So if you are visiting a relative in hospital, ensuring they get sufficient liquids and basic nutrition may be of great importance in their recovery.

Patients given nutritional support before pancreatic surgery had a complication rate of 33.8 per cent against 58 per cent for those not given supplements, and also stayed in hospital for an average of three fewer days. Intensive regimes of immunonutrition which involve supplementation including L-glutamine and n-3 fatty acids have been shown to have beneficial effects.

A note of caution – intensive supplementation should be carried out with the assistance of a nutritional therapist and after discussion with the patient's surgeon. Some nutrients such as arginine, which though it promotes wound healing might boost nitric oxide levels, will be contraindicated in some cases. It may be sensible to spend as little time in hospital as possible, as one in ten patients in UK hospitals need to be treated for infections picked up on the hospital ward (see Antibiotic Resistance, page 117).

- *Food should be nutrient-rich but easily digestible*: Soups, smoothies, light fruit salads, a small quantity of fish and steamed vegetables, or chicken soup – which has been shown to improve immune health – are all ideal. Appetite is often greatly diminished during recovery as energy is diverted away from digestion into the business of healing.
- *Hydration*: Drinking sufficient water to offset the constipating effect of anaesthetics is vital. Sip water before going in to surgery until the last moment you are permitted to do so (there will be restrictions) and make sure you sip it regularly afterwards.
- *Juices*: Naturopathic practitioners believe freshly made juices have a special part to play in recuperation. Juices are very easily digestible, are concentrated sources of nutrients and also provide a ready source of sugar for the body to use without too much metabolic effort. Juices made with a juicer or a blender are superior to shop-bought juices.
- *Foods which might be supportive*: Omega-3 fatty acids from oily fish help to regulate inflammation. Fruits and vegetables are rich in inflammation-fighting antioxidants. Yoghurt has been shown to resolve antibiotic induced diarrhoea in hospitalized patients receiving oral or intravenous antibiotics.
- *Foods which might be contraindicated*: Tomatoes are not advised before an anaesthetic, as they can interfere with its effects

and tomato juice reduces blood viscosity. High-fibre foods are not advisable in cases of abdominal surgery.

- *Supplements which might be contraindicated*: Any compound which might induce excessive bleeding during an operation should be avoided prior to admission to hospital. Some of these are fish oil supplements (but eating oily fish is fine), vitamin E (but useful afterwards), garlic supplements (but eating it is fine), and many other herbals (see Appendix IV, page 367).

## Cramp

Cramp happens from time to time for most people, most often in major muscle groups such as the leg. It is usually a passing phenomenon and can be related to cold exposure or a sudden use of those muscles, such as when swimming. However, recurrent cramps can be a strong sign of underlying nutritional imbalances and respond well to dietary intervention.

- *Magnesium*: Recurrent cramps are a strong sign of magnesium deficiency. Magnesium is used for nerve-signalling in muscles and a shortage of this essential mineral causes the nerves to be over-excited and to shorten the muscle in a spasm. Magnesium-rich foods are green leafy vegetables, nuts, seeds, wholegrains, soya beans, dried fruit, seafood, figs, mushrooms, onions and potatoes. A short-term, three-month course of 400mg daily magnesium supplements may be needed to correct the deficiency until an improved diet can have the desired effect.

- *Hydration*: Maintaining fluid is important for reducing cramp and is particularly important before, during and after exercise. Low-back pain is sometimes related to muscle spasm, which responds particularly well to drinking sufficient fluids – around two litres of water daily.

- *Period cramps*: These can also be related to nutritional deficiencies, again particularly magnesium deficiency.
- *Heart symptoms*: Any 'fluttering' heart, angina or chest pains must be checked immediately by a doctor. However, the heart is a muscle and it functions in a similar way to other muscles. Calcium-channel blockers are medication often prescribed for such symptoms. Magnesium has been described as a natural calcium-channel blocker as its chemical functioning in the body is intimately linked to calcium and they work in complementary and antagonistic ways. See the advice for magnesium above.
- *Salt*: Cramp can be a result of sodium deficiency. However, this is rare in temperate climates and most often happens in very hot climates as a result of excessive sweating (sodium is lost in sweat). Salt tablets or salty foods (salt is *sodium-*chloride) is the cure for this. Another reason for salt-depletion can be excessive bouts of diarrhoea, which leads to dehydration and is very dangerous, especially for small children; rehydration sachets containing salt (and glucose) are available from all chemists. Sodium-depletion can also happen with excessive high-intensity physical exertion over prolonged periods of time and this can lead to cramps.
- *Lettuce juice*: This is high in an anti-cramping compound, hyoscyamine. Mix the juice with a little lemon juice to improve the taste.

## Cystic Fibrosis

This is the most common serious genetic disease in children. Whilst once only a small number survived to adulthood, now a majority survive and diet can help to make life more comfortable. It involves a disorder of the gene that regulates the passage of salt and water across the cell membrane and so affects the mucus-secreting glands of the lungs, the pancreas, the mouth and the gastro-intestinal tract. This is not a disease that can be controlled by nutritional means; however, there are nutritional aspects which may be helpful.

- *Appetite*: Those with cystic fibrosis have large appetites – they are unable to digest and absorb nutrients properly and so remain hungry.
- *Digestive enzymes*: Patients are prescribed pancreatic digestive enzyme tablets to digest food and vitamin supplements, to compensate for poor uptake of nutrients from food.
- *Fat-soluble vitamins*: As fats are not absorbed properly, the fat-soluble vitamins, A, D, E and K are often deficient and a vitamin supplement is appropriate.
- *Calories*: The usual 'healthy' high fibre moderate fat diet is not appropriate, as those with cystic fibrosis need lots of calories to bypass poor digestion problems. Between 20 and 50 per cent more calories than usual is normally advised, but this will be discussed with the patient's doctor or dietician. Healthy fatty foods with high calorie contents include: oily fish, nuts, avocadoes, full-fat milk products, cheese, good quality meat, high quality sausages and burgers (home-made or top quality shop bought).
- *Liquids*: It is important to keep liquid levels up for sufficient hydration.
- *Diabetes*: This is a common complication of cystic fibrosis because of damage to the pancreas. If this is the case, then the usual advice to include lots of refined, sugary carbohydrates (advised because they are easily absorbed) will have to be moderated.
- *Fatty acids*: Patients with cystic fibrosis have altered levels of plasma fatty acids: arachidonic acid levels are increased while DHA levels are low. Whether this has treatment implications is not yet known. However, this fatty-acid

pattern is implicated in most inflammatory conditions and for other inflammatory conditions it is usually beneficial to supplement these. Supplementation should only be undertaken in the case of cystic fibrosis with the supervision of a doctor.

## Cystitis

Cystitis is a bacterial infection of the urinary tract, which results in inflammation. Symptoms are pain and burning on urination and a frequent need to urinate. It is more common during pregnancy. Cystitis should always be dealt with promptly as it can lead to infection travelling up the urethra to the bladder and kidneys. Any discharge or bleeding should be attended to by a doctor. Men with a persistent need to urinate should also read the section on prostate health, page 282.

Antibiotics are the usual treatment for cystitis and while effective in the short-term, overuse of antibiotics is unwise. In the case of recurrent infection, underlying causes such as poor immune defences need to be addressed (see Immunity, page 28). Personal hygiene is important, for women, wiping from front to back when on the toilet is vital because the infection is often spread from the anus.

- *Water*: Drink plenty of water, at least two litres daily. This keeps the urinary system 'flushed out'.
- *Dehydration*: Avoid dehydrating drinks such as coffee, excessive tea (more than three cups daily) and alcohol.
- *Cranberries and other berries*: Dark berries are rich in compounds called anthocyanidins which have been proved to stop the *E. coli* bacteria responsible for cystitis from adhering to the urinary tract. Cranberries, elderberries, blueberries and blackcurrants are effective. The easiest way to consume

these is as juices or as extracts, but you should avoid products with too much sugar as this is counterproductive. It has been established that it is necessary to drink cranberry twice daily to get 24-hour benefit, as the anti-adhesion properties start after two hours and continue up to ten hours.

- *Sugar*. Excessive amounts of sugar in the diet 'feed' bacteria, so you should moderate your intake of sweets and very sugary foods.
- *Bowel bacteria*: Eat plenty of live bio yoghurt or take acidophilus and bifidobacteria supplements to encourage healthy bacterial flora, which discourage pathogenic bacteria.

## Dairy Allergy

See Lactose Intolerance and Dairy Allergy, page 231.

## Dental and Gum Health

Gum disease, tooth decay and dental erosion are the three main preventable causes of dental problems. Brushing, flossing, regular visits to the dentist and the hygienist are obviously essential. The effect of diet on oral health is the other main tool for keeping a full set of healthy teeth. Poor dental hygiene leads to receding gums, a particular problem with ageing, where pockets of plaque and bacteria build up, leading to swollen, bleeding gums. As well as focusing on oral hygiene ask your dentist to investigate the use of Gengigel, which contains hyaluronic acid, a component of gum tissue, which helps to plump out and rebuild gums. It is actually best to brush teeth before breakfast (even better is both before and after). The reason for this is that bacteria have had a chance to build up overnight and acids begin to form within *seconds* of exposure to carbohydrates in the breakfast meal.

- *Bone nutrients*: The nutrients needed for healthy teeth are the same as for bones: calcium and magnesium rich foods are important. Adequate vitamin D, the vitamin made in skin on exposure to sunlight, helps bones and teeth to assimilate calcium.
- *Vitamin C*: One of the first signs of scurvy, or vitamin C deficiency, is soft, pulpy and bleeding gums, as vitamin C is needed to build the collagen that keeps gums firm. For vitamin C rich foods, see page 341.
- *Sugar*: Sugar and other carbohydrates act as food for mouth bacteria. What is important is the *frequency* of intake of sugar and carbohydrates. From a tooth decay point of view it is best to eat any sugary snacks with a meal rather than on their own, which increases the number of exposures. A better snack would be a small cube of cheese with some vegetable sticks.
- *Chocolate*: This treat is actually not as cariogenic – tooth decay forming – as other sweets because the cocoa butter it contains coats and protects teeth to a degree.
- *Xylitol*: Chewing gum with xylitol in it, an indigestible sugar, is a potent aid for protecting teeth. Xylitol stops bacteria adhering to the tooth surface and so reduces damage significantly.
- *Acidic foods*: Tooth erosion affects large numbers of people – particularly children – these days. Erosion is caused by the direct impact of acidic foods and drinks on the tooth enamel, causing it to soften and lose minerals, eventually eroding the whole surface of the tooth. This ultimately results in the soft under-layer of teeth, the dentine, being exposed. Signs of tooth erosion are a 'glassiness' of the teeth, sensitivity to cold, heat and sweetness, enamel fracture

and pain. It is irreversible. The main culprits are probably soft drinks such as colas and fizzy orange drinks. Eating acidic fruit between meals, consumption of fruit juices, particularly citrus fruit, and drinking fruit-based teas can all increase erosion. Modern strains of apples, such as Fuji and Braeburn, have higher sugar levels than the more traditional strains, such as Granny Smith and Cox's Orange Pippin. Healthy, but acidic, snacks such as yoghurt and pickles also contribute to tooth erosion.

- *Tooth brushing*: Oral hygiene practices can inadvertently worsen the situation because brushing teeth within an hour of exposure to acids, at the time when enamel has been softened, increases wear before the enamel has a chance to harden again. Rinse the mouth with water and avoid brushing your teeth for an hour after consuming an acidic food or drink.

- *Saliva*: Eating stimulates saliva flow, and saliva normalizes the altered acidity caused by these foods and drinks if they are taken with a meal. Eating sweet treats, fruit juices or chewable vitamin supplements with meals will not do as much harm as those taken between meals.

- *Better snacks*: It is better to eat non-eroding snacks such as vegetable sticks with dips, toast with nut butter, a cube of cheese, nuts or crispbreads instead of fruit, and drinking water, sugarless tea or milk instead of acidic drinks. (Tea naturally contains fluoride, which strengthens enamel).

- See also Bad Breath (Halitosis), page 125.

## Depression

Depression is now the most common illness in Britain, affecting one-fifth of people at some time in their lives. It can strike at any age, but is more common amongst 25–45 year-olds.

While it is normal to feel sad or low at times, depression is more intense, with a sense that the gloom will never lift. Imbalances of the brain's chemical messengers and nerve signalling are involved. Several nutritional factors have been shown to be important for brain health and normal brain function. For those on the anti-depressant medication MAOIs see Appendix IV, page 367 for food interactions. The talking therapies are important to help treat depression and a visit to your doctor to explore the available options is advisable.

- *Oily fish*: Oily fish are rich in the fatty acids DHA and EPA. Eating at least one portion a week, and preferably two to three, is recommended to counteract depression. Oily fish include: mackerel, sardines, fresh (not canned) tuna, salmon, herrings and sprats. Fatty acids in the brain form an important part of the nerve structure, the phospholipids. If the wrong fatty acids are incorporated into the brain the signalling is upset. The right fatty acids allow the neurotransmitters, serotonin, dopamine and noradrenalin, to work correctly. Seafood consumption around the world, and therefore intakes of EPA (and DHA), have been linked with rates of depression and suicide rates. People with depressive illness often have low levels of some fatty acids in their blood. For non-fish eaters there is the option of taking fish oil supplements or eating three omega-3 enriched eggs per week (equivalent to one oily fish portion). Trials have had positive results using doses of 1g daily of EPA (DHA does not seem to be effective) over three to six months for a therapeutic effect. Higher doses of 2g–4g may actually worsen depression, possibly because it then leads to an imbalance with DHA. It is hard to get such high doses from food, although the lower doses in oily fish or enriched eggs should be effective over time, as the fatty acids gradually accumulate in cell membranes.

Post-natal depression and SAD (seasonal affective disorder) may also be helped with fish-oils.

- *Blood sugar regulation*: Highs and lows of blood sugar can have an effect on mood (see page 42). Eating a diet that features protein at each meal, plenty of fresh legumes, vegetables and fruits, and which limits grains to wholegrain instead of refined, helps to maintain blood sugar balance; this seems to stabilize mood. The brain is very sensitive to sugar levels in the blood. Certain food components are thought to affect chemical messengers and signalling in the brain, in much the same way that antidepressant medication does. However, the mechanism by which it was believed proteins and carbohydrates affect serotonin – one of the major brain chemicals – does not seem to hold up to scientific scrutiny. Nevertheless, eating more protein and less sugar does have a positive effect on mood and depression, even if the mechanism is poorly understood at this time.

- *Alcohol*: Many people cope with depression by drinking alcohol, but in almost all cases this makes depression worse. There is a difference between desiring a drink at 6pm to unwind versus drinking to relieve deep sadness, self-esteem problems and mood swings. Most depressives will improve their situation if they avoid alcohol, particularly during a bout of depression. Alcohol also severely depletes B-vitamins, which are vital for healthy nerve function.

- *Caffeine*: Too much (four cups of coffee or six cups of tea) can make depression worse. It also interferes with sleep, triggering insomnia, which doesn't help.

- *Minerals*: There is some evidence that zinc deficiency is involved in depression. Zinc-rich foods include lean meat, liver, fish, nuts, seeds, oysters (the richest source), eggs and wholegrains. Selenium has been mooted as a possible mood-mineral, but research does not support this at present.

- *Supplements*: St John's wort has a good track record for alleviating mild to moderate depression, but contraindication exist if using other medication (see Appendix IV, page 367) or if planning to sunbathe, as it can increase sun sensitivity. 5HTP is a precursor of serotonin and is available as a supplement; it can be helpful, but should not be combined with other anti-depressant medication or herbs.

## Detox Diets

These have gained tremendous popularity in recent years, perhaps as concerns about pollution increase, and perhaps as a means of weight loss. The appeal of detox diets is probably also due to a 'quick-fix' mentality. There are as many detox diets as there are different books on the subject and common sense needs to be used when considering if they are of use. There is not much research to support their use, but this does not mean that people have not, in a certain number of cases, benefited. These are some general pointers:

- *Toxins*: The truth is that we have an almost permanent store of toxin residues in our fatty tissue, which result from modern exposure to chemicals in the environment, food and plastics. The only way to lose some of these is to lose weight (if it is needed) and to breast-feed (whereby chemicals are transferred to the baby – though the benefits of breast-feeding still outweigh the disadvantages).
- *Weight loss*: If weight loss is a goal, then a balanced approach to eating in tune with your metabolism (see Weight Loss, page 315) is the best approach. Detox diets may encourage yo-yo dieting in those who are not well versed in how to manage them.

- *The long run*: Detox diets usually focus on the short term (getting into a bikini for the summer, for instance) whereas a long-term commitment to eating healthily is by far the more sensible approach.

- *Eating disorders*: Detox diets often appeal to those with eating disorders. In this instance, detoxing can be very unsound and anyone with such a disorder needs professional help to overcome the condition (see page 184).

- *Diabetes*: Detox diets should not be attempted by those with diabetes, as strict diets can trigger blood sugar problems.

- *Foods to avoid*: Most detox diets advocate avoiding alcohol, coffee, wheat, dairy and red meat. None of these is harmful if good substitutes are found where necessary. Alcohol is not necessary and abstention will benefit the liver; caffeine is not necessary and abstention will benefit many conditions. Many grains such as oats and brown rice substitute well for wheat; there are many calcium-rich foods apart from dairy. Fish substitutes well for red meat. So a detox diet does not have to be deficient in nutrients.

- *Foods to include*: Detox diets also usually advocate an increase in the consumption of pulses (legumes), vegetables, fruits and fresh seeds and nuts, which no one would dispute. The only contraindications are few and are mainly for those who might have problems with increased roughage in the short term if they have digestive tract problems.

- *Short-term symptoms*: Many people who start on a detox diet will find that they get a worsening of symptoms such as headaches and spotty skin. This is not normally harmful and usually passes. If adverse symptoms go on for more than a few days, then the diet should be stopped and a GP consulted.

- *Be suspicious*: Generally a diet which advocates mono-foods (such as cabbage) or gives a long list of bad foods (such as tomatoes or bananas) should be treated with deep suspicion.

# Diabetes

Diabetes is diagnosed in about 1.4 million people in the UK, but there are estimated to be a further one million people who are undiagnosed. It is believed that the number of people with diabetes will double in the next five to ten years. It affects men and women equally, but certain ethnic groups are much more prone, including Asians and Afro-Caribbeans. Other risk factors are obesity, previous gestational diabetes (diabetes brought on by pregnancy), and a close relative already diagnosed with diabetes (genetic predispostion).

Diabetes is one of the main risk factors for heart disease, stroke, kidney failure, blindness and foot ulceration (leading eventually to lower-limb amputation). All of these relate to impaired vascular health caused by glucose build up and damage in the blood system. In normal health the hormone insulin is responsible for clearing glucose out of the blood to use it for energy or store it as fat in the cells. When this system goes awry it can lead to diabetes.

There are two types of diabetes:

*Type 1*: Also called insulin-dependent or childhood-onset diabetes. The immune system attacks the insulin producing cells in the pancreas, which cease to function. Glucose then builds up in the bloodstream. Insulin injections are needed over a lifetime to keep blood sugar levels within a normal range.

*Type 2*: Sometimes called adult-onset (though this is now outdated, as for the first time ever children are now being diagnosed with this type of diabetes). This is caused either by a shortage of insulin (because over time the insulin producing cells have been damaged) or by a fault in the way the body responds to insulin, known as insulin resistance. In insulin resistance the cells become desensitized to the effects of insulin, which can no longer do its job. The result is the same as for Type 1 diabetes and glucose builds up in the bloodstream. Type 2 diabetes can be controlled with strict dietary measures in the early stages, but if allowed to progress the person may go on to needing insulin injections.

Symptoms of diabetes include:

- Increased urination as the body attempts to get rid of glucose in urine. A urine dip-stick test is conducted by GPs as a first-line diagnosis (in earlier days it was called honey-urine, as the urine tasted and smelled sweet)
- Greatly increased thirst, as the body attempts to replace water lost in urine
- Extreme tiredness as glucose is unable to be moved into cells for energy
- Weight loss is also common, as proteins and fats are broken down to be used as alternative sources of energy.

In the case of suspected diabetes a diagnosis must be obtained from your doctor. Diet can help a diabetic to lead a normal life, but regular checks of health, and foot health, must be conducted and it is a medical decision about whether diet alone will help a Type 2 diabetic or if insulin medication is required.

- *Overweight*: This is a major risk factor for diabetes and normalizing weight is protective against Type 2 diabetes.
- *Regular meals and snacks*: Eating little and often to maintain blood sugar balance is advised. Make sure meals and snacks are healthy and well balanced. Some insulin-dependent diabetics have to eat a small amount of food every two or three hours. If hypoglycaemia happens in insulin-users 15g (0.5oz) glucose should be given as a tablet, or if necessary table sugar in solution.
- *Carbohydrates*: Eating foods at the lower end of the Glycaemic Index is advised (see Appendix I, page 350),

while cutting back on carbohydrates at the top of the GI. Sweets, sugary drinks and white bread are best avoided completely. Fruit is often avoided unnecessarily but it may be best to choose slightly less-sweet fruits or to incorporate them into meals, and to choose prepared fruit in natural juices instead of in syrup. Make sure carbohydrates are balanced out by proteins and vegetables, so avoid a huge bowl of pasta, but don't be afraid of including a small amount of pasta with salad ingredients that include egg or fish, or with vegetables and chicken. High-fibre foods generally are associated with a lowered risk of diabetes.

- *Types of fats*: Oily fish help to normalize blood pressure, cholesterol and blood fats. Eat at least once and preferably twice weekly. High levels of hydrogenated trans-fats and low levels of unsaturated fats (from fish, nuts, seeds, cold-pressed oils) are linked to increased risk of diabetes.

- *Antioxidants*: Found in vegetables and fruits, these help protect against the oxidation damage that results from unstable blood sugar. A minimum of five portions daily is advised.

- *Sweeteners*: Artificial sweeteners are aspartame, saccharine and acesulphame K. The most common bulk sweetener is sorbitol, found in diabetic sweets. While these can be useful they do nothing to curb the taste for sweetness and artificial sweetners are implicated in headaches and other problems. Fruit sugar – fructose – is tolerated by diabetics as it is very low on the GI (see page 350), but again it should not be overused. FOS is another bulk sweetener with the advantage of improving bowel bacteria health, that can be used by diabetics in moderation (see Chapter 4: Bacterial Balance, page 35).

- *Alcohol*: Keep intake to moderate levels. Low sugar diet beers and lagers tend to have more alcohol in them.

- *Physical activity*: Walking regularly and briskly reduces the risk of diabetes by about half. While it is important for weight loss and lower BMI (body mass index) it also has an independent effect. The more a person walks and the more vigorously, the more overall health benefit.

- *Evening Primrose Oil*: Neuropathy is a serious condition related to diabetes. Good results have been obtained in reversing and preventing degeneration as a result of neuropathy. EPO is rich in a fatty acid, GLA, which is involved in nerve structure and inflammation (see page 260 for more).

- *Coffee*: Coffee is a strong stimulant (caffeine is in fact an addictive drug) and has an effect on the hormone adrenaline, which triggers blood sugar. Yet some studies suggest that coffee drinkers are less at risk of Type 2 diabetes – though it is not known if this is cause or effect. It could be that coffee contains a beneficial compound, as caffeinated coffee is of more benefit than decaffeinated and tea shows no benefit. Studies have also found that physical activity is over three times more associated with better insulin sensitivity than coffee. The interpretation of this could be that if you drink coffee, it is not a risk factor, but it is not necessarily worth taking up coffee drinking. In a small recent study the exact opposite was found for caffeine (not coffee), which was found to increase blood glucose levels and insulin in Type 2 diabetics by 21 per cent and 48 per cent respectively after a meal.

- *Tomato juice*: A daily glass of 250ml tomato juice reduces blood viscosity in diabetics and should therefore reduce some of the complications associated with diabetes.

- See also Liver Health page 238.

## Diarrhoea

Diarrhoea is the body's way of eliminating the contents of the bowel because of some sort of irritation. The stools are loose or watery, usually with mucus, and there may be an increased frequency of the need to defecate. It is usually intermittent and occurs alongside other symptoms such as wind and bloating, and in the case of food poisoning possibly with vomiting. Short-term diarrhoea could be caused by bacterial, viral or protozoa infections, stress and overuse of laxatives or antibiotics. Long-term diarrhoea can be associated with infections, but also with diseases such as IBS (irritable bowel syndrome), coeliac disease, Crohn's disease or ulcerative colitis. Long-term diarrhoea, or severe short-term diarrhoea, should always be checked out by a doctor. Diarrhoea can cause the loss of large amounts of water and salts (sodium and potassium), which causes dehydration – especially in children and the elderly – and in severe cases can lead to shock and death.

- *Fluids*: Drink plenty of fluids, particularly water, to offset the effects of dehydration from liquid loss, particularly if the urine has turned dark and urine production has slowed down.
- *Rehydration*: Sachets for rehydration are available from the chemist or you can make your own by adding one teaspoon of salt and eight teaspoons of sugar to one litre of boiled water. Drink a litre over a two-hour period while diarrhoea persists.
- *Bananas, potatoes and watermelon*: These are fruit highest in potassium and ideal for repletion, though all fruit are useful sources.
- *Bowel bacteria*: Probiotic bacteria are highly effective at reducing the risk of diarrhoea from bacterial infections, especially when travelling. It is less certain that they have a therapeutic effect at the point of actually suffering diarrhoea. Yoghurt and prebiotic supplements can also help to resolve antibiotic-induced diarrhoea.

- *Food intolerance*: If it is suspected that diarrhoea is a recurring problem due to a dietary intolerance, the main culprits to investigate are milk (due to lactose intolerance – see page 231), and wheat and other gluten grains (see Coeliac Disease, page 153).
- *Fibre*: Soluble fibre from oats, cracked linseeds (flaxseeds) and psyllium husks (purchased as a fibre to add to cereals or drinks) are highly effective at bulking out stools to normalize bowel motions. Because soluble fibre is very gentle on the digestive tract and helps to normalize mucus production, its effects are much preferred over harsher insoluble fibre from wheat bran.
- *Anti-bacterial foods*: Manuka honey, garlic and ginger have strong anti-bacterial effects.
- *Herbs*: Mint and slippery elm teas are traditional soothing tonics for the digestive tract, helping to reduce inflammation. Ginger tea or raspberry-leaf tea (except in pregnancy) can help to soothe.
- *Alcohol and caffeine*: These are both dehydrating and should be avoided after a diarrhoea attack.
- *Figs, prunes, bran*: Usually used to improve digestive health and offset constipation, they can trigger diarrhoea if eaten in large amounts.

## Digestive and Bowel Health

The importance of the digestive tract and bowel health to general health is covered in detail in Chapter 4, page 35. It surprises many that this tube, which is commonly thought of as just the place where digestion takes place, is so intrinsically linked to overall health, including immune health, allergies and mood. Digestive health starts at the top, with healthy teeth and goes right throught to the end with healthy bowel movements.

- *The mouth*: Chewing food properly is fundamental to good digestion. Asking the stomach to do the work that the mouth should do is optimistic and leads to problems over time.
- *Liquid intake*: Liquid – water – helps digestion. It does not 'dilute' digestive juices as is often supposed, but actually stimulates digestion.
- *Leaky gut*: A damaged digestive tract can let compounds into the bloodstream that are not meant to be there – the condition is called, informally, leaky gut. It is implicated in a number of health problems including allergies, headaches, aching joints and ME. Eliminating food intolerances such as wheat or dairy (see pages 205 and 231) can help to reduce damage to the gut wall, allowing it to heal. Simple steps can help, such as eating more oily fish and zinc-rich foods, as well as foods rich in the antioxidant vitamins A and C. On the other hand, chronic stress, aspirin, antibiotics and too much alcohol will have a detrimental effect on the ability of the digestive tract to heal itself. Promoting healthy bowel bacteria (see below and also Bowel Bacteria, page 138) is fundamental to the integrity of the digestive tract wall.
- *Bowel bacteria*: Foods that can help to promote beneficial bowel bacteria include fibre-rich foods such as beans and pulses, live yoghurt, cabbage, garlic, onions and a useful prebiotic sugar substitute called FOS (fructo-oligosaccharides). Improving beneficial bacterial levels in the bowel has important immune modulating effects. It is even evident that infants who have a better bowel flora balance, or who are inoculated with beneficial bacteria, have a lower risk of allergies later in life.
- *Fibre*: This is vital for bowel health and helps to avoid diverticulitis (where little pockets form in the bowel) and bowel cancer. Fibre gives the bowel something to work with, encouraging peristalsis (the movement of the contents along the tract) and also slightly acidifies the contents.

Switching from a low-fibre diet to a high-fibre diet too quickly can cause discomfort and should instead be done slowly over time. Insoluble fibre, found in grains such as wheat, is often too harsh, while soluble fibre, found in oats, fruits, vegetables and linseeds, is more gentle and encourages healthy mucus production. Note that linseeds should not be used, unless ground to a powder, by those with diverticular disease as the little seeds can get stuck in the pockets and cause inflammation. See Appendix III, page 363.

- *Herbs*: Some herbal teas including mint, fennel and ginger help the digestive process. Slippery elm is the general herb of choice for most digestive problems. The herb *centaurium* helps to regulate stomach acid and stimulates digestive enzymes. Cayenne pepper is a potent stimulant of digestion and of digestive enzymes – just a pinch daily can promote digestive health.
- See also Bowel Bacteria, page 138, Indigestion, page 222, Ulcers, page 307, Constipation, page 160 and Diarrhoea, page 179.

## Diverticulitis

See Digestive and Bowel Health, page 181.

## Dyslexia and Dyspraxia

Dyslexia is a learning disorder whereby the ability to read and write are impaired. Dyspraxia is similar, but involves physical co-ordination problems making, for instance, shoelace tying, buttoning shirts, using cutlery and some sports difficult to master. It is most obvious in children who are in a learning phase of life but it affects adults as well. Dyslexics are often very intelligent but their 'brain wiring' interferes with processing written information. About 30 per cent of dyslexia or dyspraxia co-exists with attention deficit disorders or hyperactivity and some consider them to be part of the same spectrum of disorders. From a nutritional standpoint, similar interventions can make a positive difference.

- *Fish oils*: High EPA omega-3 fatty acid supplementation has shown promising results for children and adults in trials over a three- to six-month period. The evidence is for the fatty acid EPA and not DHA (though DHA is usually found with EPA and is beneficial to general health). The supplements used in studies contained about 560mg EPA, 170mg DHA and 60mg GLA (see Healthy Fats, page 17 for an explanation of these.
- *Food colourings*: These can have a tremendous effect on children with ADD or ADHD (see page 220) and even impact on children without diagnosed disorders, making them more irritable and less able to concentrate. In a child battling with dyslexia or dyspraxia the added burden of food colourings – the azo dyes such as sunset yellow and ponceau 4R – triggering attention problems is an unnecessary burden.
- *Caffeine*: This is found in colas, other soda drinks and many medications (including for headaches). Again, a child with concentration problems may find relief when caffeine is eliminated; while this is not a 'cure' for dyslexia, it can only improve the situation.

## Eating Disorders

Anorexia means, and involves, starving, while bulimia nervosa involves bingeing followed by purging using vomiting, laxatives or starving. An anorexic will often develop into a bulimic.

This is a specialized area of nutrition with many psychological aspects to consider. Eating disorders usually involve an altered body image. Food is used as a punishment, to make up for perceived failures and as a source of comfort. About 10 per cent of girls aged 12 and older show signs of eating disorders. Boys are much less frequently affected, but the numbers are on the increase. Children involved in gymnastics and other high intensity sports have a much increased risk of eating disorders and may be attracted to these sports precisely because of their body image issues. Particular danger times are puberty, exam times and times of emotional upset.

A child should never be made to feel guilty, as they are already enduring great difficulties and are often simply carried along on a wave they don't understand. Those with eating disorders can be extremely manipulative and confrontational and it often takes people outside the immediate family to enable the child to agree to seek help. It is important not to comment on appearance, body image and food intake. We should teach our children to feel good about themselves, not to set overly ambitious targets in various areas of their life (such as exercise and school achievement), to help them to adapt to their changing and developing bodies and to be critically aware of the body images portrayed in the media. Do not use food as a reward or punishment, and keep mealtimes as low-pressure, enjoyable times. If your child has a problem, you must seek professional help – and remember that children with eating disorders need a lot of love.

- *Weight and height*: If a child is not growing or putting on weight, appropriate measures must be taken to find out if an eating disorder, or other cause, is involved.
- *Healthy eating*: Emphasize the health properties of food rather than the calorie content or fat levels. Probably a

major mistake made in the standard nutritional treatment of those with eating disorders is to focus only on how much is eaten and to ignore the quality of the food. Clearly, the amount is important in the context of calorie intake, but to ignore the importance of the quality of some important nutrients in influencing brain function, behaviour and appetite in eating disorders is not making the best of what nutrition has to offer. In particular, omega-3 fatty acids, zinc and iron are important for brain health.

- *Blood sugar.* Those with eating disorders, particularly bulimia, often have blood sugar problems and this needs to be addressed – see page 136.
- *Digestive enzymes*: These are available from health food shops and may be important in increasing nutritional uptake from food and to help resolve damage to the digestive tract from long-term disordered eating.

## Eczema

Eczema is a dry skin condition, which at its most severe erupts in wet pustules. There are two main types of eczema: contact and atopic. As the name suggests, contact eczema (also called dermatitis) is triggered by contact with something to which a person is allergic such as washing powders, particular fabrics, latex (food preparation gloves for instance), sticking plasters, perfumes, a plant or chlorine in pools. Surprisingly, peanut oil is in the formula of some creams including nappy creams and even eczema creams prescribed by GPs and this can make the condition much worse. Atopic eczema has a genetic link. Commonly, atopic eczema involves an allergy to house dust mites and certain foods can be another trigger. It can be triggered by stressful events and can co-exist with other allergic conditions such as asthma, hay fever and hives.

- *Food triggers*: It is common for eczema to develop when a baby is moved from breast to cow's milk. Soya should also be suspect as it is often used instead of cow's milk, and yet 25 per cent of cow's milk intolerant children also have a problem with soya. Other common triggers are eggs, oranges and wheat. Carefully following an elimination period where these foods are avoided and re-introduced can give a clear indication of whether or not they are involved. This is not always easy and care needs to be taken in strictly following the elimination regime. If it is found that a particular food or foods need to be avoided, it is important to make substitutions that ensure your child will not end up missing out nutritionally. If oranges are to be avoided, other fruit need to be consumed. If wheat is to be avoided, then add, for instance, oats, rice and rye into the diet. See Food Intolerances, page 205.

- *Fatty acids*: Those with atopic eczema often do not metabolize fatty acids properly, or simply do not get enough of them in the diet. Piercing a capsule of evening primrose oil and gently smoothing the contents on the inflamed skin can help. One to two tablespoons of flax oil (for adults, one to three teaspoons for children) daily helps. Add it to food – to soups, smoothies, salads or vegetables – but do not cook with it as cooking destroys its beneficial properties. Keeping this up for at least six to eight weeks usually makes a difference. Eating a couple of portions of oily fish (mackerel, sardines, fresh tuna, salmon, sprats and pink trout) a week is also very beneficial.

- *Zinc and Vitamin A*: Nutrients that are important for general skin health and so help to repair skin are zinc and vitamin A. Zinc is found in all protein foods including fish, lean meat, eggs, pulses, seeds and nuts. Vitamin A is made in the body from betacarotene, which is found in orange and dark green produce including carrots, apricots, cantaloupes and spinach.

- *Bowel bacteria*: The health of the bowels is vital to consider in all skin conditions, and is even probably relevant for nappy rash (a form of dermatitis). See Bowel Bacteria, page 138.
- *Manuka honey*: The antibiotic resistant superbug *Staphylococcus aureus* (SA) is present in most eczema and it could be the toxin produced by this bacteria on the infected skin that causes the problem. Manuka honey is effective against SA (though it is sticky) and can make a soothing topical ointment. Honey is also hydrating for skin – wash it off after ten minutes. Steroid doses were reduced by 75 per cent in one study in which those with eczema or psoriasis were asked to put a mixture of honey, olive oil and beeswax on outbreaks on one side of their bodies three times daily, and inert substances on the other side as a control. Honey and olive oil have antibacterial properties, contain flavonoids and antihistamine compounds. The mixture can be made at home using equal parts of the three ingredients.
- *Water*: As with any dry skin condition it is helpful to keep daily water intake up to avoid dehydration.
- *Herbs and ointments*: Adding a handful of oats and camomile tea bags to a bath can be very soothing. Oat-based creams have a good track record for easing eczema. Zinc ointment cream can help to repair skin. Cabbage leaf poultices, made from pulverized leaves (pounded in a pestle and mortar) and held in place by bandages, are successful as a traditional remedy for relieving eczema and rashes when used morning and night for a few days. Chinese herbs have gained a reputation for helping eczema where Western medication has failed; a bitter-tasting tea is drunk, which may make it difficult for children. Find a reputable practitioner, because some suppliers have been known to add steroids to their blends.

# Endometriosis

This condition affects one in ten women, though many are symptom-free. Possible symptoms indicating endometriosis are painful periods, deep pain during sex, deep pelvic pain and fertility problems. Endometrial cells (those that line the womb) migrate outside the womb and attach themselves to other parts of the body, most commonly in surrounding abdominal and pelvic cavities, but they can also take root in other areas including joints. These cells remain sensitive to the ebb and flow of menstrual hormone fluctuations and behave as they would in the womb – in other words they swell and bleed into surrounding tissues. This can cause painful inflammation and scarring of surrounding tissues, such as blocked fallopian tubes or lesions on the digestive tract or bladder. Endometriosis needs oestrogen in order to grow. The cyclical nature of endometrial symptoms abate with the menopause; however, the scarring and tissue damage remain. Endometriosis is a common cause of infertility or sub-fertility in women.

- *Fatty acids*: Those that help to control inflammation are important. These include: oily fish once or twice a week (women who eat the most oily fish have the least painful periods); nuts and seeds and their cold-pressed oils, such as walnuts, linseeds (flax seeds) and pumpkin seeds. Three grams daily of evening primrose oil is also recommended and has good effects.
- *Red meat*: This is a source of pro-inflammatory arachidonic acid and so should be moderated. Both meat and dairy products are sources of growth hormones that might exacerbate endometriosis. However, if cutting these out of the diet it remains important to ensure sufficient iron and calcium levels. Iron is lost with heavy bleeding and calcium is linked to reducing muscle spasms. Drinking a glass of

orange juice (or eating other vitamin C-rich foods) with breakfast cereals will keep iron levels topped up and calcium-enriched milk substitutes are readily available.

- *Magnesium*: This is an important mineral for controlling period pain and works synergistically with calcium.
- *Fruits and vegetables*: These also have a modifying effect on inflammation by providing antioxidants that damp down free-radical damage. They also provide oestrogen-modulating lignans.
- *Fibre*: Oestrogens are excreted via the bowels attached to bile, which in turn attaches to fibre. Oats, brown rice, vegetables, nuts and seeds are good sources of fibre. Linseeds also provide lignans.
- *Soya*: This has a modulating effect on oestrogen. Soya is rich in phytoestrogens, which are weak forms of oestrogen and have the effect of blocking stronger environmental and body oestrogens. Modest portions of 100g four or five times weekly may help.
- *Iodine*: Low iodine status has been linked to endometriosis. Iodine-rich foods are seaweed, fish and iodized salt and kelp supplements. Seaweed is available in grinders to use as a seasoning (it does not taste 'fishy', but slightly salty).
- *Caffeine*: High caffeine intake can worsen period problems and it is advisable to cut out caffeine if you have endometriosis.
- *Herbs*: Vitex agnus castus has a progesterone-like effect, which helps to dampen oestrogen-linked effects.
- *Exercise*: Circulating oestrogens are reduced with regular exercise, at least four half-hour sessions a week, which could simply be fast-paced walking.
- *Surgery*: If having surgery to remove lesions, usually from the bowel, see Convalescence from Surgery, page 162 and pay particular attention to re-establishing healthy bowel bacteria (see Bowel Bacteria, page 138).

## Energy, Low

Low energy seems to be the epidemic of our time. The term 'Tired All The Time' has been coined, and in extreme cases Chronic Fatigue, or ME, is now a recognized condition (see page 244). Long-term fatigue must always be checked by a doctor, as it could relate to a number of medical problems including depression, iron deficiency anaemia and thyroid insufficiency. If any of these are diagnosed, see the relevant sections in this book. Obviously a major cause of low energy and tiredness is insufficient sleep (see page 295) and burning the candle at both ends. Learning relaxation techniques, yoga or meditation can help significantly, as can reducing your workload and worry, if you can. The following relates to more general tiredness and low energy.

- *Blood sugar balance*: This is usually at the root of most fatigue problems (after lack of sleep and doing too much). Try eating foods that are low on the Glycaemic Index (see Appendix I, page 350) and avoid those that are high on the list. Eat plenty of fresh vegetables and fruit and always include protein with a meal.
- *Snacks*: Eating a sugary snack to prop your energy levels up ultimately backfires, as blood sugar levels dip soon after. It is better to snack on wholesome protein-based options such as oatcakes with peanut butter, yoghurt with fruit, rye crackers with boiled egg, or a small handful of nuts with a little dried fruit. An excellent time to drink a fresh fruit or vegetable juice or smoothie is mid-afternoon, as an alternative to coffee, when low-energy slumps are common – it gives nourishment and perks up blood sugar levels without negative consequences.
- *Nutrient deficiencies*: This is a common reason for tiredness. Anaemia – iron deficiency – is dealt with on page 115.

Other important nutrients for energy production are B-vitamins found in cereals, wholegrains, brewer's yeast, liver, eggs and green leafy vegetables, magnesium also found in wholegrains, green leafy vegetables and also nuts and seeds, and vitamin C (the citric acid cycle is a fundamental part of the energy cycle found in every cell) found in fruits and vegetables (see Part 4: A–Z of Nutrients, page 331 for good sources).

- *Dehydration*: Drinking two litres of water daily aids general health and improves energy functions. Drinks such as coffee and tea are slightly dehydrating and also serve to add to blood sugar imbalance. Alcohol is another culprit.
- See also Thyroid, Underactive page 304.

## Epilepsy

This is a neurological disorder that results in fits and seizures. Imbalances in the brain's electrical impulses are sometimes inherited, caused by damage before, during or after birth, by a tumour, fever or infection. The terms petit mal and grand mal are used less often these days, but describe the range of intensity of seizures from moments of 'tuning out' with short-term memory and concentration loss (sometimes called absences), to full-scale convulsions that can occur up to a few times daily. Triggers can include menstruation, bright or flickering lights, stress, alcohol or illness. Drugs keep four-fifths of epileptics free of seizures. There is no nutritional treatment that is a 'cure' for epilepsy, but some factors may help to reduce the number of seizures.

- *Casein and gluten*: Some people find that eliminating the milk protein casein from their diet, as well as the grain protein gluten, greatly reduces the risk of seizures. For more on implementing these, see pages 153 and 231. However, if improvements are experienced, it is vital that individuals do not cease to take their anti-epilepsy medication in case of accidental exposure to the eliminated substances.

- *Ketogenic diet*: Some success has been had with controlling epilepsy with a very high fat diet, which triggers ketogenesis. When a diet is low in carbohydrates, which are the normal source of immediate energy, the body turns to using fats as a fuel source. As fat breaks down acids called ketones are produced. This must not be attempted other than with the supervision of a dietician versed in this approach.

- *Magnesium*: This mineral, which is involved in nerve transmission, helps some epileptics. See Part 4: A–Z of Nutrients, page 335 for magnesium-rich foods.

- *Deficiencies*: Some rare cases of epilepsy may result from deficiencies in vitamin D or vitamin B6. Supplements should only be used with medical supervision.

- *Blood sugar balance*: As low blood sugar (hypoglycaemia) can trigger attacks in some people, maintaining an even blood sugar is advisable. See page 136 for more.

- *Contraindications*: Evening primrose oil (and possibly borage oil and raspberry seed oil) sold as supplements as rich sources of the fatty acid GLA (gamma linolenic acid) should be avoided, as there is a possibility that these can increase the risk of seizures.

## Exercise and Sport

Only 36 per cent of men and 26 per cent of women take the amount of daily exercise that is recommended by the Department of Health: at least 30 minutes of moderate physical activity, five days a week. Aerobic exercise, which burns oxygen, such as fast walking, running or swimming, is ideal for general fitness and cardiovascular health. Strength and resistance training, using the trampoline, cycling or weight training, is ideal for maintaining muscle health as we age. For those who are overweight and find it difficult to lose weight, exercising on a regular basis will offset a lot of the negative consequences of being overweight. It has been theorized that someone getting 30–60 minutes daily exercise, say from fast walking or cycling to work, with a BMI (body mass index) of 30, may have fewer health risk factors than someone with a BMI of 24 who does no exercise.

- *Protein*: The mechanism by which muscles increase in volume involves microscopic tears that are inflicted on the muscle whilst exercising the muscle. The repairs to these tears bulks out the muscle over time. Therefore any exercise that increases muscle strength (even beneficial muscle increases such as recommended for elderly people with muscle wasting) involves necessary damage to muscle. This means that the raw materials – proteins – must be there to repair this damage.
- *Antioxidants*: Any increase in activity increases oxygen use. This is beneficial as it improves circulation around the body. However, the flip-side is that increased oxygen use means increased oxidation damage, which increases the need for dietary antioxidants to protect tissues. Eating a diet high in fruits and vegetables therefore becomes even more important.
- *Hydration*: Staying sufficiently hydrated is vital. Even a small amount of dehydration – 3 per cent – leads to a 10 per cent reduction in muscle performance. Dehydration can also contribute to muscle cramps due to mineral imbalance. Drinking water before a sporting activity and continually sipping small amounts throughout and afterwards is important. On a long walk always carry a small bottle of water

to sip from, particularly if the weather is warm. It is rarely necessary to drink sports rehydration isotonic drinks. The exception to this is when sports go on at high intensity for about 90 minutes. Sports drinks help to rehydrate the body because of the electrolyte balance of sodium and potassium provided. They also provide sugar for glycogen stores. If you are going to use a commercial product, make sure it has no more than 4–6g of sugar per 100ml.

- *Carbohydrate loading*: This is something that usually only concerns serious sports participants, although it has become something of a fashion amongst the more casual sports participant partly because of advertising for carb-loading products. Carb-loading is used to maintain the energy available for longer endurance by keeping glycogen (the body's instant energy stores) topped up, but the quality of the carbohydrate is important and a banana or low sugar cereal bar is a better option than chocolate, sweets or glucose. You only need to think about carbohydrate loading if the sport goes on at high intensity for over an hour.
- *Iron deficiency*: Anaemia can affect the ability to perform exercise. Improving iron status in deficient individuals improves oxygen uptake and respiratory exchange by 200 per cent.

## Eye Health

See Cataracts page 148 and Macular Degeneration, page 242.

## Fertility, Female

One in five couples find they cannot easily conceive. This may be related to several factors such as: the fertility of the man (see page 197); physical blockage from tissue scarring in the woman; fibroids; endometriosis; hormone disruption in the woman (such as early menopause or PCOS) *see relevant sections*; or early loss of the foetus. Fertility problems can sometimes persist for a few months after stopping the contraceptive pill. Where a physical blockage or early menopause has been ruled out in the woman, nutritional steps can greatly improve the chances of conception. Nutrition can serve to normalize hormone fluctuations and improve the conditions in the womb.

- *Underweight*: In a weight-conscious world, some women are just too thin to maximize their chances of conceiving. Underweight, and anorexia, are common reasons for lack of fertility. The theoretical energy cost of pregnancy is 80,000 calories, so women need a certain amount of fat. Fat stores are also an important source of non-ovarian oestrogen.
- *Overweight*: Weight normalization for the overweight can also increase the chance of conceiving – and may even be more effective than fertility treatment. Overweight, particularly central obesity, may indicate PCOS (see page 271).
- *Eating disorders*: With 1.2 million people in the UK suffering from eating disorders, this is a major potential problem for women of child-bearing age. Anorexia and bulimia affect pregnancy outcome and are associated with pre-term delivery, growth restriction, low birth-weight and low Apgar scores. The Apgar is a quick test performed at one and five minutes after the baby is born to determine the physical condition of the infant. Tests are done for heart rate, respiratory effort, muscle tone, reflexes and skin colour.
- *General nutritional status*: Pregnancy is a test of nutritional status. Generally, nature protects the potential mother and baby against problems by decreasing fertility in the face of poor nutrition. Because all nutrients work together it is better

to think of the overall quality of the diet. Zinc, vitamin E and B-vitamins are particularly important for fertility, but all nutrients play a role at some point in the process of fertility and pregnancy. Iodine, zinc, essential fatty acids and folic acid are important for the developing baby, amongst others. A diet based on the best quality ingredients (fruits, vegetables, pulses, lean meats, low-fat or medium-fat dairy and whole-grains, while avoiding low nutrient processed foods high in sugar, salt and hydrogenated trans-fats) is needed, not just before, but after conception.

- *Alcohol and smoking*: Apart from being contraindicated in pregnancy these also use up nutrients. Over four alcoholic drinks weekly is linked to reduced fertility. Therefore a woman who is experiencing problems conceiving will need to cut these down as much as possible.
- *Coffee*: Over three cups a day has been linked to reduced fertility and early miscarriage.
- See also Pre-conceptual Care, page 272 and Fertility, Male, below.

## Fertility, Male

Low sperm count or motility are major reasons for couples experiencing problems with conception – possibly contributing to 50 per cent of cases. The first step is to evaluate the quality of the sperm with a test. In a woman, all the eggs she will ever carry are present in her ovaries even at the point where she is a 12-week old foetus. However, in the man sperm are manu-factured throughout his life, meaning that a huge impact can be made on the health of the sperm with nutritional measures. Spermatogenesis (sperm creation) starts around three months before the sperm is ready for ejaculation. Improving diet over this time frame can make a positive difference.

- *Alcohol and smoking:* Common reasons for poor sperm health are alcohol intake, smoking and recreational drugs.
- *Zinc and folic acid:* Several studies underscore the importance of zinc to sperm production and zinc is concentrated in seminal fluid. Recent research found a 74 per cent increase in the sperm counts of sub-fertile men who were given very high doses of folic acid and zinc supplements for six months. Taking over 1mg of folic acid is not recommended long-term as it can mask a vitamin B12 deficiency, though lower levels of 400–800mcg are routinely available and considered safe.
- *Selenium:* This mineral is essential for the integrity of the sperm 'tail' and low levels of selenium reduce sperm motility.
- *Environmental chemicals:* A puzzle exists regarding a 50 per cent drop in average sperm count that seems to have occurred in the last 50 years. Danish organic farmers had twice the sperm density when compared to ordinary greenhouse workers who were exposed to herbicides and pesticides.
- *Vitamin C:* This reduces sperm agglutination, where sperm clump together, and several studies have shown that low vitamin C levels are associated with oxidation damage to sperm.
- *Amino acids:* Two amino acids (protein building blocks), L-arginine and L-carnitine, are found in high levels in the head of sperm but are best used with individual nutritional advice.
- See also Pre-conceptual Care, page 272.

## Fibroids

Fibroids often start growing in the womb in the 10–15 years before the menopause. They are non-malignant lumps of womb tissue (muscle and fibrous tissue) that grow in response to high oestrogen levels. They can grow as large as a grapefruit. Because they are non-malignant they can often be left until the menopause, when the natural reduction in oestrogen production means that they will shrink and disappear. In some cases they can cause problems, however. The two main problems are: interfering with fertility, as the foetus cannot successfully implant in the womb; and increasing the bleeding area of the womb to the point where periods become sufficiently heavy and prolonged to interfere with everyday life or lead to anaemia. In the latter case hysterectomies were often performed (fibroids being one of the main reasons for hysterectomies). Hysterectomy is no longer necessarily routine and removal of the fibroid or hormonal intervention can be considered instead.

- *Oestrogen modulation*: Nutritional intervention is aimed at dampening the effects of oestrogen. It can take some time, but can be effective at stopping fibroids from growing and over time may reduce them. The main measures to limit oestrogen levels (soya, fibre, exercise and alcohol reduction) are outlined in Endometriosis, page 189.
- *Background diet*: Women with fibroids are more likely to eat a lot of red meat and less green vegetables, fruit and fish.
- *Herbs*: dong quai and *Vitex agnus castus* (but not if you are pregnant) are the most effective herbs against fibroids.
- *Progesterone*: Progesterone cream is worth considering to dampen down the effects of oestrogen and it can be particularly effective to reduce fibroids. Progesterone cream is rubbed into skin which is a bit thinner, such as the inside of arms and thighs, to ensure good absorption. Instructions are given with the products.
- *Anaemia*: Large fibroids can cause excessive blood loss during periods which can easily lead to anaemia. For more on this, see page 115.

# Flatulence

Flatulence is entirely normal and everyone produces some each day. However, in some people it can be embarrassing and accompanied by uncomfortable bloating. Excess flatulence is always related to the condition of the digestive tract and diet, meaning that it is easy to control with dietary measures.

- *Food intolerances*: Wheat is a common problem and it is worth a trial period of avoiding wheat products for two weeks to see if this makes a difference. Wheat alternatives are rice, corn, oats, barley, rye and other grains. If symptoms increase when introducing these foods and avoiding wheat, it could be that other grains are causing a sensitivity as well. For more ideas on avoiding wheat and gluten, see Coeliac Disease and Gluten Avoidance, page 153.
- *Lactose intolerance*: This is a common cause of wind and bloating as well as flatulence. See page 231 for more.
- *Meat*: High-meat diets can cause a lot of wind and substituting more vegetarian meals can help.
- *Pulses*: These include beans, legumes, lentils, peas and chick peas. They are valuable sources of fibre, nutrients, minerals, phytoestrogens and are low fat, which make them an ideal food. Some people respond badly to them and produce too much wind, however, as they are unable properly to digest pulses. Cutting back, but not cutting out, pulses is advised and building up more slowly to increase tolerance levels. Canned beans (with the canning water drained off and the beans rinsed) are much more digestible than those that are dried and home-cooked. Soaking dried beans for several hours (up to a day) before cooking and throwing away the soaking water three or four times helps to make them more digestible.

- *Bowel bacteria*: Any problems with wind suggest that bowel bacteria are working overtime, so improving the balance of bacteria in the bowels will help. A daily carton of live yoghurt is a good starting point. See page 138 for more on this.
- *Sugar and alcohol*: These literally feed bacteria, causing them to produce more gas.
- *Digestive enzymes*: An inability to digest food fully can lead to wind. Taking digestive enzymes (available from health food shops) with meals can help resolve this.
- *Herbal teas*: Peppermint, dill, fennel, aniseed, rosemary and slippery elm are particularly useful.
- See also Digestive and Bowel Health, page 181 and Indigestion, page 222.

## Fluid Retention (Oedema)

Fluid retention is much more of a problem for women than men, though both can experience it. In women it is often related to the female hormone oestrogen and oedema might occur pre-menstrually. Often it is related to poor lymphatic drainage – the lymph system is the 'house-keeping' mechanism in the body – and some people find that lymphatic drainage massage is helpful. Oedema tends to be worse at the extremities, particularly the lower legs.

- *Salt*: A high-salt diet is the first culprit to consider with water retention. Most salt comes from convenience foods. See Appendix II, page 357.
- *Fruits and vegetables*: These are high in potassium, which counteracts sodium from salt, and are highly cleansing. A minimum of five portions daily, with at least two or three portions in the form of raw fruit or vegetables

(such as carrot or tomatoes) is good, and a bit more is even better.

- *Flavonoids*: Trials using flavonoid-rich supplements have shown reduction in 'heavy legs' sensation, leg girth, and post-operative swelling after face lifts. Flavonoid rich foods are all fruits and vegetables, particularly dark berries, onions and citrus.

- *Water*: Fluid retention can be viewed as a stagnant condition where fluid and toxins accumulate in certain parts of the body. The naturopathic approach is to 'flush out' the stagnant accumulation of water with fresh water. Drinking two litres daily of water can have a dramatic effect on dispersing oedema.

- *Food intolerances*: Puffiness and fluid retention are common signs of food intolerance, particularly to wheat or other grains. Pre-menstrual bloating and puffiness in particular are often exacerbated by wheat in sensitive individuals.

- *Alcohol and coffee*: Fluid retention is often related to a sluggish liver and so alcohol and coffee can worsen the condition. See Liver Health, page 238.

- *Dandelion*: The scourge of the gardener is actually a valuable herbal remedy for oedema as it has a restorative effect on the liver. Avoid dandelions that have been sprayed with chemicals and choose young leaves. Cover a handful of leaves for five minutes with two large cups of boiled water and allow to steep. Sip at regular intervals during the day and repeat for a few days.

## Food Allergy

True food allergies are relatively uncommon, affecting 1–2 per cent of people. The reason people think they are more common is that what are termed food allergies are more often food intolerances (see Food Intolerance, page 205), which are much more widespread. Reactions to food allergens (substances in foods that cause an allergic reaction) are fairly swift, making it fairly easy to identify the food involved. Food allergies, as in any allergy to substances such as pollen in hay fever or contact allergies to washing powders in eczema, result in an immune response (IgE). The immune system overreacts, with inflammation leading to symptoms such as hives or swollen lips. In some cases this reaction is life threatening, as it can interfere with breathing and the person can go into shock (anaphylaxis). It is impossible to tell if someone afflicted with mild allergic reactions will have a severe reaction on the next exposure. For this reason, it is vital that anyone who suffers a true food allergy carries with them an adrenaline self-injection kit at all times and is treated as soon as possible at a hospital.

- *Most common food allergens*: The most common true food allergies are to: peanuts, sesame seeds, eggs, soya, fish (particularly salmon), milk and other dairy products and tree nuts (such as cashews, hazelnuts, etc.). Kiwi fruit allergies are on the increase. Cross-reactions, where foods from the same family of foods cause a reaction, are common.
- *For life*: In most cases the allergy is for life and the foods must be rigorously avoided. Small children may grow out of an allergy, but it is risky to experiment with this.
- *Nuts and seeds*: It is fairly easy to eliminate nuts and seeds from menus. What is not so easy is identifying packaged foods, such as biscuits, which could be contaminated during production. Common foods that can include nuts or sesame seeds include: cakes, pastries, desserts, chocolates, sweets, snacks, fruit yoghurts, biscuits, salads, salad dressings, dips, curries, pre-made Asian sauces, chilli, stuffing and breakfast cereals. Others include pesto (pine nuts or walnuts), satay sauces (peanuts), marzipan (almonds), praline, nougat

(almonds), halva (sesame), hummus (sesame) and tahini (sesame). Peanuts and peanut oil (also called groundnut oil) are inexpensive ingredients and so find their way into a huge number of processed foods such as biscuits, cakes, breakfast cereals, savoury foods, Asian foods, breads and confectionery. A reaction to refined peanut oil (found mainly in processed foods) is unlikely, but unrefined peanut oil (mainly bottled oil and found in ethnic foods) carries a higher risk.

- *Labelling hazards*: Always read food labels and research problem foods in advance. Be aware that foods labelled as containing almonds, for example, may also contain peanuts, which are not labelled. Pre-made composite dishes are often not fully labelled and fall within the '25 per cent rule'. Packaging on a pizza with salami on it does not have to declare what is in the salami if the meat makes up less than 25 per cent of the pizza. But if the sausage meat is made with milk powder or ground nuts, then that could be a problem for an allergic person. Labelling is improving and many products are now labelled 'May Contain Nuts'. Manufacturers are also aware of the dangers of cross-contamination and a small number, including those who supply some of the large supermarkets, are opening segregated production lines.

## Food Aversions

Food aversions are simply when a food, or group of foods, is disliked intensely. Because reactions can be severe, including nausea and vomiting, aversions are sometimes mistaken for allergies. A food aversion is unlikely to be damaging to health if it is just to one or two foods. However, it may be a sign of the onset of an eating disorder, or if the aversion is extreme and to a whole food group, this could lead to nutritional deficiencies.

# Food Intolerance

Intolerances to foods are common. They differ from allergies in that they may or may not involve the immune system. If the immune system is involved, then it is a different 'branch' of the immune system (IgG). Reactions can also involve enzyme deficiency such as in lactose intolerance or an unspecified reaction. Food intolerances are linked to a wide variety of symptoms including: headaches, skin conditions, dark eye circles, digestive complaints, lethargy, mood swings, depression, aches and pains, hay fever and others.

- *Delayed reaction*: The main diagnostic tool that separates food intolerances from other reactions is that they are usually fairly slow to appear. It is not necessarily obvious that a reaction is linked to a food eaten shortly before and it may take hours or a day for a reaction to happen. They are also nearly always linked to commonly eaten and to favourite foods, which can make giving them up a bit difficult sometimes.
- *Food diary*: This is the best way to sort out what foods might be causing problems. When giving up a food it is necessary to give it at least two weeks, and then to reintroduce it in a normal portion size. Note what your reaction is. If giving up a food such as wheat, try introducing bread, pasta and crackers on different days to see if different reactions are observed.
- *Lactose intolerance*: This is very common – see page 231.
- *Amines*: These are found in a number of foods and are most commonly a problem for migraine sufferers. This is discussed on page 251.
- *Wheat and gluten intolerance*: This is not the same as coeliac disease; however, avoidance measures are the same and are dealt with on page 153.

- *Immune-linked intolerances*: IgG levels for intolerances to foods can be tested for with blood tests and indeed a whole industry has sprung up around this. However, what tends to come back is a long list of foods that are causing an IgG reaction, some of them quite obscure. It is important to recall that IgG levels need to be quite high before triggering the immunological and symptom response. These tests can be useful, but only if interpreted intelligently (see Useful Contacts, page 379).
- *Liver health*: Food intolerance may be linked to poor liver health. See page 238.

## Food Poisoning

Pathogenic bacteria in foods can cause food poisoning. In adults the first line of defence in the gut against pathogenic bacteria is the acid in the stomach. Those most at risk of severe or even fatal reactions include babies and children, the elderly, those with compromized immune systems and the malnourished. All cases of suspected food poisoning should be reported to your doctor.

- *Rehydration*: Replace lost fluids and minerals (see the advice in Diarrhoea, page 179).
- *Food preparation*: The most important protection against food poisoning is to use foods before their use-by dates, to store foods properly refrigerated below 5°C, avoid cross-contamination and heat foods thoroughly when cooking. Food poisoning is more common in summertime, when the warmth encourages the multiplication of bacteria – when buying food from a supermarket take cool-bags to reduce the risk.

- *Bowel bacteria*: A healthy bacterial balance in the gut can protect against food poisoning. The healthy bacteria have anti-bacterial properties, which deter the pathogenic bacteria from multiplying. Additionally, their very presence means that the pathogenic bacteria simply don't have enough space to take hold.
- *Stomach acidity*: In older people (age 50+), one in ten of whom have low stomach acidity, it may be useful to improve stomach acidity, if necessary by taking digestive enzymes and hydrochloric acid (available from health food shops) with meals. Acidity is a first line defence against food poisoning.
- *Pregnancy*: In pregnancy, food poisoning can severely damage the foetus and for this reason foods such as raw eggs and unpasteurized cheeses should be avoided. See Pregnancy, page 274 for more on this.

## Gall-Bladder, Removed

In those who have had their gall-bladder removed fat digestion is permanently impaired. The gall-bladder concentrates bile, which has been produced by the liver. Bile is squirted into the digestive tract when a meal containing fat has been eaten. The bile emulsifies fats, turning them into tiny globules that can be acted upon more easily by fat-digesting enzymes. Without a gall-bladder the bile is not concentrated but drips slowly and perpetually into the digestive tract, thus reducing the effectiveness of bile-emulsifying fats. If at all possible, it is best to seek an alternative to dealing with gall stones (see Gall stones page 208) rather than opting for surgical removal.

- *Dietary fat*: A low-fat diet is advisable, which means restricting butter, margarine, cream, oils, meat fat and fatty foods such as crisps, biscuits, chocolates, desserts and pastries.

- *Fat digestion*: Digestive enzymes containing lipases – fat-digesting enzymes – can be purchased as supplements and taken with meals containing fat.
- *Lecithin*: Another alternative is to take a teaspoonful of lecithin granules with a fat-containing meal. Lecithin is an emulsifying agent (often used in food processing and listed as a food ingredient), with the same effect as bile. It tastes quite pleasant.
- *Fat soluble vitamins*: Fat is important as a carrier of the fat-soluble vitamins A, D, E and K. On a low-fat diet or in the case of gall-bladder removal, a supplement that incorporates these vitamins with some lipid in the supplement is advised.

## Gall Stones

Gall stones are three times more common in women than in men, with one in five developing gall stones at some time. Three-quarters of gall stones are a build up of cholesterol, which forms hard stones lodged in the gall-bladder. This is related to possible oversecretion of cholesterol by the liver. Obesity, a high-fat diet and rapid weight loss are possible contributing causes. Gall stones can also contain bile pigment or calcium salts. Most people do not experience symptoms but if they do they can be very painful: pain in the upper right part of the abdomen, inflammation of the gall-bladder, pancreatitis (swelling of the adjacent pancreas) or jaundice.

Gall stones can be treated with ultrasound to break them into tiny pieces and allow them to pass easily from the gall-bladder, or in extreme cases by surgical removal of the gall-bladder. Nutritional treatment centres around avoiding gall stones forming in the first place and stopping existing stones from growing. Evidence from the ongoing Nurses

Health Study has found that physical inactivity, even after controlling for weight and weight change, contributes to the risk of gall stones.

- *Overweight*: Losing excess weight and following a low-fat, high-fibre diet is probably advisable for those with gall stones.
- *Vegetarian diet*: Vegetarians are half as likely as meat eaters to develop gall stones.
- *Fibre*: Soluble fibre in particular, found in porridge oats, beans, pulses, vegetables and fruits is very helpful. Soluble fibre permits cholesterol to be excreted instead of being reabsorbed.
- *Linseeds*: Also called flaxseeds, these are particularly high in lignans, which regulate cholesterol. One teaspoon daily, sprinkled on cereals, is sufficient to make a difference.
- *Nuts*: Women who eat nuts regularly have a reduced risk of gall stones.
- *Artichoke*: This vegetable is known for its bile-stimulating effects and its traditional use to reduce gall stone formation.

## Glue Ear

See Otitis Media, page 264.

## Glycaemic Index (GI)

Glycaemic Index is an index of carbohydrate foods that ranks such foods according to how fast they are digested and metabolized to blood glucose and the effect that they have on blood sugar levels. This becomes most important when dealing with diabetes, insulin resistance, metabolic syndrome, prevention of heart disease, weight loss, low energy levels and sometimes female hormone imbalance. A GI chart and further explanation are set out in Appendix I on page 350.

## Gout

Gout is a form of arthritis. It most frequently affects men and post-menopausal women. Gout is caused by urate, a salt from uric acid, which builds up and forms insoluble crystals in the joints, particularly in the big toe and extremities (including hands and knees), which become swollen, red and painful. It often runs in families. Aspirin should be avoided, as it leads to a build up of uric acid and use of diuretics can increase the risk of gout.

- *Weight*: Take steps to control overweight (see page 315).
- *Water*: Plenty of fluids will help to reduce the build up of excess uric acid crystals.
- *Fruits and vegetables*: Plenty are needed in the diet to encourage the excretion of uric acid – fruits and vegetables alkalise the urine, which encourages this. Celery has a diuretic action, which may also help.
- *Cherries*: 200g daily of fresh or canned cherries (this is quite a lot!) can help to reduce uric levels in the blood.
- *Purines*: Purines in the diet are converted to uric acid and may not be correctly excreted in those with gout. Purines are found in high levels in beer, yeast extracts, liver, offal, game, poultry, pulses and oily fish. High-purine vegetables are beans, cauliflower, peas, spinach, mushrooms and asparagus. Low-purine foods include eggs, dairy, fruit and most other vegetables.
- *Low-fat dairy*: Studies have found that drinking skimmed milk cuts the risk of gout by half.

- *Fish Oils*: Omega-3s from fish oils can help to reduce pain and swelling (but see the note about some oily fish above in Purines).
- *Alcohol*: Different alcoholic drinks seem to have different effects. Two or more beers daily increases the risk by 2.5 times compared to non-beer drinkers, as beer is very high in purines. Two measures of spirits daily increase the risk by 1.6. On the other hand, two glasses of wine or port daily seem to have no effect on the risk of developing gout.
- *Lead*: Mild lead poisoning has been observed to worsen gout (for instance in plumbers using lead piping). It may be prudent to check for lead water conduit pipes to the house.

## Gum Disease (Gingivitis)

See Dental and Gum Health, page 169.

## Haemorrhoids

Also called piles, haemorrhoids are dilated varicose veins in the rectum. Overweight, pregnancy and straining to pass stools can lead to piles. Symptoms can include veins bulging out of the anus, pain or a dragging sensation on passing stools, itching, mucous discharge and bleeding. You must always check with your doctor if there is blood in the stools to rule out more serious bowel conditions. Hygiene is important: washing after a bowel movement and drying thoroughly.

- *Fibre*: A high-fibre diet is needed to bulk out and soften stools and make them easier to pass. Bulky stools also help to 'massage' the digestive tract, which is important for its health and helps to promote peristalsis, the motion needed to help pass stools. Harsh fibre from added wheat bran will often not resolve the problem, as it can be a further irritant for the digestive tract. Soluble fibre from oats, brown rice, pulses, vegetables and fruits is preferred. Excellent added fibre is ground linseeds added to cereals, stews or other dishes, or psyllium husks dissolved in some fruit juice.

- *Liquids*: Sufficient water (preferably) or liquids are needed – 1.5 to 2 litres daily. This helps to keep the stools soft and easy to pass.
- *Vitamin C*: Foods rich in this vitamin, with flavonoids, help to maintain the health of the circulation system and prevent further collapse. Citrus and dark berries in particular have lots of flavonoids.
- *Horsechestnut*: This is a herb used topically in ointments to strengthen the veins to help prevent further collapse.
- See also Constipation, page 160 and Varicose Veins, page 310.

## Hay Fever and Allergic Rhinitis

Hay fever is a seasonal allergy to tree pollens (early-season), grasses and weeds (mid-season) or moulds (late-season). Symptoms can include itchy, watery eyes, a streaming and blocked nose, a tight throat, sneezing and headaches. Rising pollution levels and numbers of house dust mites worsen the condition. Hay fever commonly co-exists with asthma. The difference between hay fever and rhinitis is that hay fever is strictly seasonal, while rhinitis produces nasal allergy symptoms all year round. Allergic rhinitis may be triggered by factors other than pollens, for instance pets, house dust mites or moulds.

The usual advice for hay fever is to stay indoors at peak pollen times and to take antihistamines when affected. A simple barrier method is to apply a little Vaseline to the inside of the nostrils (taking care not to go too high). By creating a barrier between pollen and the mucus membranes of the nasal passages, this can reduce symptoms.

- *Food Sensitivities*: Reducing the amount of dairy products and/or wheat-based products during the hay fever season is effective for some people. Dairy products tend to have the effect of making susceptible people produce more nasal mucus. Oats and rye are also sometimes a problem. Occasionally there is a sensitivity to legumes including soya, peanuts, lentils and other pulses.
- *Antioxidants*: Vitamin C (best sources are blackcurrant, citrus and peppers) and quercitin, a plant flavonoid found in apples, tea and onions, are natural antihistamines. Include these in the diet, but also consider taking a supplement during the hay fever season.
- *Honey*: Locally made honey, where the bees have gathered pollen in the area, is believed, traditionally, to 'inoculate' hay fever sufferers if a tablespoon is taken daily for three months prior to the hay fever season. Make sure the honey is not pasteurized, which negates its effect (do not give honey to young babies under the age of one, as there is a risk of botulism).
- *Margarine*: Long-term margarine use is linked to hay fever, especially in boys.
- *Herbs*: Herbalists use plantain, which has impressive anti-allergy and anti-catarrhal actions and acts as a tonic for the mucus membranes of the respiratory tract. Camomile is another effective herb, though it may have to be avoided if the allergy is to ragwort, a close relative. Soothing lotions for itchy eyes include cucumber slices

rubbed over closed eyes, rosewater-steeped cotton pads and cold, used, tea-bags placed on the eyes for five minutes. Nettles are a favourite herbal help for hay fever and rhinitis. If you are gathering nettles, make sure you wear gloves, pick young leaves and that they are not sprayed with chemicals. Make a nettle soup in the same way you would a spinach soup, or use the nettles to make a tea by steeping in boiling water for a few minutes (the stings are neutralized by heating).

## Headaches

A sudden onset of recurrent headaches must always be discussed with your doctor in case of a serious cause. Most of the time headaches are related to tension, infections, your general health and, often, to diet. Recurrent headaches which interfere with everyday life are common and headache medication is one of the most frequently purchased over-the-counter medicines, with 56 per cent of painkillers bought to alleviate headaches and migraines. Yet frequent use of aspirin, paracetamol and other headache medications is often the *cause* of headaches – these are called rebound headaches. The liver is unable to process the quantity of medication sufficiently quickly and this leads to further headaches.

Finding the underlying cause of frequent headaches is much more useful in the long run than always suppressing them with medication. Tension, anxiety and stress management techniques can often help (yoga, meditation, autogenic training or cognitive therapy, for instance). A physical manipulative or body realignment therapy such as massage, yoga or Alexander technique, can work wonders. It may be appropriate to mention recurrent headaches to your dentist, since dental problems or jaw alignment may be a cause. A visit to the optician may also be a good idea. Dealing with sinusitis (see page 292) is often helpful.

- *Food sensitivities*: Wheat and dairy sensitivities are commonly linked to headaches. Eliminating these foods, and suitable substitutes, is covered in Coeliac Disease and Gluten Avoidance, page 153 and Lactose Intolerance and Milk Allergy, page 231.
- *Low blood Sugar*: This more commonly causes a feeling of spaciness or dizziness but can also lead to headaches that improve immediately upon eating something. Waking up with a headache is another strong sign of low blood sugar-induced headaches. For advice on dealing with recurrent low blood sugar problems, see page 136.
- *Alcohol*: Often people build up intolerances to particular types of alcohol. Red wine may trigger headaches, where white does not. Or one spirit may cause a headache while another leaves the person headache free. Alcohol also triggers dehydration.
- *Dehydration*: This is a common trigger for headaches, often related to alcohol intake, but also to hot weather and lack of liquids.
- *Caffeine*: Withdrawal from caffeine can cause headaches, which often happens at the weekend when office workers are not getting a constant supply from the coffee machine. This is not a reason to carry on drinking lots of coffee and strong tea, but is probably a sign that you should wean yourself off caffeine. Headache medication is often a strong source of caffeine.
- *MSG*: Monosodium glutamate (MSG), used extensively in Chinese restaurants (hence Chinese Restaurant Syndrome) and in processed foods, is a frequent cause of headaches in susceptible people. MSG is called E621 on food labels, but more often is simply referred to as 'flavouring' without

215

specifying what it is, making it difficult to eliminate. The solution is to eat less processed food.

- *Artificial sweeteners*: Aspartame in particular is commonly reported to trigger headaches in susceptible people.
- *The liver*: Poor liver function often leads to headaches. See Liver Health, page 238.
- See also Migraines, page 251. For pre-menstrual syndrome related headaches see page 279 and for menopause related headaches see page 246.

## Heart Disease

More properly called cardiovascular disease, the term covers a group of conditions that can affect the heart and the vascular system. Risk factors for heart disease include smoking, high cholesterol values, raised apolipoprotein(a), raised homocysteine and high body mass index (overweight and obesity). Half of all heart attacks occur in people with normal cholesterol levels. The evidence is accumulating that low-grade inflammation, measured via a 'marker' C-reactive protein, is implicated in heart disease (see Inflammation page 225). It is likely that the inflammation damages artery walls, which, over time, leads to an accumulation of arterial plaque.

- *Antioxidants in the diet*: Blood levels of vitamins A, C and E and the carotenoids (lutein, zeaxanthin, beta-cryptoxanthin and alphacarotene) are associated with less progression to arterial plaque, which blocks arteries and can lead to heart attacks and strokes. They also have an anti-inflammatory effect. Antioxidants are found in all fruits and vegetables, and the carotenoids give the orange colouring to, for example, carrots, apricots and cantaloupes. All dark red/ purple berries such as cherries, raspberries, blackcurrants and cranberries, are rich sources of anthocyanins, which are potent antioxidants. In Finland they had one of the worst incidences of heart disease in Europe until they introduced health measures to combat the problem, which brought about a 50 per cent drop in 20 years. One important measure was encouraging the regular consumption of berries. Cranberry juice has been shown to have the same inhibiting effect on plaque production – which adheres to artery walls and causes blockages – as red wine. Vitamin E is found in avocado, grains, nuts and seeds. Dark chocolate contains flavonoids, particularly epicatechin, which improve the function of blood vessels and prevent the build up of cholesterol. Just 1.5oz daily was sufficient in a trial to improve the diameter of the brachial artery.

- *Antioxidant from supplements*: Supplement trials with antioxidants and heart disease have had mixed results. Those who are genetically programmed to produce a particular type of a protein called haptoglobin, which helps return free haemoglobin to the liver, are likely to benefit when taking antioxidant supplements; others may receive no benefit; still others may worsen. Fourteen per cent of Caucasians and 26 per cent of African-Americans have the type of aptoglobin that may benefit from supplements.

- *Omega-3 fatty acids*: Fish oil is important to reduce the risk of heart disease. This may be because of the effect on reducing inflammation and also on thinning blood. In those who have already had strokes or heart attacks, taking fish oil supplements after their attack significantly reduced the risk of death by 42 per cent when compared to those who took placebos.

- *Background diet*: A diet high in fibre, particularly soluble fibre found in vegetables, oats and beans/pulses, and featuring polyunsaturated fats from nuts, seeds and their oils, and low-fat dairy, and reducing sources of sugar and trans-fats (found in most processed foods and some margarines) is beneficial for several aspects of heart disease. Hydrogenated trans-fats in particular are thought to fuel the high levels of heart disease. For more on this see Chapter 2 Healthy Fats.

- *Fibre*: In one study, for every 10g increase in fibre in the diet there was a 14 per cent drop in the rate of coronary events and a 27 per cent drop in deaths over six to ten years. Various studies indicate that 25g, or more, of fibre daily is the amount to aim for. Reduced blood insulin might be the key mechanism behind the success of high-fibre diets in reducing known risk factors for coronary disease.
- *Alcohol*: A modest alcohol intake, around two units daily, is protective against heart disease. This effect is seen for any alcohol, irrespective of type. Excess alcohol intake increases the risk of heart disease, however, so while a little is good, a lot is not. See Alcohol, Excessive Intake page 109 for specific information about alcohol measures.
- *Garlic*: This humble herb has several beneficial effects on the cardiovascular system: thinning blood, providing antioxidant selenium, reducing oxidative stress and LDL cholesterol. Include one clove daily per person in cooking as a minimum.
- *Overweight*: A high BMI is a risk factor. Testing for a compound called apolipoprotein(a) might serve to better assess the overall CHD risk of those with elevated BMI, leading to more intensive treatment of modifiable cardiovascular risk factors, such as diet and exercise.
- *Herbs and spices*: Hawthorn and turmeric are useful in preventing heart disease.
- See also Blood Pressure, High, page 133, Cholesterol page 149, Stroke page 301 and Homocysteine page 219.

## HIV and AIDS

Nutritional management of HIV consists of keeping the person as healthy as possible by supporting immune health and dealing with any health complications. This is a specialized area of treatment and it is advisable to make adjustments to your diet made with the help of a nutritionist who specializes in this field.

## Homocysteine

Homocysteine is an amino acid that we all produce and which circulates in the blood. High levels are toxic to various tissues and linked to a growing list of problems: arterial damage leading to stroke and heart disease, Alzheimer's disease, pre-eclampsia in pregnancy and cleft palate. The way the body deactivates homocysteine involves a cycle which is dependent on several B-vitamins: folate (folic acid), B6, B12, and B2.

In the USA flour has been fortified, by law, with folic acid for a couple of years (the UK decided against such a step). This was done because of the overwhelming evidence that folic acid reduces the number of spina bifida cases (additionally the downsides of fortification were few, and women planning a pregnancy did not generally supplement individually with folic acid). Interestingly as a result, plasma homocysteine levels in the general population in the USA have dropped as a result of this fortification of the diet.

It is estimated that a 25 per cent reduction in homocysteine will reduce strokes by one-quarter, heart disease by one-seventh and thrombosis by one-quarter. Homocysteine can be viewed as a marker of folic acid and B12 deficiency, in that increasing dietary levels, or supplementation, reduces homocysteine. Plasma homocysteine levels can easily be tested for with a blood test (see Appendix IV page 367).

Whether actual reduction in risk of these diseases occurs with lowered homocysteine is not yet certain, or whether homocysteine is itself the problem, or if it is a 'marker' for something else. Nevertheless, a multi B-supplement is inexpensive, certainly effective against a wide range of problems and non-toxic, making it a reasonably safe bet.

- *B-Complex*: Folate-rich foods are green leafy vegetables and fortified cereals. It is hard to get the amounts required unless you are prepared to eat a plate of spinach at three meals a day! This is one of those rare instances where the artificial version, folic acid, is better than the natural version, folate. A B-complex usually contains 400mcg, which is sufficient to have an impact on homocysteine and also delivers other necessary B-vitamins: B6, B12 and B2.
- *Vegans*: Vegans have the highest levels of homocysteine, probably because their levels of vitamin B12 are lower than most people's. This is because there are no sources of very absorbable B12 in a completely plant-based diet. Vegans should ensure they eat B12-enriched margarine and soya milk to compensate.
- *Caffeine*: Caffeine increases homocysteine levels, so it makes sense to cut down.

## Hyperactivity (ADD and ADHD)

Hyperactivity is now usually refered to as ADHD. ADD (Attention Deficit Disorder) and ADHD (Attention Deficit Hyperactivity Disorder) have been lumped together as ADHD, which is a shame. Attention Deficit is when a child is unable to sit still and concentrate for any period of time, while ADHD (Hyperactivity) is when a child has ADD but also is bouncing off the walls and uncontrollable. Oppositional Defiant Disorder is a pattern of ongoing defiant behaviour which seriously interferes with the child's day-to-day functioning. These behaviour disorders are much more common in boys than in girls. They are believed, from a brain biochemical point of view, to have similar causes to dyslexia and dyspraxia (see page 183) in that they are dependent on the same nervous tissue 'building blocks'. While we tend to think about hyperactivity as a childhood problem, children grow up and when they are adults the problem can sometimes become a more serious social issue (see Behavioural Disorders page 127). There is good evidence that a percentage of children diagnosed with ADHD, when taught good sleep hygiene (regular bedtimes, longer sleeping hours, restful periods in the hours before sleep instead of using computer games and watching TV) resolve their symptoms.

- *Fatty acids*: The brain and central nervous system are dependent on sufficient intakes of certain fatty acids, which are instrumental in correct neurotransmitter functioning. Fish oils, rich in EPA and DHA, when given at doses of 1–2g in trials, improved hyperactivity problems in around two-thirds of children. See Chapter 2: Healthy Fats for more.
- *Food additives*: In a government-sponsored trial, the azo-dye artificial food colourings which are commonly found in children's foods such as biscuits, jellies, sweets, puddings, yoghurts, cake and crisps, and a preservative, sodium benzoate, caused behavioural changes in a group of 277 three-year-old children even in those without a history of hyperactivity. They were consumed at 'normal' quantities of 20mg total artificial colours and 45mg preservative, the

amount you would typically find in a child's portion (if more than one such food is consumed in a day then typical intakes would be more than in the trial). The children had behaviour changes such as temper tantrums, difficulty settling to sleep, disturbing others and poor concentration when they were given these compounds. The researchers worked out that if these reactions were spread around the child population of the UK, the number of children affected by hyperactivity would drop from one in six to one in seventeen. This trial backed up previous findings. Some of the worst colourings are: Quinoline Yellow (E104), Brilliant Blue (E133), Sunset Yellow (E110), Carmoisine (E122), Ponceau 4R (E124), and Indigo Carmine (E132).

- *Other additives*: In sensitive children other additives such as artificial sweeteners (see Appendix I page 349) and caffeine can affect them. Caffeine is found in colas, chocolate, some medication (cold remedies, headache remedies), tea and coffee.
- *Sugar*: High-sugar diets can worsen hyperactivity.
- See also Thyroid, Overactive page 306.

## Immune Health

See Chapter 3: Immune Health and Inflammation.

## Indigestion

Also called dyspepsia, indigestion is a feeling of discomfort or burning sensation in the upper abdomen, in the stomach region (heartburn is felt behind the chest bone). A correct diagnosis must be sought from a doctor to rule out more serious conditions, especially if the symptoms continue for a week, or if they recur. Ulceration or hiatus hernia may be a problem, and in some cases in the 40+ age group it could be a symptom of stomach cancer. Indigestion and reflux (some of the stomach contents regurgitating slightly) is common in the later stages of pregnancy when the baby is squeezing the stomach. Propping yourself up with pillows at night can help to relieve this.

- *Large meals*: These are commonly a cause of indigestion. Eating little and often is the solution. Irregular or hurried meals don't help and nor does eating before bed.
- *Chewing food properly*: This is a very basic way of making sure the stomach doesn't have to do more than its fair share of work.
- *Weight*: Losing excess weight can help resolve the problem.
- *Diary*: Try keeping a diary to see which foods are most likely to cause the problem. Often the worst culprits are spicy dishes, fatty meals, acidic juices, coffee, alcohol and chocolate.
- *Herbals*: Mint tea is a potent after-meal digestive aid. Slippery elm is another effective herbal remedy and artichoke leaf reduces mild dyspepsia. Fennel and caraway help to reduce wind.
- *Poor digestion*: In the 40+ age-group it is common for stomach acidity to start to decline – it is estimated that 20 per cent of those over 60 have no, or very little, stomach acid and so have trouble breaking down protein foods. Digestive enzymes that digest other food components, fats and carbohydrates, can also be less effective in older age, which compromises the whole digestive process. Digestive enzyme supplements taken with meals can make a great difference to indigestion in these circumstances. Fresh pineapple and papaya are natural sources of some types of

digestive enzymes and eaten at the end of meals can guard against indigestion.

- *Cabbage juice*: Making a vegetable juice of which a quarter is cabbage juice, and drinking a small glass daily, can benefit indigestion. Cabbage juice has a strong taste, but is pleasant when mixed with carrot and apple (one-quarter cabbage to three-quarters other ingredients – a vegetable juicer is a necessary bit of equipment). It contains a compound that aids the digestive function of the gut.
- Indigestion may signal lactose intolerance (lactose is a sugar found in milk), see page 231.
- See also Ulcers, Gastric page 307.

## Infections, Frequent

Frequent infections, or infections that do not resolve particularly quickly, are linked to compromized immune health. In small children, especially under the age of five, it can seem as if they always have a cold or other infection, but this is fairly normal as this is the stage when they are acquiring immunity to a wide range of viruses that they come into contact with. This usually abates as they get older. Infections in children and the elderly should be checked by a doctor to rule out serious problems. Overuse of antibiotics can lead to a vicious cycle of inadequate response to infections – see page 117. Smoking, lack of sleep, stress and too much alcohol can all make us more susceptible to infections.

- *Antioxidant-rich foods*: A diet that features a wide variety and at least five portions daily of fruits and vegetables is vital.
- *Juices*: Making a fresh fruit and/or vegetable juice or smoothie a few days each week can be an excellent way of providing an emergency boost. It should ideally feature a

range of ingredients such as carrots, apples, berries, tropical fruit, bananas, plums, peaches or other fresh seasonal produce.

- *Bowel bacteria*: Healthy bowel bacteria can help to support immune status and reduces the risk of allergies. See page 138 for more on this. Live yoghurt has been known for a long time to have immune stimulating properties.

- *Dairy products*: Any infection which leads to mucus build up may be eased by avoiding dairy products, as these tend to be mucus forming.

- *Garlic*: The whole onion family – garlic, chives, spring onions, onions, leeks – has an excellent and well deserved reputation for being anti-viral, antibacterial and anti-fungal.

- *Fish oils*: Oily fish are rich in fatty acids, which are important for regulating inflammation – one or two portions weekly is ideal.

- *Oriental mushrooms*: Many of these have immune boosting properties which have been used traditionally very successfully. See Mushrooms in Superfoods, page 81.

- *Berries*: Dark berries contain anthodyanins which help to prevent or reduce the severity of infections such as flu. Sambucol, a tincture of elderberry, is a popular way of getting a daily dose of 15ml four times a day from the onset of symptoms.

- See also Chapter 3: Immune Health and Inflammation.

## Inflammation

Inflammation manifests as reddening and swelling of damaged tissue. While this is most evident on the surface, such as with a cut or abrasion, inflammation is also at the core of many diseases and ailments such as arthritis, bowel problems, heart disease and possibly Alzheimer's disease.

Low-level chronic inflammation can be measured via a marker, C-reactive protein (CRP), which does not normally appear in the blood. CRP can indicate any inflammatory problem including the common cold, rheumatoid arthritis, smoking, diabetes and other conditions. This marker may appear as a constant presence long before any health problems are evident, for instance in the case of heart disease. Elevated CRP is found in around a quarter of the population, with overweight and obese people up to six times more likely to have it. This may be a part of the link between overweight and heart disease. It is possible that Statin drugs reduce heart attack risk by reducing inflammation rather than by modifying cholesterol. Weight loss, stopping smoking and moderate exercise all help to reduce CRP levels. Inflammation is a major contributor to free-radical oxidation damage, which is why it is involved in so many diseases.

- *Antioxidants*: These are potent inflammation-modulating compounds. Antioxidants are found in all fruits and vegetables and a minimum of five portions are advised daily.
- *Fish oils*: Omega-3 fatty acids are precursors for substances called eicosanoids, which are involved in regulating inflammation in almost all cells. Eating one or two portions of oily fish weekly will benefit inflammatory conditions. Where inflammation is widespread it may be necessary to take more potent doses by taking supplements. Fish oils have a similar action to aspirin, (which acts on COX1) – without adverse gastro-intestinal problems that can lead to bleeding – because it acts in the same way as COX2 anti-inflammatory medicines.
- *Saturated fats*: Found in meat, butter, cheese and full- and half-fat milk as well as in convenience foods, saturated fats are rich in a compound, arachidonic acid, which has a pro-inflammatory effect and reduces the anti-inflammatory

effect of polyunsaturated fatty acids such as fish oils. Cutting back on sources of saturated fats, and substituting beans and pulses for a few meat-based meals a week can help.

- *Food intolerances*: While any food intolerance is unlikely to have a direct action on inflammation, it can 'overload' immune function, which in turn leads to unsatisfactory healing. If you have a food intolerance, it may be best to avoid that food or foods while trying to heal persistent inflammation. One way in which food intolerances can impair healing is to make the gut more 'leaky'; this in turn causes compounds to be absorbed into the bloodstream, giving the immune system more work to do.
- See also Chapter 3: Immune Health and Inflammation, Chapter 2: Healthy Fats, and Chapter 4: Bacterial Balance.

## Insulin Resistance

Insulin resistance is a condition that, if left unchecked, can lead to type 2 diabetes in a proportion of people. Carbohydrates from the diet are turned into glucose. Normally the glucose in blood is cleared by the actions of the hormone insulin which transports glucose into cells to be used as fuel. In those who are insulin resistant the cells become, as the name suggests, resistant to the effects of insulin, which results in elevated blood glucose. In an effort to lower blood glucose the pancreas produces more and more insulin in an attempt to force the glucose into cells. After a while (the time varies depending on your genetic make-up and diet) the pancreas becomes less able to function and type 2 diabetes can result. Some people are more genetically prone to the condition, particularly those of Asian, Native American or Aboriginal Australian descent. Insulin resistance is sometimes called Insulin Resistance Syndrome as an alternative to Metabolic Syndrome or

Syndrome X (rather confusingly). Insulin resistance can exist on its own, but when it becomes Metabolic Syndrome it becomes a collection of co-existing conditions that include heart disease risk factors. Insulin resistance is a condition that commonly co-exists with polycystic ovarian syndrome in women of childbearing age (see page 271). The good news is that insulin resistance can often be controlled with diet before it leads to diabetes.

- *Overweight*: This is a strong risk factor for insulin resistance, and a weight loss of just 7 per cent can reduce risk significantly.
- *Waist to hip ratio*: A higher waist to hip ratio is a risk factor for insulin resistance. This is sometimes referred to as the less protective 'apple' shape rather than the more protective 'pear' shape. To work out your waist-to-hip ratio turn to page 328.
- *Background diet*: The basic advice is to eat some protein at each meal, lots of vegetables and pulses, fibre-rich foods that are low on the GI, and to avoid sugar and refined carbohydrates. See Glycaemic Index in Appendix I page 350.
- *Exercise*: This has a moderating effect on insulin resistance even beyond its effect on weight loss.
- *Magnesium*: Low magnesium levels are common in insulin resistance. Eating magnesium rich foods (see page 335) or supplementing can improve pancreatic response and insulin resistance.
- *Cinnamon*: There is very promising evidence that one gram (one third of a teaspoon) a day of cinnamon significantly improves insulin sensitivity. This can be taken as a supplement or added to food when cooking.
- See also Metabolic Syndrome page 251 and Diabetes page 176.

## Irritable Bowel Syndrome (IBS)

Irritable bowel is very real in the sense that it is an accumulation of uncomfortable and distressing symptoms, yet from a diagnostic point of view it is a catch-all term. This diagnosis is usually made when a satisfactory precise diagnosis can't be made, but when obvious symptoms persist. It usually means diarrhoea and bloating, sometimes alternating with constipation, without an obvious pattern, and where biopsies and examinations don't lead to a diagnosis of, say, coeliac disease or ulcerative colitis. It is believed that stress plays a major part in irritable bowel problems – perhaps as much as 50 per cent in some cases. Working on stressful lifestyle factors, taking up relaxation such as autogenic training (which is very successful), yoga or tai chi, and seeking out one of the 'talking therapies' such as cognitive therapy can help. For dietary approaches see Digestive and Bowel Health page 181.

## Kidney Health

Any suspected kidney problem, such as stones or pain, or difficulty passing urine, must be checked by a doctor. Men who find it difficult to urinate may need to be checked for prostate problems (see page 282). A burning sensation on urinating may indicate cystitis (see page 168).

● *Water*: Fluid, preferably water, intake is vital for kidney health. Dehydrating drinks, particularly strong caffeine drinks, colas and other sodas and alcohol can have adverse effects on kidney function. Two litres daily will help to counter kidney stone formation. The exception to maintaining a high fluid intake is if the doctor advises against this in certain kidney conditions.

- *Calcium*: Kidney stones are mainly formed from calcium with oxalate. Calcium supplements should be avoided except with medical supervision. However, the Nurses Study found that those with high dietary levels, around 1000mg, of calcium from food sources, had a 50 per cent lower risk of developing stones (calcium supplements did not have a similar effect). Calcium in the gut binds with oxalate, which is then excreted and not absorbed.
- *Oxalate*: Oxalic acid-rich foods need to be avoided if you are at risk of forming kidney stones: spinach, Swiss chard, beans, beet greens, celery, chocolate, rhubarb, grapes, cranberries, gooseberries, strawberries and celery.
- *Vegetarian diet*: Vegetarians have a lower risk of kidney stones. Meat eating seems to increase the risk, though increasing vegetable intake in meat eaters can help to offset this. Vegetables are high in magnesium, which has a balancing effect on calcium. Magnesium supplements are also helpful to reduce risk of kidney stones.
- *Phytates*: Phytates are found in wheat bran and other cereals and bind with minerals, reducing their absorption. Phytates seem to reduce risk by 37 per cent. This may also partly explain why vegetarian women, who consume more phytates, have more protection.
- *Caffeine*: This increases calcium excretion and should be avoided.
- *Juices*: Apple juice and grapefruit juice intake is linked to kidney stone formation. Cranberry reduces the likelihood of developing kidney stones.
- *Salt*: A high sodium intake is counterproductive to kidney health and contraindicated with kidney stones in particular, as it causes calcium excretion (for Salt Reduction see Appendix II page 357).
- *Herbs*: Eating asparagus can lead to a strong smelling urine, and is said to suggest that the compound asparagine, found

in asparagus, is having a stimulating effect on the kidneys and improving their ability to filter. Dandelion is commonly used as a diuretic. Cape gooseberry may help to dissolve kidney stones. Ginger is contraindicated in kidney disease.

- *Protein*: In some kidney conditions your doctor will advise against high protein intakes.

## Lactose Intolerance and Dairy Allergy

Dairy was only introduced into the human diet around 10,000 years ago, which is when people started herding animals. As our physiology doesn't adapt all that quickly, it is no surprise that dairy remains a problem for many people. There are two main causes of dairy sensitivity: lactose (milk sugar) and proteins. There is also a more generalized, non-specific, intolerance to dairy.

Calcium enriched soya milk, rice milk and oat milk are all widely available. They are not suitable for babies under one year of age and should be a part of a balanced, mixed diet. With the advent of 'functional foods' – everyday foods which have some added nutritional content (and are often therefore a bit more expensive) – you can buy calcium enriched fruit juices which can help overcome the problem of ensuring sufficient calcium from in a dairy-free diet.

*Lactose Intolerance*: Around 70 per cent of the adult population of the world lacks the milk-digesting enzyme lactase, making it difficult for them to consume milk. It is particularly prevalent – up to 95 per cent of individuals – amongst those of African, Asian, Southern American, Jewish and Mediterranean descent. Symptoms that could indicate a lactose intolerance are: bloating, flatulence, constipation and diarrhoea. The lactose is not digested and is left in the gut to ferment. This leads to side-effects such as uncomfortable wind and bloating. Some lactose intolerant people can drink some milk without symptoms but have a threshold of intake beyond which it becomes troublesome.

- If lactose intolerant, skimmed milk or semi-skimmed are worse than whole milk as there is proportionately more milk sugar.
- Lactose-free milk is available in large supermarkets.
- Lactase enzymes can easily be found in pharmacies or health food shops. Adding a few drops to milk an hour or so before consumption will give enough time to act and break down the lactose (the milk is much sweeter as a result).
- Hard cheese does not usually cause problems for lactose intolerance, as there is little lactose left in it.
- Good quality yoghurts that have been fermented for long enough (the plain bio-yoghurts should be fine) will have little lactose, as the bacteria used in their preparation have pre-digested the milk sugar.
- Butter is well tolerated as it is just fat (with a few stray protein and lactose molecules in it). However, given that it is just fat, it does not count as a dairy portion and has no calcium in it.
- Goat's and sheep's milk have just as much lactose in them as cow's milk, making these not a good alternative for those who are lactose intolerant.

*Dairy Allergy*: A true dairy allergy could result in symptoms that are common to all food allergies that trigger an immune reaction: reddening of the skin, hives, swelling of the lips and face, vomiting, difficulty breathing and in severe cases anaphylaxis (shock which can be lethal).

- In cases of a serious cow's milk protein allergy, you will need to avoid foods that contain the following, in addition to milk, cream, cheese, butter and yoghurt: buttermilk, casein/caseinate, crème fraîche, curds, kefir, ghee, lactalbumin, lactic acid, lactobacillus, lactoglobulin, lactose, quark, rennet and whey. Bear in mind that 'protein enriched' may mean milk protein.
- About one-quarter of those who are allergic to dairy turn out to be allergic to soya – this is often discovered when you switch from cow's milk to soya milk.
- Allergy to goat's and sheep's milk proteins may or may not be a problem.
- See Food Allergies page 202 for more information.

*Dairy Intolerance*: A more generalized intolerance to dairy that may involve mechanisms other than lactose intolerance – possibly an immune response called IgG – include: catarrh, constipation, dark eye circles, diarrhoea, asthma, eczema, flatulence, glue ear, hay fever, headaches and upper respiratory tract infections. There are more than 30 proteins in cow's milk and casein is the protein most significantly linked to allergy. It is a large molecule, which is so dense that the amount is reduced in formula milk to more closely mimic breast milk. It is really designed for a calf's digestive system rather than a human's. Goat's milk contains a different type of casein which is less likely to be linked to intolerance and is easier to digest. Many children seem to adapt and grow out of a dairy intolerance over time. This, at least, is the conventional viewpoint. Another viewpoint is that the body's adaptive mechanisms overcome the problem, only for it to reappear in a different form later on. It is common to see adults reporting other allergy/ sensitivity problems such as migraines or irritable bowel syndrome. On questioning, they commonly mention dairy allergy or intolerance problems in childhood which eventually cleared up.

- It is often sufficient just to cut back on dairy products – say have cheese once a week, two yoghurts a week and a drop of milk in tea or the occasional dessert.
- Goat's or sheep's milk is often much better tolerated if you are sensitive to cow's milk. It is available from some supermarkets and many health food shops.

## Libido and Sexual Function

Sexuality is a complex and personal issue, encompassing how you feel about yourself, your emotions, self-esteem and body, how you feel about your partner, your sexual history and your physical health. Low libido can just be a passing phase. For instance, if you are too tired with the demands of a new job, lack of interest in sex may be a warning that you need to do something about achieving a better balance. Or if you have just had a baby, then your energy is likely to be channelled elsewhere – when the time is right for sex, you will know.

Libido and sexual function are two different things. Libido is your sexual desire or arousal and many things can interfere with it including tiredness, stress, ill health, relationship problems, hormone balance, pregnancy and menopause. Female sexual function problems can include dryness, pain on intercourse and poor blood or nerve supply to sex organs. These are less often discussed compared to male sexual dysfunction, perhaps because women don't exhibit obvious external symptoms as do men when they suffer from erectile dysfunction.

There is no such thing as 'normal': some people are highly sexed while others are not much interested in sex – and most people probably fall somewhere between these extremes. It is estimated that 12 per cent of women cannot achieve orgasm for physical reasons and unrealistic expectations can make this distressing. It is better to enjoy close physical contact, which gives pleasure, if not orgasm. A low sex-drive is only really a problem when it is bothering you and interfering with your relationships. It can be most stressful when your partner's enthusiasm for sex is not matched by your own desire.

Common physical problems related to low libido and sexual dysfunction include difficulty in becoming aroused, erectile dysfunction in men, finding it difficult to achieve orgasm, vaginal dryness in women, or pain with sex. If pain is a problem, the first port of call is a visit to your doctor to rule out infection, pelvic inflammatory disease, or other problems such as endometriosis or vaginismus, which is an involuntary spasm of the pelvic floor muscles. Sexual problems have a way of compounding themselves when not discussed. Transitions in a relationship can affect enjoyment and early experimentation and an adventurous approach can easily be replaced by routine and repetitiveness – not that there is anything wrong with this as the former can be difficult to sustain, while the latter can be comforting and familiar. Men and women can have different approaches to sex and are often excited by different things. Women often need more of a build up to sex and sensual touch is very important. Sensual exercise such as yoga, gymnastics, t'ai chi or dance can help to put you back in touch with your body and stimulate sexual feelings. Depression is a frequent cause of low sex-drive. Yet while prescription antidepressants can help to relieve the depression, they are also a common cause of low libido and sexual dysfunction. Age is no barrier to feeling sexy, though the experience may change with the years. Menopause may bring on vaginal dryness, easily resolved using lubrication, and it may take longer to become aroused. Embarrassment is often a major hindrance to seeking help, but relationship counsellors, doctors and therapists are happy to help.

- *Female hormones*: Oestrogen has the effect of 'plumping up' body tissues, including the vagina. Phytoestrogens, plant hormones – found in foods such as wholegrains, chickpeas, lentils, flaxseeds and soya – can help to balance out women's oestrogen levels and can be particularly useful for perimenopausal and menopausal women experiencing dryness. Oxytocin is dubbed the 'cuddle hormone' and levels of this hormone increase during sex and breast stimulation. It promotes pair-bonding, snuggling and the desire to please, and it is suggested that this is why women enjoy cuddling after making love. Oestrogen increases sensitivity to oxytocin. Women also produce testosterone, normally thought of as the male hormone, which is important for sex-drive. Prolactin, the hormone that triggers milk production after having a baby, suppresses sex-drive (probably to keep the Neolithic mother focused on her baby instead of going off to get pregnant again), but can be elevated in some women. Nipple over-stimulation, for example from jogging, can cause high levels.

- *Low energy*: If you are exhausted, then it is no surprise you don't feel like sex. Low energy can also relate to anaemia (low iron stores), symptoms of which include pale skin and listlessness, and low thyroid function, which your doctor needs to investigate (see page 304). When seeking comfort many people turn to fatty, stodgy foods, yet these can negatively impact on your energy levels. At the other extreme some people stop eating regularly when they are depressed which impacts energy levels.

- *Zinc and B-vitamins*: Zinc and B-vitamins are vital for male and female sex hormone production, and also for enhancing mood, supporting the adrenal glands (important for dealing with stress) and reducing tiredness. Zinc-rich foods include lean meats, nuts, seeds, seafood, lentils, eggs,

wholegrains, popcorn and yoghurt. Oysters have a reputation as aphrodisiacs, possibly with good reason – they are
the richest source of zinc. B-vitamin rich foods include
wholegrains, yeast extract, green leafy vegetables, figs,
dates, molasses, nuts, chicken, tuna and beans.

● *Alcohol, smoking and drugs*: While a drink or two can help to
release tensions and inhibitions, too much alcohol can just
induce sleep and erectile dysfunction in men. Excess alcohol
also severely depletes B-vitamin levels. Recreational drugs
can also interfere with sex-drive. Alcohol temporarily
increases testosterone in women and therefore libido. But
too much suppresses oxytocin and so women who drink too
much are thought to be more likely to have sex, but to enjoy
it less. Smoking reduces testosterone levels.

● *Herbs*: Horny Goat Weed, an aptly named herb, acts as a
tonic. It is thought to stimulate testosterone levels in both
women and men and stimulate sensory nerves, so improving sexual desire and satisfaction. Damiana works by stimulating oxygen flow to the sex organs and is useful when
depression or decreased physical sensitivity is linked to low
sex drive. Ginkgo biloba is known to improve blood flow
around the body, including to the sex organs, and has been
shown to improve sex drive in those whose libido was
knocked out by antidepressants. Muira puama possibly
affects brain centres, which influence the genitals. Avena
Sativa (oats) is used traditionally as a relaxant herb. It works
well combined with damiana. Black cohosh or red clover
are both useful for dryness as they have an oestrogenic
effect. Vitex agnus castus can help to even out period problems, which can help sexual desire and also lower prolactin
levels. The herb ginseng may also help libido by lowering
prolactin.

● *Chocolate*: It has a reputation for enhancing sex-drive as it
contains small quantities of phenyethylamine, which is the

chemical we produce in our brains when we fall in love. The higher cocoa content the better, so choose 60–70 per cent cocoa solid chocolate. Whether or not this actually has an effect, chocolate certainly triggers endorphins, our pleasure brain chemicals.

## Liver Health

The liver is usually forgotten about until something goes wrong with it, which can take a long time, as about 80 per cent degeneration is needed before liver failure sets in. The liver is a silent organ – it doesn't beat like a heart, gurgle with digestion, or ache upon overexertion. But it has more than 20 essential functions: it makes proteins, processes cholesterol, generates body heat, stores glucose, maintains blood sugar levels, makes bile for fat digestion, stores minerals and fat soluble vitamins, detoxifies drugs, alcohol, nicotine, poisons, food and bacterial by-products and chemicals. While the liver is remarkably forgiving, persistently taking it for granted with a high alcohol intake or a fatty diet will damage it. Early stages of liver damage could be jaundice, fatty liver, cirrhosis or sclerotic liver, leading eventually to liver failure. Maintaining liver health will improve general health.

- *Alcohol*: The liver can only process about one unit of alcohol each hour, therefore drinking in excess of this puts a burden on the liver and results in you feeling drunk. In the case of diagnosed liver disease, alcohol must be avoided completely. See Alcohol, Excessive Intake page 109.
- *Oily fish*: Omega-3 fatty acids are beneficial to liver health.
- *Saturated fats*: A diet low in saturated and hydrogenated fat is advised for good liver function.

- *Detoxification*: The liver has a number of detoxification pathways collectively called the P450 enzyme system, divided into Stage 1 and Stage 2 detoxification. Sometimes these two stages do not operate in a synchronized fashion. The intermediate metabolites of Stage 1, which are not being channelled into Stage 2 fast enough, cause a lot of free-radical damage. This is often the case with anyone who has unexplained 'environmental allergies', where they are very sensitive to perfumes, petrol fumes, sensitivity to pollution and similar. Frequent headaches, a general feeling of malaise and lethargy and ME are other signs. It is very helpful to make sure sufficient antioxidants are being consumed, with at least six to eight portions of fruits and vegetables daily. Grapefruit can adversely affect the P450 enzyme systems. In cases where 'rebound headaches' are experienced (by drugs such as paracetamol or caffeine causing rather than resolving a headache), it is an indication that the drug is not being cleared through the liver properly (indeed the biochemical tests for how well the P450 systems are working involve ingesting small doses of paracetamol and caffeine).
- *Helpful foods*: Garlic and oranges are very supportive of the P450 system. Beetroot, carrot and lemon are traditional tonics for liver function. While avoiding coffee is to be recommended dandelion coffee, sold in health food shops, is a very acceptable alternative. It is positively helpful, as it makes a useful hot drink and promotes liver health.
- *Herbs*: The most liver-specific herb is milk thistle (silymarin) which has been shown in trials to help liver tissue affected by cirrhosis to regenerate. Artichoke leaves (cynara) and dandelion are other liver supporting herbs. The herb St John's wort is contraindicated with some medicines (see page 369) for the very reason that it improves the

metabolism and clearance of drugs through the liver, and so changes dosage requirements.

- *Sulphur pathways*: Poor sulphation detoxification pathways in the liver may be linked to food intolerances. To improve this pathway in the liver, bathe regularly in a bath to which Epsom salts have been added: sulphur is absorbed in significant amounts across the skin.

## Lung Health

The lungs consist of delicate tissue and looking after them will help maintain function into older age, when it often declines. If you are ever breathless for no apparent reason (such as exertion or an upper respiratory tract infection), consult your doctor for a correct diagnosis. Smoking is the main cause of lung damage.

- *Hydration*: The lungs are organs with a high percentage of water in the tissue, and so keeping hydrated is important for lung health.
- *Antioxidants*: These are very important for lung health. Betacarotene, found in orange coloured fruits and vegetables and in dark green leafy vegetables, is needed to maintain mucus membrane integrity (mucus membranes line the lungs). Quercitin, an antioxidant found in high levels in onions, tea and apples, is highly supportive of lung health. Dark red berries, such as blackcurrants, blackberries, cherries, raspberries and strawberries, are rich in proanthocyanidins, which support lung health. Sambucol, available as lozenges or as a liquid, is an extract of elderberry traditionally used to fight off viruses. Taking three teaspoons daily during the flu season has been shown to be effective. Vitamin C-rich fruits and vegetables, as well as supplements, have been

shown to improve the lot of those with asthma. Low levels of dietary vitamin C (and zinc) correlate with increased levels of bronchitis. There may be a case for taking a daily antioxidant supplement if you live in an area of high pollution.

- *Smokers*: People who smoke should not take supplements with betacarotene in them as this has been found to worsen the prognosis for lung cancer. Why this should be is not certain, as dietary betacarotene seems to be protective; one theory is that artificial betacarotene was used in trials, and another is that smokers who took betacarotene were quite far into their disease and so it was too little, too late. Smokers need to double their dietary intake of vitamin C, as smoking destroys this vitamin.
- *Infections*: Lung damage can be caused by repeated infections. See Immune Health page 28.
- See also Asthma page 22.

## Lupus (SLE)

Lupus is an auto-immune disorder where the immune system does not recognise 'self' and attacks body tissue. A mild form, chronic discoid lupus, affects the skin. SLE (systemic lupus erythematosus) is the most prevalent form of lupus. It is more prevalent in women than in men, and the contraceptive pill and HRT can induce flare-ups. Initial symptoms are often a red rash across the face, red palms of the hands and swollen joints. These symptoms signal that more widespread inflammation is happening internally and throughout the body. Muscle aches, fever and extreme tiredness are common. If lupus attacks nervous tissue or the kidneys this is more serious. Treatments have improved, and usually consist of anti-inflammatory and immune-dampening drugs, with long phases of remission as a result.

- *Vegetarian diet*: A mainly vegetarian diet, which also includes and emphasises oily fish supports anti-inflammatory effects. Saturated fat from meat, butter, cheese and milk (apart from skimmed milk) is a source of arachidonic acid, which has a pro-inflammatory effect.
- *Immune dampening compounds*: Smoking, caffeine, alcohol and sugar have negative effects on immune health.
- *Oily fish*: When consumed regularly omega-3 fatty acids have a strong anti-inflammatory effect.
- *Fruits and vegetables*: Antioxidant-rich fruits and vegetables have an inflammation-dampening and immune-enhancing effect.
- *Supplements*: A high-dose antioxidant supplement may be advisable, but check with your doctor about possible contraindications.

## Macular Degeneration, Age Related

The macula is the part of the retina used for visual functions such as reading and recognizing faces and detail. Age-related macular degeneration (AMD) is the most common reason for blindness in the over-65s. The main reason for this degeneration is thought to be oxidation damage. This area of the eye has a rich blood network for its functioning, but this also means it is liable to oxidation damage unless protected. Diet over the long term is one of the main ways of preventing damage. Some evidence suggests that carotenoids may reverse AMD, but the standard view is that AMD is irreversible.

- *Carotenoids*: Two carotenoids, lutein and zeaxanthin, predominate in the macula of the eye and are critical to its functioning. Carotenoids are a family of nutrients that includes betacarotene, found in carrots, which have a reputation for improving eyesight. Betacarotene is made into vitamin A in the body – this is also called retinoic acid because of its function in retinal health. People with the highest intakes of carotenoids have a 60 per cent lower risk of developing AMD than individuals who consume the lowest amounts of carotenoids. Carotenoids have two important functions: they offer antioxidant protection; and the yellow colouring filters out harmful blue-spectrum light. Lutein and zeaxanthin are found mostly in spinach and dark green leafy vegetables such as kale, collards and turnip greens (the dark green colour masks the yellow/orange), as well as yellow/orange vegetables. Just taking lutein and zeaxanthin supplements is not necessarily the best option, as they probably work best with the full spectrum of carotenoids as found in foods. It may not be wise to take lutein separately from zeaxanthin in supplements, as they are always found together in foods. Lycopene is another carotenoid found particularly in tomatoes (processed tomatoes such as canned or puréed are richest), but also in papaya and watermelon. Again, those who consume most lycopene have the lowest risk of developing AMD.

- *Berries*: Bilberry (European Blueberry) have powerful blue-red pigments called anthocyanins, which increase retinal purple (rhodopsin) and increase ocular blood supply.
- *Zinc*: Low zinc levels may be linked to AMD and those with the highest consumption of zinc from foods have the lowest risk of AMD.
- *Other antioxidants*: Vitamin E (from food but not from supplements) and vitamin C (both food and supplements) may be protective. Improvements in trials were found despite the subjects not having any measurable clinical deficiencies in these nutrients.

## ME (Myalgic Encephalomyelitis)

Also known as chronic fatigue, or post-viral fatigue. This is an ailment which has only recently been recognized and accepted formally as a diagnosis. The cause is uncertain and it can be difficult to treat. It seems to affect teenagers quite often. It can be triggered (but not always) by viral infections such as Epstein Barr (glandular fever) or coxsackie, or by vaccination. Coxsackie triggers Hand-Foot-Mouth disease (not the same as foot and mouth disease in animals) and early signs are blisters in the mouth and throat – it is usually a mild disease. Symptoms may include some – but not necessarily all – of the following: extreme fatigue (lasting for at least six months); fatigue which is made worse by physical or mental demands; muscle weakness or pain (myalgia); joint pain which is free of swelling; painful lymph nodes; depression, memory problems; a 'woolly' head; headaches; nausea; digestive problems; and sleep disturbance. A correct diagnosis should be sought (some doctors are experienced in the treatment of ME, see Appendix VI).

- *Rest and multiple therapies*: Taking time to rest and heal is at the top of the list. It can be very difficult to carry on with normal life. A multi-pronged approach, covering diet, supplementation (possibly including herbs), physiotherapy, a 'touching' therapy such as light massage, and a 'listening' therapy to combat any accompanying depression can be effective.
- *Background diet*: Eating a healthy, well-balanced diet is paramount. It is very important to eat low on the Glycaemic Index – slow-release carbohydrates such as wholegrains, oats, sweet potatoes, pulses and pasta for energy, to control blood sugar, and for B-vitamins which are essential for healthy nerve function. Maintain nutrient intake by eating

plenty of vegetables and fruits. Eat a small amount of protein with each meal and snack to stabilize blood sugar and provide zinc and iron. Sugar, refined carbohydrates and sugary foods should be avoided.

- *Food-intolerances*: If a food intolerance is present, such as wheat or dairy, it will not 'cause' the problem but may reduce the ability to recuperate.
- *Bowel bacteria*: A healthy balance of bowel bacteria encourages a stronger immune system (see page 138). FOS (fructo-oligosaccharides), a natural sweetener available from health food shops, can be sprinkled on cereals and desserts, and has the dual benefit of promoting bowel health while making life without sugar more manageable (though use it moderately, as too much may induce bloating).
- *Caffeine*: This should be avoided as it stimulates the nervous system. Caffeine is found in coffee, tea, colas, dark chocolate, the herb guarana and some cold and headache medication.
- *Alcohol*: This can worsen symptoms by affecting the liver. It is important to consider the health of the liver in ME especially if there is suspicion of intolerance to pollution or other compounds found in the environment (see Liver Health page 238).
- *Candida*: It may also be necessary to deal with Candida, which as an opportunistic yeast, can get the upper hand in ME as the immune system is depressed (see Candida page 146 and Immune Health page 28).
- *Supplements*: A general supplement programme, which includes a multi-B complex, evening primrose and fish oils may be advised. The mineral magnesium is probably also going to be of help, and CoQ10, an energy boosting antioxidant, can also be valuable. Herbal adaptogens including ginseng, astragalus and liquorice may be helpful. However, you should consult a herbalist with experience of treating ME, as there are subtleties of use that can be

individual (for example, liquorice can help some people but worsen the condition for others – it raises blood pressure – and is best used short term with the introduction of another adaptogen after the initial use of liquorice). Trials have shown that milk thistle is useful for promoting liver health.

## Menopausal Symptoms

What is commonly called the menopause is actually the peri-menopause. This is the – usually – five to ten years before periods actually stop. The menopause itself is the time of the last period, when ovulation ceases completely. At the menopause the ovaries stop producing oestrogens and as an egg follicle is no longer being produced, progesterone is also no longer made. Oestrogen continues to be produced by the adrenal glands and fat cells, but at a lower rate than pre-menopausally. In the peri-menopausal phase, levels of these hormones fluctuate and drop. The most common age for menopause is the mid-fifties, but it can happen any time from the mid-thirties onwards. In a few women very early menopause happens in their twenties. Testing for the menopause is done by assessing levels of FSH hormone. FSH (follicle stimulating hormone) is elevated as the body attempts to stimulate the ovaries to produce eggs (from ripening follicles). Some women sail through the menopause without many signs or symptoms, and others are plagued by a range of problems including hot flushes, vaginal dryness, weight gain, headaches or depression.

The attitude towards menopause differs from woman to woman – some see it as a release from the monthly problems of menstruating and look forward to a rewarding and active phase of their lives; others see it as the beginning of a time of decline. One thing is now certain: whereas at one time women on average lived only a few years beyond the menopause, increased life span means that women can now expect to live almost half their lives after the menopause. This means that having a positive attitude and eating healthily are more vital than ever in ensuring a long life which is as free as possible of adverse health problems. Some post-menopausal health concerns are dealt with in more detail in other sections of this book. These include: libido, heart disease, stroke, osteoporosis, cancer (particularly of the breast, which is of concern post-menopausally).

Many concerns have been raised about the use of HRT (hormone replacement therapy) in relation to the risk of stroke and breast cancer and some women prefer to take a dietary and herbal approach to managing the menopause. HRT also does not suit some women, who prefer not to menstruate. The protective effect on bone health only lasts as long as the medication is taken. This means that addressing long-term bone health with dietary management becomes even more important.

- *Fruits and vegetables*: Considerably more than the usually recommended five portions – seven to ten portions daily – are highly protective of bone health, cardiovascular complications and breast cancer.
- *Soya*: Soya protein has been shown to be protective against heart disease. Additionally, the phytoestrogens (plant oestrogens) contained in soya foods are believed to be protective against osteoporosis and breast cancer. This effect on bone health comes about as a gentle form of oestrogen replacement; the protection against breast cancer is because the mild plant oestrogens are thought to block the damaging effects of more potent forms of oestrogen, which are probably involved in breast cancer – so these phytoestrogens have a dual, or balancing, effect.

Around five portions a week should be beneficial. Soya milk is a popular choice and soya yoghurts, soya snacks, tofu and other soya-based foods are available in health food shops. Other phytoestrogen rich foods are chickpeas, linseeds and linseed-enriched bread. Eat pulse-based dishes at least three times a week. Japanese women, who eat plenty of soya foods, have very few problems with menopausal symptoms (there is no word for hot flushes in Japanese).

- *Fibre*: While fibre protects against digestive and bowel problems, it also has a potent effect in protecting against heart disease, weight gain and breast cancer. Fruits, vegetables, legumes (pulses and beans), wholegrains (oats and rye are particularly beneficial), nuts and seeds are fibre rich. Linseeds have compounds called lignans in them, which have particular benefit against breast cancer as they assist in the removal of oestrogens.

- *Hot flushes*: These can be very troublesome for some women, who experience them several times daily, and they can be worse at night. To reduce their severity eat a diet which features soya products (see above) and whole-wheat foods – studies show an effect after four to eight weeks. Hot flushes are less of a problem in vegetarians so a diet high in legumes, pulses and vegetables may help. Caffeine and alcohol are frequent triggers. Regular exercise has a short-term worsening effect, but a longer-term dampening effect on hot flushes. High levels of vitamin E (800ius) have been reported to help, though avoid this if you are taking blood thining medication such as Warfarin. Sage is a prime herbal remedy for reducing night sweats; drink a sage tea made from leaves steeped in boiling water for five minutes, three times daily. Black cohosh and dong quai are the herbs most frequently taken during the peri-menopause, which have a wide range of beneficial effects on symptoms. As with all herbs, it is best to seek professional advice from a herbalist, especially if you are taking other medications.

- *Mood swings or depression*: Balancing blood sugar levels can help. To achieve this, eat more fibre-rich foods (see below). St John's wort is well known for its effectiveness against mild to moderate depression, but it must not be taken with other medications and it can increase sensitivity to sunlight. Avena sativa, better known as porridge oats (or use the herbal tincture) is used traditionally as a relaxant herb.

- *Memory*: Many women complain of worsening memory at this time. B-vitamins are important for mental function and are rich in cereals, or take a Brewer's yeast supplement. The herb Gingko biloba improves circulation and helps short-term memory problems.

- *Headaches or migraines*: These often start, or get worse, during the menopause. Caffeine is a frequent trigger, as are amine-rich foods such as wine, beer, chocolate, cheese, pickles and salami. Ginger can help to reduce headaches and migraines by dilating the blood vessels to the head.

- *Vaginal dryness*: This can begin to be a problem in the peri-menopause, but is worse after periods cease (oestrogen keeps tissues 'plumped out'). Many lubrication choices are available including those enriched with oestrogen – for short-term use – from your doctor. Again, a diet that features soya (see below) can help. The popular menopausal herbs Black cohosh and Red clover are useful to alleviate dryness.

- *Weight management*: This can become a problem around and after the menopause. Muscle to fat ratios lean towards more fat as we age and hormonal shifts predispose menopausal women to a more apple than pear shape as they age (see page 328). This fat distribution becomes a greater risk for heart disease. If weight management is a problem, then at least ensure you take enough exercise; it helps to keep weight in check and has other additional benefits. Half an hour minimum, up to one hour, brisk walking daily is the general suggestion.

- *Libido*: Sex-drive is a very personal thing and there can be anxiety about decreasing libido. With the advent of Viagra for male partners, there may be a feeling that we all need to 'perform' into our later years. Certainly age is no barrier to feeling sexy, but it is a very personal choice. See Libido and Sexual Function page 234.

- *Breast Cancer*: Risk of this cancer increases significantly after the menopause. However, breast cancer takes an average of ten years to develop from a single cell to a detectable lump. Therefore it is likely that health measures taken before the menopause are of greatest importance in prevention. See earlier comments about soya, fruit and vegetable intake and linseeds. Oily fish is also protective.

- *Osteoporosis*: The risk of thinning bones increases after the menopause, but the health of bones is established long beforehand. For this reason a healthy diet in earlier years is of most importance. But there is still a lot that can be done after the menopause to significantly help matters including weight bearing exercise and vitamin D supplementation. For Osteroporosis see page 261.

- *Cardiovascular risk*: Women are protected to a large degree from cardiovascular problems prior to the menopause by oestrogen. After the menopause their risk profile increases to similar levels to men, although there remain some differences (such as in the type of heart attacks they tend to have). Steps for reducing heart disease and stroke risk are covered on pages 216 and 301. A moderate intake of wine – one or two units a day – probably reduces risk after the menopause in women (though not pre-menopausally, when alcohol increases damaging oestrogens and breast cancer risk).

- *Herbs*: Popular herbs for managing the menopause are vitex agnus castus, black cohosh (for hot flushes), dong quai (a general modifier of female hormones), St John's wort (for mild depression) and valerian (to improve sleep).

## Metabolic Syndrome

Metabolic syndrome, also called Syndrome X, is a group of conditions related to insulin resistance. Apart from leading to poor blood sugar control and eventually, in many cases, to diabetes, insulin resistance also causes other metabolic disturbances in the body. Metabolic syndrome consists of increased blood fats, blood viscosity, blood urate levels, blood coagulability and blood pressure (all risk factors for heart disease). It is this collection of symptoms that has been given the names Metabolic Syndrome or Syndrome X. See Insulin Resistance page 227 for treatment.

## Migraine

About one in eight people experience migraines, of which there are two main types. One-fifth involve an 'aura' of visual disturbances such as flashes and zig zags, while most – four-fifths – do not involve an aura. Migraines are often characterized by one-sided head pain and it is common to experience nausea. Triggers for migraines can include stressful episodes, strong smells such as petrol or perfumes, irregular meals, changes in the weather and too little sleep. Women are three times more likely to suffer from migraines than men, and menstruation, menopause and taking the oral contraceptive can all trigger attacks.

- *Blood sugar balance*: The most important dietary trigger is missed or delayed meals. This is most evident in children, but is just as important for adults. Slow-releasing carbohydrates such as wholegrains are best. It can help to eat a bowl of breakfast cereal or a banana before bed to head off the potential effect of a whole night without food.
- *Diary*: Keeping a migraine diary, which records all foods consumed and significant events that lead up to migraine attacks, can help to pinpoint culprits.
- *Trigger foods*: Migraines are often linked to specific foods, most commonly the 'Five-Cs' – chocolate, cheese (and other dairy foods), claret (wine), coffee and citrus fruit. Some substances in foods act directly as triggers for migraines, for example octopamine in oranges and tyranine in cheese. It is thought that people who react to these foods may be deficient in an enzyme, PST (phenol-sulphotransferase), which normally inactivates the compounds called amines, abundant in most of these foods. The rise in levels of amines seems to stimulate blood platelets in the brain to clump together, which then release a chemical messenger – serotonin – so triggering a migraine. Other amine-rich foods include Marmite, Horlicks, liver, sausages, broad beans, pickled herrings and beer.
- *Nitrates and nitrites*: These are used to cure meats such as bacon and salami and can trigger attacks in some people.
- *Aspartame*: This artificial sweetener is also a possible trigger. One study looking at adverse reactions to aspartame reported to the Food and Drug Administration in the US that 45 per cent of the cases involved headaches and migraines, though more usually around one in 12 people identify it as a trigger.
- *MSG*: Another common food additive trigger is MSG (monosodium glutamate, or E621). It is important to

realize that not all foods will cause attacks in all people and the response can be very individual.

- *Food intolerances*: Commonly eaten foods such as wheat and dairy products trigger migraines in sensitive people. If other symptoms co-exist, such as bloating or lethargy, it is worth a trial of two weeks in which you replace suspect foods with others that do not cause reactions (see page 205 for more).

- *Magnesium*: According to several studies, magnesium deficiency seems to be linked to migraine attacks, particularly for women whose migraines are triggered by menstruation. Magnesium-rich foods include all green leafy vegetables, nuts, sunflower and pumpkin seeds, dried fruit, brewer's yeast, seafood and wholegrains.

- *Herbs*: Feverfew, which reduces platelet clumping, and butterbur root (*Petasites hybridus*), which reduces muscle tension, are both very successful in treating migraines. If you prefer foods to supplements, you can keep a feverfew plant on your window-ledge and add one or two leaves daily (no more) to your salads or sandwiches. Make sure you have the right variety: *Tanacetum parthenium*. For migraines triggered by the onset of periods the herb chasteberry (Vitex agnus castus) taken for two to three months can help to balance out the hormonal fluctuations, which can be triggers.

- *Omega-3*: Fatty acids from fish oils do not seem to be helpful in migraine.

- See also Headaches page 214.

## Mood Swings

Mood swings can be linked to a wide variety of potential factors. It is not always a problem that needs to be addressed with medicine, or for that matter nutrition. It is, after all, normal to feel better on some days than others, and worse as a result of factors that affect all of us at some time or other. It is normal to feel sad, anxious, frustrated or at the other end of the scale, joyous, elated and happy – when circumstances and our mood dictate it. Anxiety and depressive disorders are fairly unremitting, and for these the talking therapies can be very useful, and nutritional strategies can make a difference (see Depression page 171). But mood swings is another thing, where seemingly unreasonable changes in behaviour are not linked to specific events. A person who suffers from this, or a person who lives with them, will be aware of how it impacts on daily life. The common factor with mood swings is likely to be how the brain's neurochemical balance is behaving. Serotonin, noradrenaline and dopamine can all be affected by diet. Serotonin in particular seems to play an important role and low levels are commonly experienced when a person is subject to one or some of the following: premenstrual food cravings, sleep disturbance, depression and alcohol cravings. For this reason, SSRI antidepressant medication has found some limited success with treating all of these conditions. But many people don't want to take medication for these conditions, it is not always successful and, of course, potentially has side-effects. Nutritional measures can offer a viable and sustainable approach.

- *Blood Sugar:* Poor blood sugar imbalance is probably the main problem behind mood swings and this impacts on how the brain functions. Eating foods low on the Glycaemic Index (GI) and restricting foods high on the GI is sensible (see page 350). A little protein with each meal helps to slow down the impact that carbohydrates have on blood sugar. Choosing a snack is a particularly vulnerable time: a piece of fruit with a small handful of unsalted nuts, some cottage cheese on a rye cracker, nut butter on an oat cake or a yoghurt with fruit all provide protein as well as fairly low-GI options. Coffee has an affect on stress hormones and so inadvertently makes blood sugar control more difficult – drink decaffeinated coffee or weak teas, or switch to caffeine-free herbal or fruit teas.

- *Hormone Imbalance*: In women it is common to have mood swings premenstrually or peri-menopausally. Evening out hormone fluctuations with diet can help. See Premenstrual Problems page 279 and Menopause page 246. An under-active or overactive thyroid can predispose a person to mood irregularities – thyroid health can be checked by your doctor (see Thyroid, Underactive page 304 and Thyroid, Overactive page 306).

- *Alcohol*: This can make controlling mood swings more difficult and imbalances blood sugar. Alcohol is not actu-ally a stimulant but a depressant and it has a negative effect on the nervous system.

- *Food intolerances*: An intolerance to certain foods can have wide but non-specific effect on health. Occasionally, in some people, this extends to making mood swings worse – the most likely culprit is wheat. It is worth avoiding wheat for a couple of weeks at a vulnerable time to test if this is the case, particularly if you are experiencing digestive upset such as bloating and wind. See Food Intolerance page 205.

- *Aggression*: Adults can suffer from hyperactivity problems, as can children (see Hyperactivity page 220). Food additives such as food colourings, preservatives, sweeteners and flavourings, and deficiencies of fish oils, can all have an effect on this condition.

- *Calming foods*: Oats, calcium-rich foods (such as low-fat milk), B-vitamin rich foods (such as wholegrain cereals and liver), potassium rich foods (bananas, potatoes and water melon) are all helpful. Chocolate promotes the 'pleasure chemicals' endorphins. See also Chapter 5: Food and Mood.

## Morning Sickness

See Nausea, page 259, and also Pregnancy, page 274.

## Mouth Ulcers

Recurrent ulceration in the mouth can be linked to a number of potential problems. It is often simply a sign of being 'run down', but a correct diagnosis from a doctor is needed in cases of persistent ulceration in case it is linked to coeliac disease, inflammatory bowel disease, lupus or other immune insufficiency problems, including mouth cancer. Cold sores (see page 156) can also be mistaken for mouth ulcers. Mouth ulcers have been linked to toothpaste containing a strong detergent SLS (sodium laureth sulphate) and mouthwashes containing alcohol. These compounds dry out the mucus membranes of the mouth and trigger ulcers in sensitive people. Mouth ulcers are also a known side-effect to some medications, especially some forms of chemotherapy. Smoking also causes mucus membranes to dry out. A jagged tooth can ulcerate the mouth, in which case visit your dentist.

- *Vitamin C*: One of the first observed nutritional deficiency signs was scurvy resulting from lack of vitamin C. This manifests as ulcerated gums and mouth – vitamin C is a key nutrient in forming collagen. Eating vitamin C-rich fruits and vegetables is vital. Smokers need about twice as much vitamin C as non-smokers.

- *Zinc*: This mineral is vital for healing ulcerated tissue. See Part 4: A–Z of Nutrients page 337 for food sources or consider zinc lozenges.
- *Mouth bacteria*: Mouth ulcers can be linked to hypersensitivity to a bacteria commonly found in the mouth, *haemolytic streptococcus*. Anti-bacterial herbs such as cloves and sage can be used as a mouthwash by steeping them in boiling water for five minutes. A garlic clove each day, included in cooking or salads, has a general immune boosting effect and a specific anti-bacterial action (do not apply to an ulcer directly, however, as this will sting).
- *Iron deficiency*: Recurrent mouth ulcers can be a sign of iron-deficiency. If this is suspected, your GP can run a test. See Anaemia page 115.
- *Digestive tract ulceration*: Mouth ulcers that recur can also be a sign of ulceration further down the digestive tract, as in coeliac disease (see page 153) or Crohn's disease (see page 157). In these instances it is necessary to get a correct diagnosis from your doctor.
- *Helicobacter pylori*: For information on this see Ulcers, Oral, Gastric and Duodenal page 307.

## Multiple Sclerosis (MS)

Multiple sclerosis (MS) is a breakdown of the protective myelin sheath around nerve fibres. As the sheath becomes 'demyelinated', nerve degeneration can cause problems with co-ordination, sensation in the limbs, walking, eyesight and speech. MS affects more women than men and the causes are unknown – there is an assumption that it has an autoimmune link where the body breaks down its own tissue, but this is not certain. There is often unpredictable progression and remission from the disease over many years and symptoms may be mild or moderate or, in one-fifth of cases, severe.

- *Low saturated-fat diet*: This is one of the regimes that has attracted most attention. Patients who followed a very low saturated-fat diet of less than 20g (3/4oz) daily of saturated fat with high polyunsaturated fats had a reduction in relapses, better energy levels, and improved life expectancy. As this diet is well balanced and does not contravene healthy eating guidelines, it is unlikely to be of any risk.
- *GLA*: A fatty acid called GLA, which is found in evening primrose oil and borage (starflower) oil, is normally made in the body, but some people do not do this efficiently. High doses of GLA from supplements may offer relief of symptoms for some people, but this is not yet proved.
- *Omega-3s*: Supplementation is unlikely to do harm, but the latest research has found that it is unlikely to be of benefit. The hope was that as polyunsaturated fatty acids form part of the myelin sheath, supplementation would help, but this has not proved to be the case.
- *Vitamin D*: Supplementation (but not from food intake) has been linked to a 40 per cent reduced incidence of developing MS, and it is notable that those who live in sunnier climates (and so manufacture more vitamin D in their skins) have a reduced risk of developing MS (their risk increases when they move to northern hemisphere climates). It is not certain if this information can be extrapolated to treatment for existing MS.
- *Health Problems*: Health problems for those with MS who are immobile or who lose function can be supported with nutritional measures. See the relevant sections such as Leg Ulcers, page 309, Cystitis (which can result from incontinence), page 168, and Constipation, page 160. Fatigue can severely affect those with MS and eating plenty of low-fat

complex carbohydrates such as oats, brown rice, rye bread and pasta will help.

## Nausea

Nausea is usually an indication of a more full-blown digestive illness such as food poisoning. If reflux (food or digestive acids coming up from the stomach) is a regular feature, this needs to be checked by a doctor as it may indicate an incompetent sphincter at the top of the stomach and stomach acids can cause problems with dentition. Motion sickness is another common reason for nausea. Unexpected nausea may accompany dizziness, which can be a sign of low blood pressure or an ear infection. Avoid bending forwards, as this can stimulate the vagus nerve leading to the stomach. Nausea sometimes provides the first inkling for a woman that she is pregnant.

- *Ginger*: This is a highly effective anti-nausea treatment even for chemotherapy-induced nausea and is also safe to take during pregnancy. It can be taken as ginger tea, ginger beer or by nibbling on crystallized ginger (a particularly pleasant option). Mint is also calming for the digestive system and is effective against nausea and travel sickness.
- *Pregnancy nausea*: Morning sickness (though it can happen at any time of the day or night) can be a transient nuisance, which usually clears up during the second trimester. In extreme cases morning sickness can be severe, however, and it can be worrying and debilitating to be vomiting regularly during pregnancy. It is rarely a cause of malnutrition, or harms the baby or mother.
- *Vomiting*: If vomiting, you should always consult your doctor, and it is important to stay hydrated by drinking

sufficient water, or if in danger of dehydration, to take rehydration salts.

- *Smells*: Avoid smells that make you feel nauseous, nausea can be a sign of food aversion (see page 204).
- *Acupressure point*: pressing the acupuncture point P6 located just inside the wristbone is particularly effective – wristbands are available from chemists which make this easier).
- See also Balance, page 126.

## Neuropathy

Neuropathy is a loss of sensation in the nerves (most commonly the extremities – the legs, feet and hands). It is different to neuromyalgia, which is pain in the nerves. Neuropathy can be experienced as prickling, tingling, aches, pain or loss of sensation in the carpal tunnel/hand area and in the feet/legs.

- *Vitamins and minerals*: Many nutrients, especially B-vitamins and magnesium, are essential for proper nerve functioning. Improving your diet to include lots of wholegrains can help to overcome this. Taking a multivitamin and multimineral supplement can speed up improvement in the condition and give diet time to take effect.
- *Diabetes*: Neuropathy is a major complication of diabetes. Success in treatment with evening primrose oil (EPO), a source of GLA (gamma linolenic acid) has been noted in two trials, particularly when used alongside the antioxidant alpha-lipoic acid. Starflower oil (also called borage oil), which is a much richer source of GLA, does not have the same therapeutic advantage of EPO, possibly because the GLA structure is slightly different.
- *B-vitamins*: Reversible neuropathy can be induced by excessively high doses (200mg+) of vitamin B6 supplements

over a prolonged time (over six months). Vitamin B6 is an effective treatment used by many for period problems, to reduce homocysteine levels (along with other B-vitamins: B2, B6 and B12). Because of the risk of (reversible) neuropathy, an upper limit for B6 use has been set at 50mg, though in reality higher levels can be tolerated by most people over the short term, particularly when taken along with other B-vitamins.

- *Herbs*: Gingko biloba, ginger and garlic are all herbs known to improve blood flow to the extremities.
- See also Carpal Tunnel Syndrome page 147.

## Osteoporosis

Osteoporosis is thinning of the bones. Bone is not static and is constantly remodelling itself. Calcium is turned over and minerals are lost from the bone (for use elsewhere in the body) and replaced all the time, but osteoporosis develops when this balance is interrupted. In the UK one in three women and one in 12 men over 50 endure osteoporotic fractures, and in the elderly this frequently leads to death. It is not just a female problem, with 30 per cent of hip fractures occurring in men.

Osteoporosis is largely preventable and it has a number of causes. Weight-bearing exercise is vital for building up bone density (however, those with active osteoporosis should check with their doctors, as some types of exercise may induce fractures in vulnerable bones). Weight-bearing exercise is anything that 'stresses' the bones, such as running, dancing and using a mini-trampoline. Non weight-bearing exercise is, for example, swimming or cycling. Smoking seriously affects bone density. Certain drugs also thin bones, particularly long-term use of corticosteroids, and use of excessively high doses of the hormone thyroxin to correct underactive thyroid problems.

- *Peak bone density*: Maximum density is achieved in bones around the late teens. This is a critical time for bone development, as it is this reserve of minerals that will set the scene for how easily bone is lost in later years. Unfortunately, many negative health habits are common amongst children and teenagers who are building up to this critical stage. This is becoming a serious problem, with teenagers now experiencing soaring rates of bone fracture due to poor bone density. If avoiding dairy at this age, then it is important to use other calcium-enriched sources or foods. See information below regarding soft drinks, salt and exercise.

- *Calcium and magnesium*: Many people, including doctors, often only think of calcium in relation to bone health. In reality, several minerals are needed for bone health; magnesium is particularly important, as it works in close collaboration with calcium. There is much dispute about the amount of calcium needed for optimum bone health: in the US around 1,000mg daily is advised; in the UK around 700mg; and in Eastern populations (who have lower levels of osteoporosis) around 400mg can be the typical intake. It is likely that not taking the co-minerals into account leads to this diverse opinion and that a diet featuring more magnesium (from wholegrains, nuts, seeds and leafy green vegetables) permits a lower calcium intake. For calcium- and magnesium-rich foods see Part 4: A–Z of Nutrients page 331. When taking a supplement, it is important to choose one that has a ratio of 2:1, or even 1:1, calcium to magnesium and also includes vitamin D.

- *Vitamin D*: This vitamin is commonly deficient in UK populations, particularly in the elderly. We get most of our vitamin D from sun exposure, but some from foods. Vitamin D-rich foods include oily fish, liver and fortified margarine. In the elderly, deficiency is exacerbated by a reduced ability to synthesize vitamin D upon exposure to the sun, a greater tendency to cover up and reduced exposure due to invalid status. Supplemented levels of 800ius (20mcg) have been shown to be of great benefit. Increasing vitamin-D intake can increase bone density, reduce bone loss/turnover, and has been shown to reduce the incidence of (non-vertebral) hip fractures by 30–40 per cent. A secondary means by which osteoporotic fracture risk is reduced by vitamin-D supplementation is an improvement in body sway and muscle function, reducing the risk of falls.

- *Plant oestrogens*: In women, the menopause heralds a large reduction (but not total loss) of oestrogen. Oestrogen has a protective effect against bone loss. Some oestrogen continues to be made from fat cells and this is one instance where heavier women have the upper hand, as the oestrogen produced can help bone health. Foods rich in plant oestrogens may help maintain bone density. These are: soya, chickpeas, wholegrains, beans and pulses and vegetables.

- *Fruits and vegetables*: Several new studies are focusing on the effects of fruit and vegetable intake. It is early days, but it looks as if an intake of eight to ten portions of fruits and vegetables daily could be more important for bone health than calcium intake.

- *Fish oils*: These have been shown to improve bone density. One or two portions of oily fish weekly is advised.

- *Reducing mineral loss from bones*: In addition to smoking and the use of some drugs such as steroids, fizzy drinks are thought to be one of the major reasons why young women and men are not building up peak bone density. Fizzy drinks have a lot of phosphoric acid in them, which leaches minerals from bone.

- *Salt*: Excess dietary salt is responsible for calcium leaching from bone, conversely reducing dietary salt results in lowered quantities of bone reabsorption markers.

- *Anorexia*: This is a major hazard for bone density. It is common for young anorectic women to have active osteoporosis and even fractures. The ground can rarely be fully made up in later years.
- *Protein*: It has been of concern that high protein in the diet induces calcium loss in the urine, with an assumption that this involved leaching of calcium from bones due to an excess of acidic metabolism needed to process proteins. However, this theory has not stood up to the rigours of research, which has found that protein increases bone density as long as it is in the presence of a high fruit and vegetable intake (see point above).
- *Beer and silicon*: Silicon is linked to improved bone health and beer (in moderation) is a good source of silicon. Other good sources of silicon are wholegrain cereals and green beans.
- See also Balance, page 126.

## Otitis Media (Glue Ear)

Otitis media is a build up of sticky mucus in the ear, usually due to an infection. It is a problem for children who have small ear canals, which can get totally blocked. It is often mistaken for inattention, when they are actually not hearing properly. All ear infections should be taken seriously and checked by your doctor, as they can progress and lead to permanent damage. Otitis media is usually treated with antibiotics or, if it persists, with a minor (but still stressful) operation to insert grommets to open up the ear canal. Breast-feeding is protective against otitis media. The problem often responds very well indeed to dietary changes.

- *Sugar*: A high sugar diet will often increase the risk of inflammation, making glue ear worse.

- *Food intolerances*: Dairy is most commonly a problem and children with glue ear are often 'addicted' to their milk. When using milk-substitutes such as soya milk or rice milk for children, make sure they are calcium-enriched. Wheat is another common food intolerance involved in glue ear.
- *Liquids*: Drinking plenty of water helps to keep mucus more clear and free running. Six to 8 glasses daily are recommended for children, two litres for adults.
- *Bowel bacteria*: If given a few concurrent courses of antibiotics for repeat problems with glue ear it is very important to re-establish a healthy bacteria balance with pro- and prebiotics. See page 138 for more on this.
- *Xylitol*: This bulk sweetener is now added to a number of brands of chewing gum because of its impressive record of reducing mouth bacteria responsible for tooth decay. It has also been shown to reduce incidences of otitis media when used regularly.

## Pain Management

Pain is a messenger. The pain from a sprained ankle tells you not to put weight on that foot. Toothache is a warning that a visit to the dentist cannot be delayed. An arthritic twinge is telling you to find out what might be causing the inflammation. But the fact that pain may provide an important message does not make the messenger any more welcome, and the market for painkillers stands at more than £270 million annually.

Not everyone can take over-the-counter (OTC) painkillers – aspirin can cause gastritis or ulcers and if you are asthmatic, it can trigger an attack; and those who take paracetamol just once a week increase their risk of developing asthma. Prescription steroids that suppress inflammation can have far-reaching consequences from long-term use, including osteoporosis. While OTC painkillers may be useful for relief of short-term acute pain, they have a disappointing track record for long-term pain. After checking with your doctor to ensure that there are not more serious health problems, the nutritional approach may offer long-term relief. There are several important ways in which dietary manipulation and supplements might help. The first is to affect leukotrienes and prostaglandins, hormone-like chemicals produced in the body, which regulate inflammation. The second is to lower levels of histamine, an irritating chemical, which is implicated in inflammation and allergies. Other important mechanisms for regulating pain include breaking up fibrin, a substance that collects in areas of inflammation and contributes to swelling and pain, as well as blocking substance P, a neurotransmitter partly responsible for the pain message.

- *Saturated fats*: Changing the type of fats that you eat is usually the first step in a nutritional programme. Saturated fats, found in meat, butter, eggs, cheese and full- and half-fat milk, are rich in a substance called arachidonic acid, which produces leukotrienes. These in turn promote inflammation.
- *Unsaturated fats*: Those found in oily fish, fresh nuts and seeds – for example walnuts, almonds, pecans, pumpkin seeds, sunflower seeds and evening primrose oil – are rich in omega-3 and omega-6 fats, which promote anti-inflammatory prostaglandins. Fish oils and cod liver oil switch off the COX-2 enzyme (aspirin inhibits COX-1 to stop pain, but also triggers gastrointestinal upset, while COX-2 inhibition kills joint pain without this side-effect).
- *Food sensitivities*: Some people find that inflammation is worsened by certain foods to which they are sensitive, such as wheat, dairy products, citrus fruit, coffee, sugar and alcohol.

Food sensitivities have been associated with headaches, migraines and arthritic pain.

- *Cherries*: Twenty cherries contain between 12–25mg of salycilates, which has the same painkilling capability as an aspirin tablet.
- *Enzymes*: The enzymes bromelain, found in pineapple, and papain, from papayas, can also ease pain. These are proteolytic enzymes (which digest proteins) and can be taken in capsule form, fairly high doses of which have been used successfully to treat back and joint problems. Capsules are normally taken with meals to aid digestion, but when taken away from meals it is believed that they remove waste products and fibrin in the area of the injury, reducing swelling and helping to speed up the healing process. Bromelain also seems to block the formation of inflammatory prostaglandins. (Do not take enzymes if you have ulcers or gastritis.)
- *Antioxidants*: These have a mild histamine-reducing effect and also appear to help stabilize the structure of cartilage. Another antioxidant substance, quercitin, found in apples, tea and onions and also available in capsule form, blocks histamine release as well as stopping the release of leukotrienes and is often used alongside vitamin C for pain relief.
- *Minerals*: The minerals magnesium and calcium help to relax muscles, which can be involved in back spasm. While both minerals are important the bias is often towards needing magnesium at around 400mg daily to relax muscle tension. It has a marked effect on cramped leg muscles, can be effective at treating back pain and is very useful for migraines. Food sources of magnesium include wholegrains, fresh nuts and seeds and green leafy vegetables.
- *Hydrations*: Low back pain can be related to dehydration, which affects the strength of the muscles, and drinking two

or three litres of water daily, while cutting back on dehydrating caffeine and alcohol, can make all the difference.

- *Spices*: Ginger has a long history as an anti-inflammatory compound (do not use if you have stomach or duodenal ulcers) and also acts as an antihistamine. The active agent in turmeric, curcumin, is a potent antioxidant, which gives the spice its dark yellow colour and is said to work as well as the steroid drug cortisone in relieving acute inflammation, by inhibiting inflammatory prostaglandins and by depleting substance P. Curcumin and ginger also promote the breakdown of fibrin.

- *Herbs*: Devil's claw is a herb used successfully for pain management, including arthritic pain. Another useful antispasmodic and muscle relaxant is the herb cramp bark, which can be taken as a tea or in capsule form.

- See Inflammation, page 225.

## Pancreatitis

This is an inflammation of the pancreas, which is mostly linked to gall-stone formation or to excessive alcohol intake. The pancreas is the gland which secretes insulin for blood sugar control and also digestive enzymes for digestion. It is a serious condition with far-reaching health consequences.

- *Alcohol*: All alcohol must be avoided totally.

- *General diet*: A low-fat, low-sugar, high fibre diet is recommended. Caffeine should be avoided.

- *Antioxidants*: One possible explanation for unexplained pancreatitis is a lack of antioxidants. The resulting free-radical damage allows the inflammation of the pancreas to progress unchecked. Fruits and vegetables are our sources of antioxidants and a minimum of five portions and ideally seven or eight portions is advised daily. Another antioxidant nutrient, the mineral selenium, probably also has a role to play against pancreatitis.

- *Green tea*: The active constituents in green tea have been shown to improve pancreatitis. Drink seven to ten cups daily for effect.
- *Olive oil*: Use cold-pressed extra-virgin oil in preference to other oils to dress salads and cooked vegetables. Avoid cooking with it at high temperatures, as this causes it to smoke, thus destroying valuable antioxidant compounds. Olive oil seems to stimulate the production of pancreatic enzymes.
- *Omega-3s*: Fish oils support pancreatic health and reduce inflammation.
- *Digestive enzymes*: These may be prescribed by your doctor, or are available from health food shops, to take with meals when pancreatic function is impaired.

## Parkinson's Disease

Parkinson's Disease occurs when cells in an area of the brain, called the *substantia nigra*, are damaged leading to low levels of the neurotransmitter dopamine, which is normally produced by these cells. It mainly affects elderly people, but early onset Parkinson's is not uncommon from the age of 40+. Tremor is the most obvious outward sign, fine motor control is impaired, with rigidity and slowness of movement, sometimes accompanied by aggression and disorientation. Medical treatment involves a drug called Levodopa, which is actually an amino acid (protein building block). Treatment with nutrition is not curative, but may make life more comfortable and allay symptoms. It should only be undertaken with medical supervision.

- *Medication and protein*: Some people with Parkinson's find that too much protein interferes with their medication – in these cases medication should be taken between meals with their doctor's approval.

- *Appetite and digestive tract*: This is often poor and small, frequent meals may be better tolerated than three 'square' meals daily. Eating may be more difficult with Parkinson's when the tongue and chewing ability are affected. In this case make meals leisurely and comfortable. Constipation is also often a problem – see page 160 for more on this.

- *Protein and vitamin B2*: Those with Parkinson's have been found to have higher than normal intakes of red meat, often influencing the choice of meals in the family by this craving. A low-red-meat diet has been advocated in one trial, which was combined with vitamin B2 supplementation. A significant reduction in tremor was observed, though it is unclear how much of this was attributable to avoiding red meat. Vitamin B2 (riboflavin) supplementation at high doses of 30mg every eight hours for six months seems to help control tremor, with improvements noted after 20 days of treatment. Aggression and agitation were reduced or disappeared after three months. Milk is particularly rich in B2.

- *Antioxidants*: Those with a diet highest in antioxidant-rich foods, particularly vitamin E, are least likely to develop Parkinson's. When affected by Parkinson's it is sensible to maintain fruit and vegetable intake for its general health benefits and to ease constipation.

- *Iron supplements*: These may negatively affect Levodopa medication.

- *NADH*: NADH stands for nicotinamide adenine dinucleotide, it is a coenzyme which plays a key role in cellular energy production and stimulates dopamine production. It is available as oral supplements. NADH supplements may help the medication Levodopa to work more effectively, particularly for those with early-onset Parkinson's, but this approach is controversial.

## PCOS (Polycystic Ovarian Syndrome)

PCOS is believed to affect around six per cent of women of reproductive age but diagnosis of the condition is considerably lower than this, meaning that many women suffer health concerns for which they do not have a diagnosis. As the name suggests, PCOS is when there are many egg follicles in the ovaries that do not mature correctly and, not released, produce cysts around the periphery of the ovaries. Symptoms of PCOS are mainly irregular periods, due to lack of regular ovulation, and higher than normal levels of 'male' androgen hormones (all women produce testosterone, as indeed all men produce oestrogen, but in both cases usually at low levels). The high level of androgens can produce male-like symptoms including acne, facial hair and (rarely) an enlarged clitoris. The first signs are often in teenage years with acne and facial hair, but interrupted periods and poor fertility follow. An over-abundance of the hormone insulin is also produced, leading to Insulin Resistance (see page 227). Women with PCOS often have trouble controlling their weight, may be more apple-shaped (see page 328) and have an accompanying risk of heart disease and stroke.

- *Insulin resistance*: The most important measure is to get insulin resistance under control, which can ameliorate many of the symptoms of weight gain and disease risk. For more on this see page 227. You should eat foods low on the Glycaemic Index (GI) and avoid those high on the GI (see Appendix I page 350), or follow a moderate-carbohydrate diet (see Weight Loss Diets, pages 315–327).

- *Exercise*: This is an important factor in reducing insulin resistance. Brisk walking for half an hour five times weekly is the minimum advised.
- *Calcium and vitamin D*: Abnormal calcium metabolism may be a feature of PCOS. In one small trial supplementing vitamin D (which affects calcium metabolism) and calcium resulted in over half of the women returning to normal menstruation within two months (and two pregnancies from normalization of egg follicle maturation).
- *Herbs*: Saw palmetto (*seranoa repens*) is a herb traditionally used to moderate testosterone hormone production in men with prostate problems. It has also found a use in women with PCOS to help interrupt the conversion of testosterone into dihydrotestosterone, which is responsible for the male hormone-related symptoms such as facial hair.

## Piles

See Haemorrhoids, page 211.

## Post-natal Depression

See Depression, page 171, and Pregnancy, page 274.

## Pre-conceptual Care

Many couples only start to think about adjusting their diet and lifestyle once they know they are pregnant. At best this can be two weeks after conception, though often it can be two, three or even four months into the pregnancy. However, the first three months of the pregnancy is when the baby is developing from a fertilized egg into a fully formed human being. The most important organ and nervous tissue developments take place in the first trimester. From then on it is mostly a matter of further maturation and growth. It is therefore much better to plan ahead, if you can, to optimize the environment for your baby in those first crucial weeks, which means starting with the healthiest possible egg and sperm. Nevertheless, the reality is that three-quarters of pregnancies are not planned, so it is important to not panic but to simply eat as well as possible from now on.

- *Six months prior to conception*: Stop taking the contraceptive pill and use barrier methods of contraception. Chlamydia and other STDs (sexually transmitted diseases) can be the cause of impaired fertility and miscarriage. Chlamydia can also lie dormant and symptomless meaning that it is a good idea to check for this before embarking on pregnancy. Both partners can benefit from screening. Other check-ups should ideally include testing for toxoplasmosis, German measles, diabetes and thyroid function. Stop smoking. Start following a wholefood diet, minimizing refined, packaged and junk food. Start to avoid unnecessary exposure to chemicals in the house and garden, and in foods and drinks – the womb should, as far as possible, be a pollution-free zone.
- *Three months prior to conception*: Reduce your alcohol intake to a bare minimum, but certainly to no more than four measures per week. Start taking a vitamin and mineral supplement specially formulated for pregnancy, which includes 400mcg of folic acid. Try to reduce stress and improve fitness levels.
- *One month prior to conception*: Avoid all alcohol. If using an IUD for contraception, you should have it removed, and

use barrier methods until you are ready to try for a baby. Avoid over-the-counter drugs. Speak to your doctor about the effects of any prescription medication you are taking (do not stop taking prescribed medication without discussing with your doctor). Moderate or cut out caffeine. Continue to eat a wholefood diet and take your pregnancy formulated vitamins and minerals up to and throughout your pregnancy.

## Pre-eclampsia

See Pregnancy, below.

## Pregnancy

Pregnancy is a time when well-intentioned aims at improving diet can't be put off any longer. Food, drink and activity levels during those vital nine months will affect the pregnancy and, more importantly, the developing baby. Try to stay physically active and to incorporate sensible exercise such as walking or swimming into your daily routine.

### First trimester

Many women do not know that they have conceived until they are several weeks into the pregnancy and may have carried on drinking, or even smoking, at this time. At 12 weeks the baby is fully formed, but is still only the size of a small plum. These first weeks are crucial in nutritional terms, so it is best to think about lifestyle changes as early as possible, ideally pre-conceptually. Some substances cross the placenta and, unfortunately, this includes many things that do not serve the baby well. In particular alcohol, caffeine and drugs (prescription or over-the-counter) can affect the baby – check with your doctor to see if you really need medication.

## Second trimester

The mother-to-be has got used to changing hormone levels, the baby is not yet big enough to hamper activity and energy levels are often improved by adrenaline from the baby.

## Third trimester:

The final three months is when the baby is putting on most of its weight.

- *Folic acid*: Despite all the publicity about the need for adequate folic acid to avoid neural tube defects such as spina bifida, 39 per cent of women are still unaware that government guidelines advise taking 400mcg supplementally 12 weeks prior to conception and for the first 12 weeks of pregnancy. Folic acid is unequivocally needed to reduce the chances of neural tube defects (spina bifida) in babies – where the spine does not fully close up. This is one instance where you cannot get sufficient amounts from food and where the supplemented form (folic acid) is preferable to the food form (folate) to achieve the effect. Even greater protection may be afforded by taking the folic acid in with a general B-vitamin supplement which gives co-vitamins B2, B6 and B12, which help folic acid to work more effectively. In one study vitamin B12 levels were found to be significantly lower in mothers with spina bifida children than in women with non-spina bifida children. In the US flour is fortified with folic acid for this reason, in the UK flour is not fortified by law but many breakfast cereals are. Green leafy vegetables are good sources of folic acid (though so much needs to be eaten that this is not practical on a daily basis). Supplementation is still needed.

- *Foods to avoid*: Soft cheeses, unpasteurized milk, soft whip ice cream and uncooked eggs may harbour listeria or salmonella, which can be dangerous to a developing baby. Undercooked or raw meat or fish can harbour parasites. Liver has levels of vitamin A which could be harmful to the baby. Betacarotene in orange coloured fruit and vegetables – carrots, cantaloupes, squash – is safe as it converts to vitamin A as needed. Peanuts should probably be avoided as they may establish a peanut allergy in the baby. Alcohol and caffeine deplete zinc, low levels of which are linked to nerve abnormalities and low birth weight. Maternal caffeine intake has been linked to infant cot death syndrome in some studies. Pregnant women should not have more than 300mg of caffeine daily (about equivalent to three cups of coffee).
- *Calorie intake*: A pregnant woman needs around 2,000 calories a day to feed both her and her baby in the first two trimesters and an extra 200 calories in the last trimester. Pregnancy is not a time to lose weight or restrict calories, but it is a time to eat healthily. A nutrient-rich diet will also help to ensure that breast milk quality is good, and to speed post-natal recovery. Eat plenty of fresh fruit and vegetables – five to seven portions a day. Fibre-rich foods are beans, pulses, wholegrains, brown rice, oats and dried fruit. See Chapter 6: Changing Dietary Needs for more on calorie intakes.
- *Snacks*: Make snacks as healthy as possible. Try oatcakes, a slice of wholemeal bread, a yoghurt, some dried fruit or some pumpkin and sunflower seed mixture or fresh almonds and walnuts. These will help to maintain energy levels and have good levels of nutrients such as beneficial oils, zinc, calcium and magnesium for the developing child.
- *Oily fish*: Eat one or two portions a week of oily fish, as the oils they contain are used for brain development in the

developing baby. However, as certain fish have unacceptably high mercury levels for pregnant women, they are advised to avoid shark, marlin and swordfish completely and to limit tuna to one fresh steak a week, or two cans. Fish such as mackerel, sardines, pilchards, anchovies and sea trout are fine. Salmon is also a first-rate source of omega-3s, but it may be advisable to eat wild salmon while pregnant as farmed salmon may have higher levels of contaminants.

- *Caffeine and alcohol*: Caffeine increases homocysteine levels (see page 219), a risk factor for pre-eclampsia and possibly other birth defects. Substitute caffeine-free and fruit teas and coffees for the regular sort and avoid alcohol. Herbal teas should be avoided unless you know they are safe in pregnancy. Safe teas include camomile, mint and vervaine. Dandelion and barley 'coffees' are good options.

- *Supplements*: Before and during pregnancy it is probably a good idea to take a supplement specially formulated for pregnancy as a form of health insurance; these will always contain sufficient folic acid (see above point). It is important to avoid taking a normal formula, as this may contain components that are not advised during pregnancy such as high levels of vitamin A or some herbs. Magnesium supplementation may help with muscle cramps, which are quite common in the last trimester.

- *Calcium*: No increase in calcium is needed during pregnancy above the 700mg women are advised to take normally, but it is a good idea to make sure that intakes are sufficient. During breast-feeding an extra 550mg is advised and an extra couple of plain, live yoghurts and 25g/1oz piece of cheese a day will help reach this target. Good sources of calcium include: green leafy vegetables, nuts and seeds, tinned sardines and salmon, eggs, figs, carrots, broccoli, soya beans, dates and raisins, bread and fruit such as oranges, blackberries and apples.

- *Morning sickness*: This is often a problem in the first trimester and is probably related to hormonal swings. An excellent anti-nausea tip is to drink ginger tea: grate a bit of fresh ginger root into a cup, poor boiling water over it and let it steep for about three minutes. See Nausea, page 259.

- *Fluid retention*: Some women will develop water retention problems and this should be dealt with to avoid discomfort. You should drink lots of water, avoid coffee, tea and soft drinks, and avoid salt and packaged products as much as possible (a bowl of cornflakes has twice as much salt as a packet of crisps). See Appendix II, page 357.

- *Pregnancy diabetes*: If you are at risk of pregnancy-related diabetes, cut out soft drinks, sweets and sugar (these are best minimized anyway) and indulge yourself with mixed dried apricots or prunes and nuts, yoghurt with chopped fruit, baked apples or oatcakes with 100 per cent fruit jam. This form of diabetes usually disappears, but is an early warning sign of an increased risk of diabetes later in life.

- *Food cravings*: Some say that these are signs of nutritional deficiency, but this is not substantiated. However, listen to your body and if in doubt, get your doctor to check your health. Traditional lore says that, for instance, craving for spinach or red meat may mean a need for iron, a craving to eat chalk (it does happen) could indicate a need for calcium.

- *Anaemia*: Iron deficiency during the last trimester is a possible complication, but it may not be advisable to take iron supplements or tonics unless a doctor has confirmed that iron is needed (blood volume naturally increases meaning iron is typically lower than normal). Iron is vital at this stage and may well be necessary, but an excess can interfere with zinc levels, which are equally important for growth of the baby.

- *Constipation*: The majority of pregnancy-related problems in the last trimester relate to the sheer bulk of a baby pushing up against organs, and a mother may notice heartburn and changes in bowel habits. It is best to eat little and often so as not to have too full a stomach, and if constipation is a problem, avoid added wheatbran, opting instead for gentler psyllium husks or linseeds.
- *Fluid intake*: Drink at least two litres of water or liquids a day; this will offset constipation from the baby pressing on the gut and extra liquid will be needed after the birth for milk production.
- *Pre-eclampsia*: This is a serious condition encountered by 5–10 per cent of pregnant women and your doctor will check for it. Supplementation to reduce the risk of pre-eclampsia may be advised if a previous pregnancy has been affected. Research tells us that the risk may be reduced by supplementing with vitamins C and E, selenium and possibly magnesium during the pregnancy. Supplementation needs to start as early as the 16th week of pregnancy, long before mothers who have not already had a pre-eclamptic pregnancy know they might be at risk. Pre-eclampsia is also linked to high homocysteine levels, which are controlled by taking folic acid (preferably mixed with the B-vitamins B12, B6 and B2), see Homocysteine, page 219.

## Pre-menstrual Symptoms

PMS is a cluster of symptoms, which are unified in that they occur in the time from ovulation (mid-cycle) to the onset of a period and stop when a period starts, only to return with the next cycle. It is also called Premenstrual Dysphoric Disorder, but the old term pre-menstrual tension (PMT) has fallen into disuse as this only referred to emotional symptoms.

PMS has been clustered into four main categories according to symptoms:

| | |
|---|---|
| PMS-A (Anxiety) | Anxiety, irritability, mood swings, nervous tension |
| PMS-B (Bloating) | Weight gain, abdominal bloating, breast tenderness, swelling of extremities (oedema) |
| PMS-C (Craving) | Increased appetite, craving for sweets, fatigue, palpitation, headaches |
| PMS-D (Depression) | Depression, withdrawal, lethargy, forgetfulness, confusion, insomnia |

- *Carbohydrate cravings*: Starchy or sugary carbohydrates can make you feel better, but usually only in the short term. It is most useful to regulate blood sugar imbalance by basing meals on proteins (fish, meat, eggs, cheese) and lots of vegetables, salads and fruits and small amounts of complex carbohydrates, while restricting refined carbohydrates and sugars.
- *Lignans*: Women who eat high-vegetable, wholegrain and fruit diets seem to experience less PMS, which may be related to the higher lignan (and isoflavone) content of their diets. Linseeds are particularly rich in lignans and a tablespoon daily sprinkled onto breakfast cereals can be highly beneficial.
- *Phytoestrogens*: Soya is rich in mildly-oestrogenic isoflavones, which counteract more aggressive oestrogens found in the body. Consumed at the rate of four or five portions weekly, soya can help to alleviate symptoms over time and helps slightly to increase the length between periods. This is a good thing, as it reduces the negative effects of oestrogen on body tissues and is related to lower breast cancer risk.
- *Caffeine*: High doses have been implicated in premenstrual breast tenderness. Other PMS symptoms have

been linked to high caffeine intake (four to ten cups a day of strong tea or coffee) and those with PMS may well be more sensitive to caffeine than women who are free of PMS. A trial period of three cycles without caffeine is worth trying.

- *Fish oils*: Omega-3s are strongly anti-inflammatory and a low-omega-3 fatty acids in the diet has been linked to a variety of menstrual symptoms. Two or three portions weekly can help.
- *Calcium*: A large-scale study of women taking 1,200mg calcium over two cycles had significantly fewer pre-menstrual problems such as low mood, pain, fluid retention and food cravings. See Part 4: A–Z of Nutrients page 332 for calcium-rich foods, or if taking a supplement use an easily absorbed form such as calcium citrate.
- *Magnesium*: Deficiency is commonly linked to PMS and magnesium works with calcium. It has the effect of normalizing nervous/muscular contractions, acting as a relaxant, and so seems to help nervous symptoms, pre-menstrual cramps, headaches and low back pain. Favouring magnesium-rich foods can help, but some women may need short-term (3 months) supplementation of 350mg magnesium daily.
- *Vitamin B6*: (Pyridoxal phosphate) B6 is important for serotonin and dopamine production in the brain and high oestrogen levels may lead to B6 depletion. It is also involved in magnesium metabolism. Most common symptoms of PMS have been shown in trials to be alleviated by supplementing B6; however, high doses over long periods are linked to (reversible) neuropathy side-effects. Consequently a maximum of 50mg is now advised for the long term and increasing food sources is wise.
- *GLA*: (From evening primrose oil) is a common prescription item to alleviate PMS symptoms, particularly breast tenderness and heavy periods (menorrhagia). It is

probably effective because it increases the production of anti-inflammatory compounds. However, insufficient amounts are commonly prescribed and at least 4g daily are needed for 3 months then cut back to 1g daily thereafter.

- *Herbs*: Those used to regulate PMS symptoms are chaste-berry (Vitex agnus castus), dong quai, and black cohosh (*Cimicifuga racemosa*).
- See also Endometriosis page 189, PCOS page 271 and Oedema page 201.

## Prostate Health

Most men over the age of 50 suffer some degree of enlargement of the prostate gland. The prostate is shaped like a ring-doughnut and is about the size of a walnut. It surrounds the top of the urethra (the urine duct), just under the bladder. Its job is to secrete a slightly acidic fluid, which contributes to seminal fluid and improves the viability of sperm. The two conditions of concern are BHP and prostate cancer.

### BHP (Benign prostate hypertrophy)
This is a non-malignant (non-cancerous) increase in volume in the prostate sufficient to cause problems (usually two to four times its original size). Enlargement can also be due to infection or inflammation (prostatitis). Signs of prostate problems usually come about as the urine flow is constricted through the urethra because the enlarged prostate is pinching it off. There is normally an increased urgency to urinate, but often there is reduced flow, dribbling and a feeling of not having finished. If the blockage is prolonged or total, then this needs urgent surgical attention. Serious blockage can also lead to infections, kidney damage, bladder stones or retention of urine in the blood.

## Prostate Cancer

Prostate problems often go unchecked for quite a long time as many men are embarrassed to report problems to their GP, or may even believe that they have some sort of venereal disease. Investigation involves a rectal examination and, while the majority of problems turn out to be BHP, the delay in diagnosis means that cases that turn out to be cancer are frequently diagnosed at a later stage than they could have been. PSA levels can be checked by the doctor with a blood test to assess risk of prostate cancer. It is not a perfect test and works best if taken at regular intervals to assess levels on an individual basis.

- *Hormones*: Testosterone, the male hormone, is broken down into DHT (dihydrotestosterone) and it is DHT that is the main hormonal culprit in enlarged prostate problems. It has recently been suggested that we are living in a sea of man-made oestrogens called xenoestrogens. These man-made oestrogens result from obvious sources such as the Pill and HRT being excreted into the water, but also from less obvious sources including farm chemicals and plastics. These chemical xenoestrogens are thought to increase the amount of testosterone that is converted into DHT, which is a factor in both BHP and prostate cancer.
- *Water*: Liquids are important for keeping the whole urinary tract healthy, and the temptation to cut back when experiencing difficulty urinating because of BHP is a false economy.
- *Tomatoes*: These fruits are the richest source of a powerful antioxidant called lycopene. The higher your intake of this member of the carotene family, the lower your risk of prostate cancer. Ten portions weekly of tomatoes and tomato products is the recommended amount. Interestingly,

cooked and processed tomato products (particularly when cooked with a little oil) are considerably richer sources of available lycopene than fresh tomatoes. This is because it is liberated from the 'bonds' in which it is held. Ideas for getting your weekly quota include: tomato soup; tomato sauce on pasta; tomato salad; tomato juice; tomato salsa dip; grilled or stuffed tomatoes; chopped sun-dried tomatoes on toast; canned tomatoes in stews or chillis; tomato topping on pizzas; ketchup (sugar and sweetener-free is best).

- *Soya*: Eastern men who consume soya regularly have a much lower incidence of prostate cancer (this changes when they adopt a Western diet). Soya has been shown mildly to mimic the female hormone oestrogen, with compounds called phytoestrogens, which have a beneficial effect on the prostate by interfering with the conversion of testosterone to DHT. Soya sources include: soya beans cooked and added to stews; mashed tofu added to mashed potato or other root vegetables; marinated tofu; soya milk in cooking and on cereals and soya baked beans. Soya yoghurt is indistinguishable from ordinary yoghurt and makes a delicious dessert with chopped fruit. Try adding soya flakes to muesli in the morning and make milk shakes using soya milk and silken tofu mixed with soft fruit.

- *Vegetarian diets*: Vegetarians get prostate cancer at half the rate of meat-eaters and this could be because soya beans, high-fibre diets and tomato products can be protective.

- *Saturated fats*: There is a link between high meat and animal fat consumption and the development of prostate cancer. Switching from the typical Western level of 38 per cent of calories from fat to 30 per cent has been shown to lower levels of troublesome male androgen hormones. To cut back on fat levels, favour lean meats such as skinless chicken and game over other cuts, eat more fish and low-fat dairy products (or use soya alternatives, which have healthy fats).

You can also reduce your reliance on butter, full-fat milk and processed foods, especially convenience snacks.

- *Polyunsaturated fatty acids*: Evening primrose oil (EPO), which is rich in a compound called GLA, seems to reduce the risk of BHP and prostate cancer. It may do this by stopping testosterone from adhering to prostate cells and by stopping the conversion of testosterone into DHT. Cold-pressed flax oil is rich in omega-3 essential fatty acids and this may also be helpful. Two grams of EPO or a tablespoon of flax oil daily could be a wise investment. You can even get delicious garlic and chilli flavoured flax oil now. Oily fish, such as mackerel, sardines, tuna and salmon are also rich sources of the omega-3 fats that inhibit prostate cancer.

- *Fibre*: Studies of Seventh-Day Adventist men have shown that the more fibre consumed, the greater the amounts of troublesome testosterone excreted. Seventh-Day Adventists eat high quantities of beans, lentils, peas and dried fruit, all of which are rich sources of fibre. It is easy to incorporate more beans and pulses into your diet, in familiar and tasty ways: chunky lentil soup; baked beans on wholemeal toast; hummus and other bean dips; Tex-Mex refried beans with tortillas; chickpea curry; green peas; red kidney beans in chilli; butter beans as a side vegetable; and flageolet beans added to salads.

- *Zinc*: The prostate gland is the tissue with the highest concentration of zinc in the human body. Each ejaculation uses up about two or three milligrams of zinc and the portion of seminal fluid contributed by the prostate gland is the source of this mineral. Zinc is required for producing male sex hormones and low levels may have a part to play in the change in ratio of testosterone to female sex hormones in men after the age of about 40. Men with BHP and prostate cancer routinely have lower levels of zinc than men who do not have these problems. Zinc-rich foods include most nuts (unroasted and unsalted are best), sunflower and pumpkin seeds, turkey, crab meat, soya beans and eggs. Up to fifty grams daily of pumpkin seeds, as snacks or sprinkled on dishes either whole or ground, are favoured for prostate health because they also contain healthy fats and lots of fibre in addition to the zinc. A supplement of 15mg daily may be a wise investment for prevention, but 50mg daily, over several months, has been shown in trials to return BHP to normal in 70 per cent of cases. Zinc supplements should have a 10:1 ratio with copper.

- *Selenium*: This is one of the most important antioxidant minerals, which helps to fight most cancers. It also seems to protect against the toxic heavy metal cadmium (which we get mainly from cigarette smoke and cookware) which appears to stimulate prostatic tissue in BHP. Selenium-rich foods include wheatgerm and bran, tuna, rice, tomatoes, broccoli and nuts. Two Brazil nuts daily should provide the amount needed. Smokers have a higher incidence of prostate cancer, especially if they also have low blood levels of vitamin E, which works alongside selenium.

- *Herbs*: Saw palmetto (*Serenoa repens*) is used in the prevention of BHP as it interferes with the conversion of testosterone to DHT. Studies have shown that it is effective at shrinking the prostate, without side-effects. About 300mg of standardized extract in supplement form daily is the dose that has been used successfully in several trials. There are a number of products that combine saw palmetto with zinc and EPO. Some products also contain beta-sitosterol, which is found in plant oils and is also rich in saw palmetto. Other herbs that may be included in supplements formulated for prostate health are stinging nettle extract and *pygeum africanum* extract. Parsley is a traditional remedy for BHP.

- *Sunshine*: In areas of the world where people get more sun exposure there are also lower prostate cancer levels, due to the vitamin D that we manufacture in our skin.

Supplementing with vitamin D may not necessarily have the same effect. This does not mean baking in the sun sporadically on holiday, but regularly getting half-an-hour sun exposure at times of the day when burn is least likely. Even weak winter sun can be beneficial.

- *Sex*: Men who have regular sex, or at least who ejaculate most often, are less likely to develop prostate cancer.
- *Tea*: One interesting study showed that prostate cancer cells grew more slowly when exposed to blood from tea drinkers (both black and green tea), than when exposed to blood of non-tea drinkers.

## Psoriasis

In healthy skin the superficial dead skin cells are sloughed off and replaced. In psoriasis the cells do not die off and so they build up, creating chronic scaling of the skin from high levels of keratinocytes (surface skin cells). It is a fairly common condition, affecting around 2 per cent of Western populations and usually first comes to light between the ages of ten and 30. Symptoms can vary and the scaly patches, sometimes bright red, can be anything from very small to very large plaques. Other types apart from the plaque-type are guttate psoriasis, which often starts after a throat infection in children and may not lead to plaques; erythrodermic (pustular) psoriasis, where secondary infections are a possible complication; and psoriatic arthropathy, which is a form of arthritis. There is a genetic link in about three-quarters of psoriasis cases.

Psoriasis is not the easiest condition to treat, but careful management can certainly increase the length of remission between outbreaks and reduce the severity of symptoms. Pregnancy often improves the condition, which suggests that hormonal shifts may influence the situation. Others find that psoriasis appears for the first time after pregnancy, which might suggest that nutritional deficiencies, stress or tiredness – exacerbated by pregnancy – are involved. Standard treatments can include ultraviolet light (this helps some, but worsens the condition in others), emollient creams, coal tar extract and anti-inflammatory medication. Stress is a frequent trigger and keeping stress levels under control can help.

- *Fish oils*: This is the most promising help for psoriasis. Eating two or three portions weekly will help, but the quantities needed probably mean taking supplements, around 2 or 3g daily.
- *Saturated fats*: These contain arachidonic acid, which is pro-inflammatory and can tip the balance away from the anti-inflammatory effects of fish oils. Eating up to three fish meals a week will reduce reliance on saturated fats from meat and one or two vegetarian based meals can help improve the balance. Other sources of saturated fats are butter, cheese, semi-skimmed and full-fat milk. Hydrogenated fats should also be avoided and are found in convenience foods and some margarines. See Chapter 2: Healthy Fats.
- *Antioxidants*: These are needed for healthy skin. Eating at least five portions of fruits and vegetables daily should help.
- *Food intolerances*: These can sometimes be involved in exacerbating symptoms. Gluten is a relatively common culprit, as is dairy.
- *Alcohol*: Alcohol and smoking can induce flare-ups.
- *Selenium*: Those with psoriasis were shown to have low selenium status in several trials, which would suggest that supplements might be effective. Yet trials supplementing selenium in psoriasis have had mixed and not very encouraging results, however, these were small trials and some for fairly short periods of time. It is unlikely to be detrimental to eat two Brazil nuts daily and it may indeed be beneficial.

- *Bee products and olive oil*: Steroid doses were reduced by 75 per cent in one study that asked those with eczema or psoriasis to put a mixture of honey, olive oil and beeswax on outbreaks on one side of their bodies three times daily and inert substances on the other side as a control. Honey and olive oil have antibacterial properties, and contain flavonoids and antihistamine compounds. The mixture can be made at home using equal parts of the three ingredients.
- *Water*: As with any dry skin condition, hydration is important for psoriasis.

## Raynaud's Syndrome

This is extreme sensitivity of the fingers and toes to cold, due to the small arteries in the extremities constricting, thus cutting off the blood supply. Symptoms are numbness and tingling, and sometimes pain and a burning sensation, accompanied by a whitish colour to the fingers and toes. As circulation is restored the extremities take on a blueish colour, followed by a bright red colour. Women are more susceptible to Raynaud's than men. Occasionally it can be caused by repetitive movement over the long term, such as is involved in typing or playing the piano, but mainly it relates to atherosclerosis, blood clotting disorders, rheumatoid arthritis, lupus and certain drugs such as beta-blockers. Smoking dramatically limits the blood supply to the extremities – easily seen on a heat-sensitive scan – and so should be stopped. It is also important to avoid sudden changes in temperature and to wear gloves and thick socks when needed.

- *Blood thinning*: Omega-3 fatty acids from oily fish help to keep the blood flowing by reducing blood stickiness. Garlic is another blood thinning agent and one clove daily included in cooking helps.

- *Ginger*: This spice has a warming effect and can be taken in teas or used in salads, or in cooking.
- *Vitamin C and its flavanoids*: Flavonoids and vitamin C from fruits and vegetables, particularly the flavanoid rutin found in orange pith, improves vascular integrity.
- *Herb*: Gingko biloba has been used in trials to reduce the number of attacks in Raynaud's, and may be enhanced if used alongside garlic and ginger.
- *Magnesium*: This mineral has anti-spasmodic effects on the arterial system and vitamin E supplements as a blood thinning agent. Magnesium levels are low in winter in those with Raynaud's.

## Rhinitis

See Hay Fever and Allergic Rhinitis, page 212.

## Salt Restriction

See Appendix II, page 357.

## Seasonal Affective Disorder (SAD)

SAD (Seasonal Affective Disorder) is a problem for large numbers of people in the Northern Hemisphere. It is a strictly seasonal event, in autumn and winter, which is what distinguishes it from other problems. Common symptoms are depression, anxiety, sleep problems, extreme tiredness and lethargy and a tendency to overeat. Other symptoms include loss of libido, mood swings, pre-menstrual syndrome, comfort eating, palpitations and a low resistance to stress. Symptoms are relieved in the spring when days begin to get longer. The standard treatment for SAD is full spectrum light-boxes, which help around three-quarters of those affected. Full spectrum light includes ultra violet light, which can penetrate the skin sufficiently to trigger vitamin D production – indoor lighting cannot do this. Those with SAD are also advised to make a point of getting out of doors during the daytime, whatever the weather, to increase their exposure to light.

- *Antioxidants*: Light increases levels of the hormone melatonin, which governs our wake/sleep cycles and is probably disturbed in those with SAD. Whilst light is the most important element, a diet rich in antioxidants also boosts melatonin levels. Antioxidants are found in vegetables, fruits, legumes such as beans, dark green olive oil, tea, green tea, rosehip tea, red bush tea and good quality chocolate.
- *Fish oils*: Countries where the most fish is eaten suffer from the lowest levels of SAD. Iceland, which has high oily fish consumption and is a Northern Hemisphere country, has much lower rates than similar countries with lower fish consumption.
- *Comfort eating and cravings*: Increased eating, comfort eating and carbohydrate cravings are common effects of SAD. If carbohydrate cravings are a problem, then following an eating plan that minimizes this by featuring proteins, vegetables, fruits and limited amounts of grains will help to control the cravings. Others with SAD do not crave carbohydrates, but crave protein instead. Identifying your eating pattern is the first step to dealing with this. Eating too many fatty proteins without sufficient vegetables can make you feel sluggish. Cravings for alcohol, coffee, sugar and chocolate are also common.

- *Diary*: Keeping a diary of meals eaten and the response to meals can help. Over a few days, keep a diary when eating protein-based meals (with vegetables, but not with dense carbohydrates such as potato, bread, rice or pasta), or a carbohydrate meal (eating the previously mentioned carbo-hydrates with vegetables and fruits, but avoiding dense proteins such as meat, eggs or cheese). Record the effect on your moods:

  - Note if you feel any of the following: alert, calm, refreshed, relaxed, energetic, enthusiastic, able to concentrate
  - Or the following: lethargic, tired, 'woolly' brained, anxious, depressed, agitated, tearful.

By understanding your emotional response to foods and the effect on your energy levels, you can better choose meals that make you feel lively during the daytime and sleepy towards evening, thus improving the natural rhythms and cycles.

## Schizophrenia

See Behavioural Disorders, page 127.

## Sinusitis

Sinusitis is inflammation of the sinuses leading to a blocked feeling and sometimes post-nasal drip. If the inflammation is severe, pain can refer down to the teeth – dentists are com-monly called upon for toothache that turns out to be sinusitis. In severe cases involving bacterial infection antibiotics may be needed. Travelling in an airplane or driving at high altitudes in mountains with blocked sinuses can be very painful. Inhaling steam over a basin of boiling water with a towel over the head (taking care not to burn) can provide short-term relief and loosen mucus very effectively.

- *Food Intolerances*: Wheat and dairy intolerances are often implicated in recurrent sinusitis problems. Diary intolerances tend to be mucus producing, making the situation worse.
- *Garlic*: This herb has natural antibiotic properties and when included regularly in the diet (one clove a day) has a preventive effect.
- *High-histamine drinks*: Wine and beer can bring about sinusitis in sensitive people, as the histamine increases inflammation.
- See also Hay Fever and Allergic Rhinitis, page 212 and Otitis Media, page 264.

## Skin, Hair, Nails

Hair, nails and the top layer of skin are all dead, but spring from live tissue. The quality of the live basal tissue determines the quality of skin, hair and nails. After making nutritional changes, a reasonable amount of time is needed to see a difference in the quality of these tissues. Skin takes around six weeks to replace itself, nails between two and six months, and hair grows at around the rate of one inch (2.5 centimetres) per month. Hair-loss patterns are largely governed by genetics and scarring of skin, or trauma to nail beds, are likely to result in long-term damage.

- *Fruits and vegetables*: Vitamin C is vital for collagen manufacture and repair. Eating vitamin C-rich foods helps skin health. Betacarotene, found in orange coloured fruits and vegetables and in dark green leafy vegetables, is converted into vitamin A. Both nutrients are needed for skin and mucus membrane health.

- *Collagen damage*: A low-GI diet (see Appendix I page 350) is protective of many of the effects of ageing. Sugars interact with collagen, causing glycosylation (damage). This is visible in skin as the collagen cross-links, robbing it of its natural elasticity. Age spots (lipofuscin) are caused by skin pigment getting trapped in cross-linked collagen fibres. Copper is a mineral needed for melanin pigment formation, which protects against sun damage and protects collagen and ellastin, making skin springy and youthful looking. (See Travel Advice, page 375 for more information on protection against the sun.)

- *Silica*: This mineral is important for hair and nails. In skin it maintains the structure between collagen and elastin fibres and prevents cross-linking. It is found in beer, oats, muesli, parsley and certain mineral waters (Fiji and San Pelegrino) in good quantities. The herb Horsetail is an excellent source of silica, selenium and zinc and supplements formulated for hair and nail health usually include this herb.

- *Zinc and essential fatty acids*: These are necessary for skin health and are vital to reduce scarring after operations. Both promote wound healing. Good dietary sources are in Part 4: A–Z of Nutrients, page 331, but if healing needs to be promoted as an urgent measure, such as for a burn or an operation, then supplements may be advised.

- *Fungal infections*: These can usually be helped by following the recommendations for Candida (see page 146). Tea tree oil applied topically can help.

- *Dandruff*: Rinse your hair with rosemary, sage or thyme steeped in hot water for ten minutes.

- See also Acne, page 102, Eczema, page 186 and Psoriasis, page 287.

# Sleep

Sleep is vital for optimal health and allows the body to repair tissues. In particular, children need sufficient sleep, but often do not get it as their routine is not fully established and they play computer games and watch television late at night. Good sleep hygiene includes: getting to bed at a similar time each night, at least one or two hours before midnight; being physically active during the day, but not exercising just before bed (as this boosts metabolism); avoiding over-stimulating television late at night; and finding ways to reduce sources of anxiety or stress. Some children diagnosed with ADHD resolve their behavioural problems when taught good sleep hygiene. Adults do not all need the same amount of sleep and older people often need less than younger people. This can cause anxiety, which in turn leads to interrupted sleep, as people believe they 'need' a certain amount of sleep.

- *Late-night eating*: During sleep, digestion is quiet – in fact since a meal takes about four hours to digest, and we rarely allow that much time between meals and snacks, night-time is the only time when food is not being digested. Digestion takes up lots of energy and so this reduction on the call on energy reserves allows this energy to be diverted to repair and maintenance activities. This is one of the reasons why it is unwise to eat a heavy meal late at night.
- *Shift work*: Night-shift work and eating at the wrong times interrupts normal circadian rhythms. Shift workers have twice the incidence of peptic ulcers. Structured light, carbohydrate-based meals is best, avoiding ad-hoc snacking on high-fat foods.
- *Blood sugar*: A common reason for waking in the middle of the night is poor blood sugar regulation. If this is the case,

keep a small snack such as half a banana or an oatcake easily to hand to eat if needed.

- *Alcohol*: Alcohol is often used as a nightcap, which can be a mistake. A small drink may make you feel soporific and relaxed and may be beneficial. However, even a moderate amount more than this can severely interrupt sleep patterns. While you may get to sleep, alcohol interferes with the ability to enter deep REM sleep, which means that you stay at the more fitful, and less deep, level of dreaming sleep.
- *Caffeine*: This drug is well known for interfering with sleep. Even those who think that they are acclimatized and can tolerate caffeine, find that giving up – after the initial 'withdrawal' period – makes a great difference to their sleep patterns. Caffeine is found in coffee, tea, dark chocolate, guarana (a herb) and some medications (such as headache pills).
- *Oats and calcium*: Oats have a long traditional history as a soporific herb. Calcium also has a calming effect on the nervous system. This is why oat-based milky drinks have been used for centuries as a nightcap. However, most popular modern products are also very high in sugar (much more than in the past), which has a stimulating effect. To make a nightcap, use very finely milled oats, warm milk (or calcium-enriched milk substitute such as soya milk) and a teaspoonful of honey.
- *Herbs*: Valerian is the herb most widely used to aid sleep without the side-effects of other sleep remedies.
- *Lettuce*: Lettuce, raw or juiced or taken as the herb wild lettuce, has a long-standing reputation for promoting sleep. It is high in an alkaloid, lactucarium, which has similar properties to opium. If taking juice, mix with a little lemon juice for flavour.
- *Weight*: Snoring is often exacerbated by excess weight.

## Smoking Cessation

Smoking-related diseases include heart disease, stroke and cancer, but smokers who give up in their thirties avoid most of the risks of smoking-related diseases and quitting at 50 still halves the risks. Smoking cessation options are mainly nicotine-based therapies such as gum, patches and inhalators. While these devices might deal with the immediate chemical addiction, they don't address the underlying addictive tendency, nor do they help to resolve some of the damage that smoking has inflicted. While nicotine is the addictive compound in cigarettes, it is not the most harmful ingredient. There are around 4,000 other compounds in cigarette smoke such as arsenic, carbon monoxide, hydrogen cyanide and formaldehyde, which are highly toxic. Some people find that counselling, acupuncture and hypnotism work. Regular, brisk exercise helps to alleviate cravings by releasing endorphins.

● *Blood sugar.* The most important strategy is to balance blood sugar levels. It doesn't help that cigarette manufacturers add sugary compounds such as sucrose, caramel, sorbitol, maple syrup and honey, to low-tar cigarettes. Smoking raises blood sugar levels by triggering stress hormones, and when these levels fall, this increases the desire for another cigarette. This yo-yo assault on blood sugar is one reason why so many ex-smokers exchange one fix, tobacco, for another, sweets, when they give up. The way to maintain even blood sugar levels is to concentrate on eating wholegrains such as wholemeal bread and brown rice, vegetables and proteins, and to avoid sugary drinks, snacks and cereals, refined carbohydrates such as white bread and rice, and caffeine-laden drinks and alcohol. See Appendix I Glycaemic Index, page 350.

- *Alcohol*: This is a natural accompaniment to smoking and it is best to avoid situations that the smoker associates with having a cigarette. Many people light up when they have an alcoholic drink or a coffee. Sticking to herbal teas such as green tea or peppermint, or a drink of tonic and angostura bitters, helps to avoid the habitual link.

- *Dairy*: Excessive use of dairy products can be curbed to reduce the mucus that builds up when you first quit.

- *Fruits and vegetables*: An antioxidant-rich diet that features fruits and vegetables can help to undo some of the damage. Smokers need about twice the amount of vitamin C as non-smokers, as smoking actively destroys this nutrient. In countries where there is a high consumption of fruits and vegetables, such as Greece, Italy and Spain, it is noticeable that though many people are heavy smokers, there is a surprisingly low incidence of heart disease when compared to countries where smokers eat less fruits and vegetables.

- *Supplements*: Smokers should not take an antioxidant supplement that includes betacarotene, as this has been linked to increasing the risk of fatal cancer – though betacarotene from foods is likely to be beneficial and should probably be emphasized.

- *Herbs*: Medical herbalists have a number of possible aids to stopping smoking, though these should not be self-prescribed. Lobelia, also called Indian tobacco and only available via herbalists, has the active compound lobeline, which is sufficiently similar to nicotine to make the transition to giving up tobacco easier. Wild oats, *Avena sativa*, have a calming effect on the mind and *Acorus culamus* was used by miners in times gone by to keep their lungs clear (though it should not be used for long). St John's wort helps to ease the depression and low moods associated with giving up nicotine. Levels of the brain chemicals serotonin and dopamine fall when people quit smoking and it is possible that St John's wort may go some way to alleviating this.

## Stress

There are many types of stress and often they work together to compound health problems. Each person's reaction to stresses is different, depending on their personal make-up. If a person is prone to headaches, backache, eczema, or digestive upset, then that is how stress is likely to manifest. Such symptoms are usually a strong hint that some lifestyle changes may be needed. Ignoring the stress is usually detrimental in the long run. We subject our bodies to many different types of stress: emotional, lifestyle (having too much to do, lack of sleep, over-exercising, under-exercising, etc.), pollution (smoking, living in cities, chemicals used in the home), and nutritional stresses (relying on stimulants, sugar, high fat diets, salt, etc.), and these can have a compound effect. From a nutritional perspective there are several important means of reducing the effects of stress on the body.

- *Anti-stress nutrients*: When we feel stress we produce stress hormones, which have an evolutionary role to play in protecting us. This is called the 'fight or flight' syndrome. Because it is an emergency reaction, the rush of adrenaline takes priority over other body processes. For instance, the digestion of food shuts down at this time, which is one reason why so many digestive disturbances are linked to stress. Stress hormones use up large amounts of vitamin C, zinc, magnesium and B-vitamins as a priority. Because these nutrients are so important for healing skin, producing energy and other body functions, when they are diverted to deal with stress these other functions begin to break down. This makes it easy to understand why stress is also involved in conditions such as poor wound healing, eczema, psoriasis and low energy levels. Eating foods rich in these nutrients can offset some of this. See Part 4: A–Z of Nutrients, page 332 for sources of these nutrients.

- *B-vitamins*: These are considered the main anti-stress nutrients, as they are needed for smooth nerve function and are also required by the adrenal glands. As most are water soluble, they need to be replenished daily. Eating a bowl of fortified cereal can help, plenty of wholegrains and liver occasionally (unless pregnant).

- *Caffeine*: Reaching for the coffee pot is a common reaction to stress, but caffeine increases adrenaline levels beyond that normally experienced in the stress reaction. This makes it harder to normalize hormone levels and can lead to a feeling of jitteriness, so caffeine is best avoided. Calming drinks to substitute include vervaine herbal tea, camomile and oat drinks.

- *Sugar*: This is a stimulant and again is commonly eaten to offset feelings of stress. Eating foods low on the Glycaemic Index (see Appendix I, page 350) is more beneficial.

- *Antioxidants*: If under constant stress, then this will take a toll on the body by increasing oxidation damage. Eating plenty of antioxidant rich fruits and vegetables can help to offset this.

- *Time to eat*: When stressed it is common to eat on the run. However, as digestion is rarely working well when stressed, this compounds any problems of poor digestion and absorption. Taking the time to eat calmly can help to break this cycle and provide a welcome break in the day.

- *Herbs*: Herbalists use a group of herbs called adaptogens for times of stress. These help the body to adapt to the demands of stress and to balance stress hormone output. Ginseng is a well known adaptogen and Ashwagandha is gaining popularity, as it is so effective. Valerian is calming and can help to induce sleep.

- See also Chapter 5: Food and Mood, and Depression, page 171.

## Stroke

Strokes are part of a group of problems that are included in the general term cardiovascular disease (see Heart Disease, page 216). Ischaemic stroke happens when the brain does not receive enough oxygen, usually due to a blood clot. Strokes can also involve the vasculature leaking blood into the brain. Congenital weaknesses in the vasculature can lead to strokes when no other risk factors for cardiovascular disease are present. Strokes are life-threatening events that can also lead to severe disability. Immigrants to the West quickly take on the stroke incidence of their adopted country, which suggests lifestyle and diet are important factors. Smoking, high blood pressure, diabetes and irregular heart beat are all important risk factors for stroke.

- *Other countries*: The 'Mediterranean Paradox' is that people in countries such as Spain, Italy and France have only one-third of the risk of coronary events, including stroke, as Northern European countries such as Denmark and the UK. This has been put down partly to the overall differences in diet, including fish consumption, olive oil, fruits and vegetables. In Finland over a 20-year-period, they experienced a dramatic drop in the mortality rate, by around 50 per cent, from strokes when public health measures were taken to improve diet, including recommending the eating of fresh fruits and vegetables (especially including berries).

- *Fruits and vegetables*: A diet high in fruits and vegetables is important to reduce the risk of stroke. These are good sources of vitamin C, which strengthens arteries. The flavonoids they contain are also protective against stroke.
- *Salt*: High salt intake is a major determinant of increased blood pressure, which is linked to stroke, and also independently a risk factor for stroke. Potassium acts to oppose the negative effects of sodium (from salt) and again fruits and vegetables are dietary sources of potassium. The higher the potassium intake, the lower the risk of stroke.
- *Omega-3s*: Oily fish consumption is important for keeping blood thin and preventing strokes. However, those at immediate risk of stroke should avoid fish supplements, as they can thin the blood too much and increase the risk of cerebral haemorrhage.
- *Homocysteine*: High homocysteine levels are probably linked to risk of stroke, and stroke shares many risk factors with heart disease. For information on homocysteine, see page 219.
- *High cholesterol*: There may be a link between high cholesterol levels and stroke. See Cholesterol, page 149.
- *Alcohol*: Excess alcohol intake has a strong link to stroke, while a little (one or two modest-sized glasses daily for men and post-menopausal women) may be protective, much more than this increases risk. The risk goes up dramatically with binge drinking.
- *Metabolic syndrome*: Insulin resistance, reflected by waist-to-hip ratios and blood sugar regulation problems, increases the risk of stroke (see page 251).

## Sugar Intake and Sugar Substitutes

See Appendix 1, page 349.

## Syndrome X

See Metabolic Syndrome, page 251.

## Taste, Loss of (Ageusia)

Loss of taste (ageusia) can severely impact on nutritional status, particularly in the elderly, in whom loss of taste is common. It makes the person less interested in fresh delicately flavoured foods and people then often compensate by using too much salt. Smoking is a common cause of loss of taste. Chemotherapy can also induce differences in taste perception. Loss of taste is closely linked to smell, and a cold can induce short-term loss of taste.

- *Salting food*: Avoid salting food as a response to loss of taste. This creates a vicious cycle, where the taste buds are further blunted and expect more salt. Use a seaweed grinder, or get into the habit of using herbs, which can help to reduce a dependency on salty foods. Excess salt is a major cause of high blood pressure and so can induce additional problems. The taste of fresh foods is impaired by excessive use of salt and it may take a couple of months to begin to enjoy unsalted foods – initially they taste bland, but eventually the subtleties of delicate flavours wins through. See Appendix II: Salt: Reducing Intakes, page 357.
- *Zinc*: A sign of zinc deficiency is loss of taste. This is easily corrected with the use of 10-15mg zinc daily (ensure that the zinc supplement has a 10:1 ratio to copper). Zinc-rich foods may be preferred by those who wish to avoid supplements; however, zinc is also needed to produce digestive enzymes, which liberate zinc from proteins. In a deficiency

state, this system may not be working correctly, which is common in the elderly.

- *Sense of smell*: The senses of smell and taste are closely linked. Blocked sinuses, or a nose that is frequently blocked, will impair taste sensation. For Allergic Rhinitis and Hay Fever, see page 212.

## Thyroid, Overactive

Symptoms of an excess of thyroid hormones include hyper-activity, rapid pulse, palpitations, sweating, weight loss, period problems and bulging eyes. Hyperthyroidism often runs in families and is more common in women than in men. Medical treatment often impairs the thyroid gland, to the point where the opposite – hypothyroidism – results.

- *Iodine*: Avoid supplements that include iodine, iodized salt and kelp.
- *Goitrogens*: Increase your intake of goitrogens, which interfere with thyroid hormone function. Goitrogenous foods are: the cruciferous family (broccoli, cabbage, cauliflower, Brussels sprouts, turnip, swede and cress), soya beans and peanuts.
- *Stimulants*: Reduce any dependency on stimulants such as coffee, strong tea and caffeinated fizzy drinks, which can worsen hyperactivity and nervousness. Drink Rooibosch (red bush) tea, which is naturally caffeine-free but is a source of fluoride. This may block iodine receptors in the thyroid gland.
- *Speedy metabolism*: An elevated metabolic rate means that nutrients are used up that much more quickly. It is then more important to eat nutrient-rich foods such as fruits and vege-tables, and possibly also to take a multi-vitamin/mineral supplement.

- *Antioxidants*: Graves disease is the most common cause of hyperthyroidism. Antioxidant supplements (vitamin C, E, betacarotene and selenium) seem to normalize thyroid function faster when taken in addition to medication, compared to medication alone.
- *Herbs*: Various herbs have adaptogenic properties, which help the body to adapt to stressful situations. If considering these, it is best to consult a medical herbalist, who can help you make the correct choice of the numerous herbs available. Avoid the herb, and the confectionery, liquorice.

## Thyroid, Underactive

The thyroid gland, located in the neck, produces thyroxin (T4) a hormone that, with its active version tertroxin (T3), controls metabolism. It does this by controlling the rate at which glucose is used by cells. So important is the thyroid hormone to the health of every cell that it is tested for at birth in all babies. A lack of thyroid hormone leads to a slowing down of all body processes: symptoms include fatigue, drowsiness, feeling cold, weight gain and skin thickening. Thyroid disease affects about one in 100 people. There are several possible reasons for thyroid problems, including disease, auto-immune problems (where the immune system attacks the gland) and a reduced ability to convert one hormone into the other. If suspected, a doctor will run several tests looking for TSH levels (which are elevated when the thyroid is underperforming), T4, possibly T3 and possibly thyroid antibodies. There are several possible nutritional aspects to thyroid insufficiency. Subclinical hypothyroidism is now recognized as a condition, which is monitored to see if it develops into a condition that needs thyroid hormone treatment.

- *When iodine may help*: One of the major forms of thyroid insufficiency relates to iodine deficiency. This has largely ceased to be a problem in the West, due to iodized salt and iodine cleaning machinery used in food production, but it still prevails in mountainous areas of the world with low iodine levels. These areas are called 'goitre belts', due to the manifestation of iodine deficiency as goitre, or enlarged neck due to an overgrown thyroid gland. In developed countries goitre is more likely to be a result of auto-immune disease. Nevertheless, iodine deficiency is making a comeback, probably because of complacency due to the belief that this is a problem that has previously been conquered. There is particular concern that pregnant women should get sufficient iodine, as thyroid insufficiency can impact on the foetus. The richest sources of iodine are iodized salt, seaweed (kelp), fish, milk and bread (the iodine comes from the cleaning of the machinery), meat and eggs (the iodine comes from supplementation given to promote livestock health) and even sea air (living by the coast ensures about 15-20mcg iodine intake daily).
- *When to avoid iodine*: If a person has previously been more seriously iodine deficient but moves to an area of high iodine intake (or starts taking iodine supplements), this can lead to thyrotoxicosis. This in turn leads to an overactive thyroid – a condition called Jod-Basedow.
- *Foods which don't help*: Goitrogens are vegetables containing glucosinolate compounds, which interfere with thyroid function. In cases of thyroid insufficiency these foods should be eaten in moderation, perhaps only three or four times weekly in total. Goitrogenous foods include the cruciferous family (broccoli, cabbage, cauliflower, Brussels sprouts, turnip, swede and cress), soya beans (fermented soya is fine) and peanuts. Cooking partly destroys goitrogens. It is important not to completely

avoid vegetables from the cruciferous family, as they have such potent anti-cancer properties (see Cancer, page 142).

- *Selenium and zinc*: Where T4 is not being adequately converted to T3 (the active hormone), this can be a 'hidden' reason for an apparently underactive thyroid where tests seem to show otherwise. This can be helped by eating the daily recommended amounts of selenium and zinc. Both are involved in the enzymes responsible for the conversion. The liver is instrumental in the conversion from one hormone to the other and improving liver health may be a good idea (see page 238).

- *Fluoride*: If too much is ingested from toothpaste, mouth rinses and fluoridated water, this may interfere with thyroid function.

- *Vitamin A*: An underactive thyroid impairs the conversion of betacarotene (from orange coloured fruits and vegetables such as apricots, cantaloupe melon, carrots and peppers) into vitamin A. Signs of vitamin A deficiency may include poor skin health or poor vision.

## Ulcers – Leg

Leg ulcers are open sores that resist healing and are a common problem with ageing. They are linked to poor circulation in the lower limbs and are a particular problem with diabetes. A blocked artery, varicose veins and poor lymphatic drainage can all be linked to leg ulceration. In these circumstances a leg ulcer can be triggered by as small an injury as a scratch. Standard treatment includes compression stockings, keeping legs propped up when sitting or lying to encourage drainage away from the area and using anti-bacterial creams or powders.

- *Water*: Despite the tissues often being affected by oedema (accumulated fluids), drinking plenty of water – up to two litres daily – is an important measure. This helps to 'flush' through and restore correct hydration. In bedridden elderly nursing home residents, just the simple measure of leaving a full glass of water by the bedside – thus making drinking water constantly available and within easy reach (i.e. not in a jug that has to be poured out and that the frail can find difficult) – had the effect of dramatically improving bed-ulcer healing.

- *Vitamin C*: This nutrient is vital for repairing skin tissue, as it is involved in collagen formation. Vitamin C-rich fruit and vegetables, such as citrus, kiwi, strawberries, blackcurrants, broccoli, cabbage, peppers, cauliflower and Brussels sprouts are important.

- *Zinc*: This is also essential for skin and wound healing. In the elderly, mineral absorption can be impaired, so while it helps to increase dietary zinc, a multi-supplement with 100 per cent of the RNI for zinc is advised. Zinc paste bandages are available from doctors.

- *Omega-3s*: Oily fish twice a week, or fish oil supplements, helps to thin the blood and improve circulation. If you are already taking blood-thinning medication, do not take supplements without consulting your doctor, but favour dietary oily fish instead.

- *Manuka honey*: This particular honey applied to the wound (not eaten) is a standard and highly effective treatment for leg ulcers in Australia and New Zealand. It has strong antibacterial properties, even against *Staphylococcus aureus*, the skin bacteria superbug, but also hydrates the skin and stimulates skin growth. It is applied under bandages and dressings and changed three times daily. This treatment should be supervised by a medical practitioner.

# Ulcers – Oral, Gastric and Duodenal

Ulcers in the upper part of the digestive tract can cause symptoms of indigestion or a burning sensation. The environment of the stomach is extremely acid and the stomach lining is normally protected from this by a thick layer of mucus. In the duodenum (the first part of the small intestines, just after the stomach) alkaline digestive juices normally de-acidify the food mass as it passes through. Virtually everyone with gastric or duodenal ulcers is infected with the bacteria *Helicobacter pylori*. *Helicobacter* burrows into the mucus lining, which allows the acidity to damage the lining. *Helicobacter* protects itself from the acid by secreting alkaline ammonia. Standard treatment involves antibiotics to eliminate the bacteria infestation, along with acid-reducing medication.

- *Mouth ulcers*: These can be linked to a generally poor nutritional status, particularly deficiency of the antioxidant nutrients, vitamins A, C and E, which protect mucus membrane health. Some are caused by sodium lauryl sulphate (SLS), a foaming agent found in most toothpastes (sodium *laureth sulphate* is a slightly different compound). SLS is the same compound used in industrial cleaning agents and it can damage the delicate membranes in the mouth of sensitive people. Mouth ulcers can respond favourably to regular consumption of cranberry juice (choose a sugar free version such as Biona, though you should avoid drinking fruit juices separately from meals, as they are sugary anyway) and chewable liquorice tablets (not the confectionery, but those available from health food shops). Both of these combat *Helicobacter pylori*. Good quality tea tree oil rubbed onto gums affected by gingivitis and onto ulcers can also speed up healing. For more, see Mouth Ulcers, page 256.

- *Cranberry juice*: Cranberry contains a potent bacterial anti-adherent. In addition to its better known ability to stop the bacteria that causes cystitis from clinging to the urinary tract, it has the same effect on *Helicobacter* in the stomach.
- *Manuka honey*: This is a specific honey that comes from New Zealand. It has a proven track record of being able to kill off *Helicobacter* (as well as the super-bug MRSA). Four teaspoons, four times daily, on an empty stomach, is the recommended dose. However, make sure you buy a certified product that has sufficient bio-active effects.
- *Bowel bacteria*: Probiotic bacteria found in live yoghurt (*Bifidobacteria* and *Lactobacillus acidophilus*) inhibit the growth of *Helicobacter*. Supplements containing probiotics are another alternative.
- *Herbs*: Slippery elm, fenugreek tea, peppermint oil and diluted aloe vera juice all help to heal ulceration. Do not use ginger if you have stomach or duodenal ulcers.
- *Shift workers*: Shift workers have twice the incidence of peptic ulcers, probably due to eating at times of the 24-hour cycle when digestion is not geared up to receiving food. Have structured, light, carbohydrate-based meals and try not to snack on high-fat foods.
- See also information on ulcerative colitis, page 157.

## Varicose Veins

Varicose veins are caused by the valves in leg veins collapsing, causing a pooling of blood in the veins. Valves in the veins are there to keep the blood moving upwards to return it to the heart against the force of gravity. When the valves collapse in superficial veins, the blood pools and the vein can become dilated and twisted, which is easy to see. Other symptoms are tired legs and swollen ankles and legs. If left untreated, varicose eczema can develop – dry, itchy skin resulting from poor circulation to the area – and this can lead in turn to ulceration (see page 309). Pregnancy increases the risk of varicose veins. Varicose veins can also develop in the groin area in pregnancy, and haemorrhoids (also called piles) are varicose veins in the rectum area. Support stockings can help to keep legs comfortable and reduce the progression of the problem. Elevating legs whenever possible helps, for instance adding a wedge or pillow under the bottom of the mattress at night.

- *Weight*: If excess weight needs to be lost, this is important to reduce progression of the problem.
- *Hydration*: Sufficient hydration is important and drinking up to two litres of water daily is advisable.
- *Fibre*: Dietary fibre is important to avoid haemorrhoids (see page 363 for further advice).
- *Thinning blood*: Blood flow can be improved by eating oily fish regularly, two or three times weekly. Garlic is another important agent to improve blood flow – add one clove to cooking daily.
- *Fruit*: The flavanoids in the pith of citrus fruit, rutin and hesperidin, help to strengthen blood vessels, as does vitamin C, so when you eat citrus fruit, avoid peeling away every last bit of pith. Flavonoids in dark red berries also have a similar effect of strengthening blood vessels.
- *Herbs*: Creams containing horsechestnut and gotu kola massaged into the area of varicose veins help to strengthen veins and capillaries.

## Vegetarianism and Veganism

A vegetarian avoids meat, fish and fowl and their by-products. The advantages of a well-planned vegetarian diet include

lower saturated fat intake and more fibre for a healthy digestive tract. It will do no harm, and probably a lot of good, for
everyone to eat a vegetarian meal at least once or twice a
week. Some people describe themselves as vegetarians but eat
fish, so are really 'fishitarians'. These diets are virtually identical, or superior, to meat eating.

Vegans avoid all animal products, including eggs and dairy,
and sometimes honey.

Those following a vegan diet need to be careful that their
children get sufficient calories and nutrients. Vegan diets can
be very bulky because a lot of plant food is eaten, but since
children have small appetites this can fill them up without
quite providing sufficient calories. It is therefore important to
provide sources of fat, including fortified vegan margarines,
vegan milks, nuts and seeds and their oils, and avocadoes.

● *Important nutrients*: Meat in the diet is an easy way of obtaining iron, zinc (both very commonly deficient) and vitamin-
B12, which are needed for blood and brain function, growth
and bone health. Oily fish provides vitamin D, as well as
essential fats and selenium – all of which are, in any event,
commonly deficient in the average diet and not just in vegetarians.

● *Vitamin B12*: There are no sources of very absorbable B12
   in a completely plant-based diet. B12 is important for a
   number of functions: making protein, DNA and RNA for
   cell division, the myelin insulating sheath that protects
   nerves and brain tissue, and working with folic acid to lower
   homocysteine (see page 219). Vegans should ensure they
   eat B12-enriched margarine and soya milk to compensate.
   Vegetarians can obtain B12 from eggs and dairy.

● *Iron absorption*: Serve a source of vitamin C, such as a small
   glass of orange juice, a portion of vitamin-C rich fruit (kiwi,
   strawberries, blackcurrant, citrus) or vegetables (peppers,

broccoli, cabbage, Brussels sprouts) with plant-based meals. This doubles the absorption of iron from plant sources. Vegetarian sources of iron are much less absorbable than from meat and this simple step helps to overcome this problem. The most common sign of iron-deficiency anaemia is being pale or listless. An inability to concentrate may also be a sign to watch out for (see Anaemia, page 115).

- *Protein*: From a nutritional viewpoint, meat protein sources are easily replaced with vegetarian sources of protein such as beans, lentils, peas, chickpeas, nuts, seeds, eggs and dairy, which provide valuable iron and zinc. Plant protein sources provide most, but not all, of the amino acids (protein building blocks) and need to be combined with grains (wholegrain rice, wholewheat, corn, etc.) for the other necessary amino acids. (However, it is not essential that these are eaten at the same meal.) This is why classic vegetarian dishes feature both elements, such as beans and rice or beans and tortilla.

- *Omega 3s*: Oily fish such as mackerel, sardines, salmon and fresh (not canned) tuna provide omega-3 fats for brain and immune health. Vegetarian sources of fats in the same family include flax, walnut, hemp and canola oil, which can be added to dishes, and eating pumpkin seeds and walnuts is a good idea. However, while these fatty acids are metabolized (inefficiently) to EPA, they are not converted to DHA. Vegetarian source DHA (but not EPA) is from algae and supplements are available (see Chapter 2: Healthy Fats page 17 for an explanation of DHA and EPA).

- *Soya*: While this is a good source of lean protein, avoid giving too much to children, as an excess may affect hormonal balance. A modest portion, three to four times a week is fine for children, and five portions weekly for adults.

- We get vitamin D from exposure to sunlight. In winter and if regularly covered up (as is common with some ethnic groups) and fish is not eaten, fortified margarine should be used and vitamin supplements are usually needed.

## Vegetarian catering

Meat-eating parents of vegetarian children or teenagers can find the prospect of catering healthy meals somewhat daunting, especially if they are concerned about the child achieving sufficient nutrition. Vegetarian cooking does not require any special skills and often it is straightforward simply to substitute one ingredient for another – for instance making a Shepherdess pie (beans, mushrooms and vegetables in a rich tomato sauce with a potato crust) instead of a Shepherd's pie, or a vegetable-based spaghetti sauce. Other simple ideas include pea or lentil soup with crusty bread, Caribbean rice and bean dishes, potato, cheese and vegetable pie, mild bean and vegetable curry, bean burgers, hummus dip or spread on sandwiches, pea and vegetable samosas, falaefel (made from packet mix) or egg dishes. Vegetarian foods to keep available include:

- Soya dairy alternatives: milk, cheese, yoghurt, cream, desserts
- Quorn or soya mince to substitute for minced meat
- Protein sources such as beans (baked, butter, flageolet, pinto, chickpeas), lentils (ideal for soups and casseroles) and tofu (available in a range of flavours and textures such as dips and for kebabs)
- Rice and pasta are good sources of energy. Other dried grains such as oats, corn and millet. Also potatoes, yams and sweet potatoes
- Vegetable stock cubes, bouillon or yeast extract (though all of these are too salty for babies). Tomato or garlic purées add lots of flavour
- Nuts and seeds are very nutritious. Ground nuts can be added to dishes such as pesto, nut butters (such as almond)

can be used as spreads and tahini (sesame paste found in hummus) are some suggestions

- Products that are suitable for vegetarians carry the vegetarian society symbol on packages.

## Non-vegetarian foods

Foods which might easily trip up the good intentions of a vegetarian, or someone catering for a vegetarian, include:

- All stock cubes other than vegetable
- Worcestershire-style sauces which can contain anchovies
- Animal fats can be found in pastries, cakes, biscuits and desserts – check the labels
- Non-vegetarian cheese can contain animal rennet from calves' stomachs
- Gelatine used in jellies, sweets and some biscuits. Products are available using non-animal gelling agents and vege-gel is a good option when making jellies from fruit juice, as it also helps to avoid the colourings that are common in jellies. Gelatine can also be found in drinks containing beta-carotene (not in foods containing betacarotene). Many supplements, especially fat-based ones are encased in gelatine
- Finings, used to clarify apple juice, may not be suitable for vegetarians.

## Weight-loss Diets

This is one of the ongoing problems in nutrition. In earlier times the science of nutrition concerned itself with the problems of under-nutrition in vulnerable groups – particularly children, the elderly and the underprivileged. Now, in the West exactly these groups, and all other groups in between, have the opposite problem – of over-nourishment. At least in terms of choices of foods and calories, as we live in a time of plentiful supply of food. The race is on to find a successful weight-loss system – and most people would like to find one that does not have to over-restrict food intake! To this end, we now have a wide range of available diets: low fat, low carbohydrate, high carbohydrate, high protein, and so on. Advocates for one system over the other will 'prove' their viewpoint very convincingly.

Whichever way you look at it, if you are prone to putting on weight, it is undoubtedly easier to put weight on than to lose it. In the controversial film *Super Size Me*, Morgan Spurlock, for one month, only ate the food available at a major fast food outlet. He gained 11.4kg (25lbs) in that time, but it then took him 14 months to lose the weight, even though his partner is a vegan chef. At the same time, his skin became blotchy, he became depressed, headachy and lost his sex drive. His doctor implored him to stop the experiment as his cholesterol rose to dangerous levels and his liver became fatty. Two things obviously ultimately happened: his metabolism adjusted to the new weight, which explained why it took so long to shift; and he became severely deficient in vitamins and minerals, resulting in the symptoms he experienced.

So which diet is the best weight loss diet? We will probably, in the course of time, find that different individuals with different genetic make-ups respond to different diets and that the 'one-diet-fits-all' approach is naïve. Having said this, by restricting one major nutrient group (usually fat or carbohydrates), as most of the following diets do, it is inevitable that calories are also restricted, and it is the calorie equation that is most likely to have an effect, however it is achieved. Calories-in need to equal calories-out. In other words, either calorie intake has to be restricted, or exercise levels increased, or – preferably – both need to happen at the same time. The significant difference in the success of each approach as outlined below is probably to do with what suits a person's individual metabolism and lifestyle, and which approach is likely to be easiest to stick with in the long term.

Weight-loss diets should not be used when you are pregnant or breast-feeding. Calorie restriction, or restriction of any food group, should also be used with great caution in children, as they need energy and nutrients for growth and development. It is more appropriate, usually, to look at the quality of foods they eat, the amount of sugar, possibly of fat, and levels of physical activity.

## Calorie counting

### Main approach

Sticking to calorie intakes that are less than energy (calorie) expenditure. It is recommended that a woman of average weight and height eats 2,000 calories daily, and that a man of average weight and height eats 2,500 calories daily. A low-calorie weight loss programme will usually entail eating around 10–20 per cent less calories. Some well-known weight loss clubs work with a points system that assigns points to particular foods and makes calorie counting easier. Low-calorie diets, below 1,300 calories (for women) are usually not advised, as they overly restrict nutrient intakes. Very low-caloric diets have been used with success for extremely obese individuals (around 800–1,000 calories), but this should never be attempted without supervision by a registered dietician who specializes in this approach and who can monitor for potential adverse health effects and the risk of eating disorders and nutritional deficiencies.

### Advantages

Negative energy balance can be further enhanced by exercising (see Exercise below).

### Disadvantages

One of the main problems with low-calorie diets is that they can signal the body to hang on to excess fat by down-tuning metabolism. This can make it difficult for some people to maintain weight loss and people often have to battle with the 'plateau' effect, where weight ceases to be lost for a while, and which can result in a loss of motivation. Exercise can help to counter this. Low-calorie products are often low in fat, but have increased levels of sugar to compensate (see Low-Fat diets below). Calories are not the only thing at stake and eating healthily is just as, if not more, important. Therefore eating a chocolate bar instead of three pieces of fruit will give a similar calorie count but will not aid weight loss or be a healthy approach.

### Evidence to back it up

Calorie counting has the most research behind it and it is an approach that usually works. But the number of calories is not the only factor (see Evidence to back it up in Low-GI Diet below).

## Low fat

### Main approach

How low is low fat? It is certainly not 'no fat' (which would be very unhealthy, as we need a certain amount of fat to function). Generally, low fat is under 30 per cent of calories from fat: in the 20–29 per cent range. Most people on a Western diet eat 35–38 per cent of calories from fat. A woman eating 2,000 calories daily will need to eat 70 grams of fat to get 30 per cent of her calories from fat, and a man eating 2,500 calories daily will need to eat 95 grams of fat to get 30 per cent of his calories from fat. To eat less than 30 per cent of calories from fat, amounts lower than 70g and 95g need to be eaten daily. Fat counts are given on many packaged foods in grams. Keeping a tally of fat eaten in grams is the easiest way to achieve this goal. Fat quantities in fresh foods are to be found in tables readily available. All the following give 5 grams of fat: 25g/1oz avocado, 1 teaspoon any oil, butter, margarine or mayonnaise, 8.5–2.5g/⅓–½ oz cheese, ½ one egg yolk, 70–100g/2.5–4oz very lean poultry or meat, 310ml/10 fl oz semi-skimmed milk (skimmed has almost none), 2 teaspoons nuts, seeds or nut/seed butters, 1 scoop ice cream.

### Advantages

Fat is energy dense (provides a lot of calories). Fat provides 9 calories per gram, while protein and carbohydrate provides around 4 calories per gram. Avoiding fat means that more of other foods can be eaten for the same calorie count. If done properly, this should lead to an increase in high-fibre, low-fat foods such as fruits, vegetables, pulses and grains.

### Disadvantages

Fat is very satiating and avoiding fat in favour of carbohydrates will not suit some people, as it will trigger the desire to eat refined carbohydrates more often. Commercially produced low-fat foods are often fairly high in sugar, as sugar replaces fat for taste and 'mouth feel'. This can put foods on a collision course with the low-GI approach (see below). Reducing fat too much without paying attention to the quality of the fat could result in deficiency of the essential fatty acids (vital to health in the same way that vitamins are). Nuts, seeds, their oils and oily fish provide essential fatty acids.

### Evidence to back it up

There is fairly good evidence, as societies that eat little fat, such as those on traditional Eastern diets and rural African diets, are rarely overweight or obese. However, societies that eat higher-fat diets, such as some Mediterranean countries, while having more overweight people also have low incidences of what we consider to be fat-related health problems, such as heart disease and some cancers. At stake is likely to be the quality of the fats and not just the quantity. High-fat diets will probably pre-dispose to overweight, but the quality of the fats will protect from, or predispose to, disease.

## High-carbohydrate

### Main approach
A high-carbohydrate diet features bread, rice, pasta, vegetables and fruit, restricts fat intake and keeps a normal protein intake. In essence these end up with the same dietary profile as low fat (see above).

### Advantages
High-carbohydrate diets that feature high-fibre foods tend to be satisfying, as they are bulky.

### Disadvantages
The types of carbohydrates are important for health and focusing on fresh foods and complex carbohydrates is important. See Low GI below.

### Evidence to back it up
In one study, a high carbohydrate diet that did not restrict calorie intake found that participants ate more than 2,200 calories daily, 63 per cent from carbohydrates and only 18 per cent from fats (very low fat). Foods and supplements provided up to 60 grams of fibre. Participants did not feel hungry, they had more food than they could eat, and they lost about 5 kgs and body fat over 12 weeks. Metabolic rates did not decrease.

### High fibre

*Main approach*
A daily fibre intake of around 30–35 grams of fibre is the basis for this diet. Average daily fibre intakes are about 9–12 grams, while the UK health authorities advise around 18 grams. The US health authorities advise around 25 grams.

*Advantages*
High-fibre foods arc highly satiating (curb food cravings). Fibre, particularly soluble fibre found in fruits, vegetables, pulses and oats, is important for a healthy bowel.

*Disadvantages*
Switching from a low-fibre to a high-fibre diet too quickly can lead to adverse digestive symptoms, including bloating, constipation, trapped wind and, in severe cases, blockages. It is advised that slow increments of between 2–5 grams daily be added to the diet each week – if adverse effects are noted, eat a little less fibre and build up more slowly.

*Evidence to back it up*
There is a lot of evidence to tell us that high-fibre diets are beneficial for cutting cholesterol levels, stabilizing blood sugar, cutting the risk of some cancers and helping weight reduction. On average, those who consume 25 grams of fibre daily weigh 3.5 kilos (8 lbs) less than those who eat 12 grams.

### Food combining

*Main approach*
Foods classified as 'dense' protein foods (such as meat, eggs, fish, cheese) are not eaten at the same time as 'dense'

carbohydrate foods (such as bread, rice, pasta, potatoes). They are eaten separately from each other, but each can be combined with vegetables or salads. This means that a meal would consist of, for example, meat and vegetables/salad, or potato and vegetables/salad. But the meal would not consist of meat *and* potatoes and vegetables/salad. Additionally, fruits are eaten separately from other foods and given time to digest (they pass through the stomach quite quickly when no other food is present). Therefore a meal might consist of a piece of fruit, with about 20 minutes allowed for digestion, followed by the main course. Four hours is allowed for a protein meal to digest before eating again, and two hours for a carbohydrate meal. The theory behind this approach is to work with the digestive system and the different digestive juices that are produced along the length of the digestive tract. Some well-known diet plans allow for red days and green days (protein days and carbohydrate days) to make it an easier system to follow.

### Advantages
By restricting what foods can be eaten and when, almost inevitably less food is likely to be consumed.

### Disadvantages
It is an approach that requires some knowledge in terms of how to apply it. In practice it is not too difficult and, if eating out for instance, it is easy to leave the rice or potatoes on the side uneaten.

### Evidence to back it up
This approach has little or no scientific evidence to back it up; however, many people swear by this approach and find that it helps digestion, bloating and weight loss.

## Low carbohydrate

### Main approach

Low carbohydrate diets have become popular recently. Normal carbohydrate intakes are around 300 grams per day. A low-carb approach is around 80–100 grams of carbohydrates per day. Some very-low carbohydrate diets (also sometimes called high-protein/fat diets – see below) start off at 20 grams of carbohydrates daily during the induction phase of about 2–4 weeks, and then build up carbohydrate levels slowly until the individual tolerance level is found. Very low-carbohydrate diets aim to trigger ketogenesis, a state where the body is no longer able to draw on the very limited stores of sugar (in the form of glycogen stored in muscles and the liver), forcing it to use fat stores as fuel, a process that produces ketones used for energy. A ketogenic diet has less than 20 grams of carbohydrates daily.

### Advantages

Cravings for carbohydrates are quickly subdued. Despite often being described as a high-fat diet, in practice this is not the case, as it is hard to eat too much fat in the absence of carbohydrates. This means that after an initial high-fat phase for a week or two, fat levels drop to normal levels quite quickly.

### Disadvantages

Fibre levels can be too low on this approach and it is advised that a fibre supplement, such as ground psyllium husks, is taken to compensate. Low fruit intake is likely to result in low intakes of antioxidants, which is a concern. It is unknown what the effects on bone health are, in the long term, of such a diet.

### Evidence to back it up

When compared to low-fat diets, low-carb diets seem to be more successful in the first six months, with participants losing more weight. However, over a year this evens out and those on low-carb diets don't lose further weight, while those on low-fat diets continue to lose weight slowly. At the end of a year, the amount of weight loss seems to be about the same. What does seem to give low-carb the edge over low-fat at the end of a year is that those on low-carb have better blood triglyceride (fat) levels and for many, HDL-cholesterol profiles are improved.

## High protein/high fat

### Main approach
This is, for all intents and purposes, the same as a low-carbohydrate diet. However, some of the more relaxed low-carbohydrate diets do at least permit a middling range of carbohydrates, while more stringent low-carb diets work on the basis of very little carbohydrate. In practice this means they are more high protein/fat. See above for more information.

### Advantages
Cuts cravings for carbohydrates quite quickly, as the fats that accompany proteins are very satiating (reduces cravings).

### Disadvantages
Not advised in cases of kidney disease. Such a diet may be difficult to stick to over the long term. Choosing healthier fats is advised, therefore eating more oily fish instead of meats (especially cured meats) is sensible.

### Evidence to back it up
See low-carbohydrate diets above.

## Low GI (Glycaemic Index)

*Main approach*
Eating foods at the lower end of the GI scale (see Appendix I, page 350) instead of foods at the higher end of the GI scale.

*Advantages*
Foods from all food groups are included and substitutions can be made with practice.

*Disadvantages*
Taken purely at face value, a food such as a chocolate bar is lower on the GI than a fruit such as watermelon. Interpreted in this way the approach would result in no weight loss, probable weight gain, and an unhealthy diet. Followed correctly, it will probably work for most people.

*Evidence to back it up*
In one study two groups ate a low-calorie diet. One group ate high-GI foods such as bread and potatoes within their calorie count. The other group (who were eating exactly the same amount of calories and balance of proteins and fats) ate low-GI foods such as lentils, pasta, porridge and corn (instead of the bread and potatoes). After 12 weeks the low GI group had lost 2kg (4.4 lbs) more than the high GI group (9kg versus 7kg). So for the same effort they lost more weight, and the defining difference was the insulin levels measured between the two groups.

## Exercise

*Main approach*
The other factor in any weight-loss equation is activity levels. We are increasingly sedentary, with many labour-saving

gadgets and pastimes such as TV-watching. Our forbears had to be very active in their every day lives and so there was no need to 'exercise'. It is recommended that children get one hour of physical activity daily and adults at least half-an-hour of exercise daily if of normal weight, and one hour if overweight. Calories burned per hour by various activities are:

| Number of calories | Activity |
| --- | --- |
| Under 100 | Sitting, Standing |
| 100–150 | Driving a car |
| 150–200 | Strolling |
| 200–250 | Bowling, gardening (moderate) |
| 250–300 | Gardening (strenuous), swimming, golf |
| 300–350 | Brisk walking, dancing |
| 500–600 | Jogging, tennis |
| 600–650 | Cycling |

### Advantages
Exercise does not necessarily mean going to the gym. Movement can be incorporated into everyday life, including walking, cycling and housework. Regular physical activity is linked to an improvement in outcome for almost all health problems.

### Disadvantages
A regular exercise regime requires consistency of approach. Medical advice must be sought before starting an exercise programme if you have medical problems, particularly heart disease, joint or back problems or are already diagnosed with osteoporosis.

### Evidence to back it up
Studies show that exercise, even in the absence of dieting, leads to weight loss. In one study, middle-aged individuals,

over three years, increased their exercise levels without altering diet. They took two to three months to work up to their assigned activity levels, and the minimum was equivalent to walking for 30 minutes daily. This led to a 2kg weight loss, which while it may not sound like much, was statistically significant. More activity led to more weight loss. At the same time, physical activity improves fat/muscle ratio, and leaner body mass has an improved metabolic rate. Depending on the type of exercise undertaken, cardiovascular health can also be improved.

## Weight, Overweight

One in four people in the UK are overweight or obese. Overweight is a risk factor for heart disease, diabetes and some cancers. Too much weight increases pressure on supporting joints (hips, knees and ankles) as well as making surgery more risky. It is more difficult to lose weight as we age, as muscle to lean tissue ratios change unfavourably. If you are overweight, it is ideal to lose the excess slowly; however, if this is not manageable, it is important to compensate by staying fit and, at least, walking fairly briskly for half-an-hour each day.

BMI refers to Body Mass Index. It is the (fairly crude) device used to work out if a person fits into the normal, underweight or overweight ranges. It works most of the time, but if someone is not of typical build then the figures can be skewed: it is said that the actors Danny de Vito and Arnold Schwarzenegger, who have starred together on film and who have totally different body fat/lean ratios both would work out to have the same BMI of 30+.

To work out your BMI (for adults, not for children):

|  | EXAMPLE | YOUR STATISTICS |
| --- | --- | --- |
| Your height in metres | 1.60m | |
| Your weight in kilograms | 63kg | |
| Times your height by itself | 1.60 x 1.60 = 2.56 | |
| Your weight divided by the answer to the sum above (2.56 in the example) | 63kg / 2.56 = 24.60 | |
| BMI: The answer is | 24.60 | |

A BMI of less than 20 is in the underweight range.
A BMI of 20–25 is in the healthy range.
A BMI of 25–30 is in the overweight range.
A BMI of 30–40+ is in the obese range.

BMIs are not used for children. Instead, there are centile charts available from doctors and health visitors to work out if the child's height and weight are normal for the child's age and if they are growing normally.

## Waist-to-hip Ratio

Apple shapes (android) have more risk of health problems than pear shapes (gynoid). Men are more typically apple shape and carry weight around their middles; women tend to move from pear shape, where they carry weight around their hips, towards apple shape as they progress past the menopause.

To find your waist-to-hip ratio, divide your waist measurement by your hip measurement (both in centimetres).

| Example |
| --- |
| Waist = 75cm |
| Hips = 100cm |
| Waist to Hip ratio – 75/100 – 0.75 |

Women are classified as apple-shaped if the waist to hip ratio is greater than 0.85, while men are classified as apple-shaped if their waist to hip ratio is greater than 0.95.

## Weight, Underweight

To assess if you are underweight, work out your BMI with the information on page 328. If a sudden loss of weight is experienced for no apparent reason, consult your doctor as a priority in case it is a symptom of a more serious condition. Underweight is a risk factor for reduced fertility in women, and when severely underweight periods can stop altogether (amenorrhoea) as production of hormones is interrupted. This is nature's way of protecting against the demands of a developing baby on an undernourished body (see Fertility, page 195). Underweight is also a risk factor for Osteoporosis (see page 261). Putting on weight, if prone to underweight, can be surprisingly difficult. Resistance weight training can be needed over at least a year to make a difference to muscle mass. Underweight in the elderly is a common problem – see Ageing page 106.

- *Healthy eating*: If you are aiming to put on weight, it is desirable to put on lean as well as fat tissue and so healthy eating is just as important – low-nutrient, high-calorie foods such as sweets, crisps and pastries are adverse to health. High-calorie foods that are nutrient-dense include full-fat milk, cheese, avocadoes, nuts, seeds, vegetable dishes cooked in olive oil and oily fish.
- *Cachexia*: Weight loss as a result of illness, for example in cancer patients, needs careful handling and your medical team should advise. Omega-3 fatty acids have a good track record of aiding weight gain in cachexic patients.
- See also Eating Disorders, page 184.

# PART 4:

# A–Z OF NUTRIENTS, SIGNS OF INSUFFICIENCY AND FOOD SOURCES

Overt nutrient deficiency diseases, such as scurvy resulting from vitamin C deficiency or anaemia resulting from iron deficiency, are well established. More insidious are vague signs of nutritional insufficiency, which might manifest in a variety of possible symptoms, some of which are listed here. Of course, symptoms could be due to other causes and it is important to get a correct diagnosis from your doctor. Just one symptom is unlikely to indicate insufficiency or deficiency, but a cluster might lead to increased suspicion. Biochemical tests (blood, serum, sweat, saliva) can be done by a doctor or suitably trained nutritionist to assess actual status.

Good food sources of these nutrients are also listed. As ever, a well-balanced diet features a wide variety of foods.

## Minerals

### Calcium
Possible signs of insufficiency:

- Osteoporosis
- Tooth decay
- Nervous tension
- Insomnia
- High blood pressure
- PMS
- Poor wound healing

Good sources:

| Source | Average serving | Amount of mineral per serving | Amount per 100g food |
|---|---|---|---|
| Almonds | 10 | 25mg | 240mg |
| Bread | 1 slice | 35mg | 135mg |

| Source | Average serving | Amount of mineral per serving | Amount per 100g food |
|---|---|---|---|
| Broccoli | 50g | 28mg | 56mg |
| Cheddar cheese/Edam | 25g | 180mg | 720mg |
| Chickpeas | 50g | 35mg | 70mg |
| Chocolate, milk | 10g | 24mg | 48mg |
| Figs | 25g | 65mg | 260mg |
| Greens/spinach | 25g | 45mg | 180mg |
| Legume beans | 100g | 128mg | 128mg |
| Milk | 100ml | 120mg | 120mg |
| Molasses | 10g | 50mg | 500mg |
| Orange | 1 | 60mg | 47mg |
| Sardines, canned | 35g | 175mg | 540mg |
| Salmon, canned | 50g | 50mg | 100mg |
| Sesame seeds, whole (i.e. dark tahini) | 10g | 120mg | 1,200mg |
| Prawns | 50g | 55mg | 110mg |
| Tofu | 60g | 300mg | 510mg |
| Whitebait/sprats | 50g | 290mg | 860mg |

## Chromium

Possible signs of insufficiency:

- Insulin resistance or diabetes
- Sugar cravings
- Need for frequent meals or snacks
- Feeling cold
- Need for sleep or drowsiness in daytime
- Frequent excessive thirst

Good sources:

| Source |
|---|
| Beans/pulses |
| Brewer's yeast (best source) |
| Brown rice |

| Source |
| --- |
| Liver |
| Meat and chicken |
| Nuts |
| Rye bread |
| Shellfish |
| Wholegrains |

*NB: Nutrition charts do not quantify amounts*

## Iron

Possible signs of insufficiency:

- Pallor of skin tone
- Listlessness
- Heavy menstruation
- Poor concentration
- Reduced resistance to infections
- Poor appetite
- Mouth ulcers, sore tongue, cracks at the side of the mouth
- Hair loss

Good sources:

| Source | Average serving | Amount of mineral per serving | Amount per 100g food |
| --- | --- | --- | --- |
| Beef | 50g | 2.5mg | 5.0mg |
| Liver | 50g | 4.4mg | 8.8mg |
| Mussels | 40g | 3.0mg | 8.0mg |
| Sardines | 35g | 1.5mg | 4.5mg |
| Chicken, light meat | 50g | 0.3mg | 0.6mg |
| Chicken, dark meat | 50g | 0.95mg | 1.9mg |

*NB: The most absorbable form of iron is found in meats*

| Source | Average serving | Amount og mineral per serving | Amount per 100g food |
|---|---|---|---|
| Apricots, dried | 25g | 1.2mg | 4.8mg |
| Baked beans | 200g (small can) | 3.0mg | 1.5mg |
| Beetroot | 25g | 0.3mg | 1.2mg |
| Bran flakes | 30g | 6.0mg | 20.0mg |
| Chickpeas | 50g | 1.75mg | 3.5mg |
| Cocoa powder | 10g | 1mg | 10.0mg |
| Figs, dried | 2 | 1.25mg | 4.2mg |
| Molasses | 10g | 2mg | 20.0mg |
| Mushrooms, raw | 25g | 0.2mg | 0.8mg |
| Rice, brown, boiled | 50g | 0.25mg | 0.5mg |

*NB: Plant sources are not as well absorbed but, quantity-wise, provide most of our iron*

## Magnesium

Possible signs of insufficiency:

- Heart palpitations
- Muscle cramps or spasms
- Tension headaches
- Muscle twitching (e.g.: around the eyes)
- PMS
- Nervousness/irritability
- Wheezing
- Insomnia
- Constipation
- High blood pressure
- Pre-eclampsia in pregnancy
- Osteoporosis

Good sources:

| Source | Average serving | Amount of mineral per serving | Amount per 100g food |
|---|---|---|---|
| Bread, white | 50g | 12mg | 24mg |
| Bread, wholemeal | 50g | 38mg | 76mg |
| Brussels sprouts, boiled | 50g | 7mg | 14mg |
| Peanuts | 25g | 48mg | 190mg |
| Okra, boiled | 50g | 28mg | 56mg |
| Brown rice, cooked | 50g | 20mg | 40mg |
| Legume beans | 100g | 50mg | 50mg |
| Millet, cooked | 50g | 60mg | 120mg |
| Muesli | 50g | 45mg | 90mg |
| Prawns | 40g | 25mg | 63mg |
| Sardines in tomato sauce | 50g | 25mg | 50mg |
| Taco shells | 25g | 26mg | 104mg |
| Weetabix | 2 | 50mg | 120mg |

## Selenium

Possible signs of insufficiency:

- Frequent infections
- Low thyroid hormone function
- Fertility
    Women: spontaneous abortions
    Men: sperm motility problems
- Asthma
- Acne
- Family history cancer
- Pre-eclampsia

Good sources:

| Source | Average serving | Amount of mineral per serving | Amount per 100g food |
| --- | --- | --- | --- |
| Baked beans | 200g (small can) | 4µg | 2µg |
| Bread | 50g | 3µg | 6µg |
| Brazil nuts | 2 | 40µg | 254µg |
| Cashews | 25g | 9µg | 34µg |
| Chicken | 50g | 4µg | 8µg |
| Clams (cockles) | 25g | 12µg | 48µg |
| Cornflakes | 50g | 2.5µg | 5µg |
| Fish, white | 50g | 15µg | 30µg |
| Molasses | 10g | 14µg | 140µg |
| Mushrooms, cooked | 25g | 3µg | 12µg |
| Rice, white, cooked | 50g | 2µg | 4µg |

## Zinc

Possible signs of insufficiency:

- Frequent infections
- Poor wound healing
- Impaired digestion
- Acne
- Depression
- Stretch marks

Good sources:

| Source | Average serving | Amount of mineral per serving | Amount per 100g food |
| --- | --- | --- | --- |
| All Bran | 30g | 2mg | 6mg |
| Bran flakes | 30g | 0.8mg | 2.5mg |
| Bread, wholemeal | 2 slices | 1.3mg | 1.6mg |
| Cheddar cheese | 25g | 1mg | 4mg |
| Chickpeas, cooked | 50g | 0.6mg | 1.2mg |

| Source | Average serving | Amount of mineral per serving | Amount per 100g food |
|---|---|---|---|
| Lentils, cooked | 50g | 0.7mg | 1.4mg |
| Muesli | 50g | 1mg | 2mg |
| Oyster | 1 | 8mg | 80mg |
| Popcorn | 25g | 2mg | 8mg |
| Sardines | 35g | 1mg | 3mg |
| Sunflower seeds | 25g | 1.2mg | 5mg |
| Steak | 50g | 1.7mg | 3.5mg |
| Walnuts, shelled | 30g | 1mg | 3mg |

# Water-soluble Vitamins

## B-vitamin group

Possible signs of insufficiency:

- Low energy
- Difficulty concentrating/poor memory
- Cardiovascular disease
- High alcohol intake
- Depression/anxiety/irritability
- Neuropathy or 'prickly legs'

Good sources:

### Thiamine (vitamin B1)

| Source | Average serving | Amount of vitamin per serving | Amount per 100g food |
|---|---|---|---|
| Bacon, grilled | 25g | 10.7mg | 0.43mg |
| Bran flakes | 35g | 0.3mg | 1.0mg |
| Chips, homemade | 100g | 0.24mg | 0.24mg |
| Fortified cereals | 35g | 0.3mg | 1.0mg |

| Source | Average serving | Amount of vitamin per serving | Amount per 100g food |
|---|---|---|---|
| Kidney | 15g | 5.3mg | 0.32mg |
| Liver | 50g | 0.13mg | 0.26mg |
| Marmite | 10g | 0.32mg | 3.2mg |
| Oats, raw | 15g | 0.15mg | 0.9mg |
| Peas | 50g | 0.13mg | 0.26mg |
| Pork chop | 100g | 0.66mg | 0.66mg |
| Potatoes, boiled | 100g | 0.18mg | 0.18mg |
| Quorn | 50g | 18.3mg | 36.6mg |
| Lentils, cooked | 50g | 0.5mg | 0.11mg |
| Wholemeal bread | 50g | 0.17mg | 0.34mg |

## Riboflavin (vitamin B2)

| Source | Average serving | Amount of vitamin per serving | Amount per 100g food |
|---|---|---|---|
| Beef | 100g | 0.33mg | 0.33mg |
| Cereals, fortified | 35g | 0.43mg | 1.3mg |
| Cheddar cheese | 25g | 0.1mg | 0.40mg |
| Chicken, lean | 100g | 0.19mg | 0.19mg |
| Eggs | 1 | 0.11mg | 0.35mg |
| Liver | 50g | 2.2mg | 4.4mg |
| Marmite | 10g | 1.1mg | 11.0mg |
| Mushrooms, cooked | 50g | 0.17mg | 0.34mg |

## Niacin* (vitamin B3) (* equivalent)

| Source | Average serving | Amount of vitamin per serving | Amount per 100g food |
|---|---|---|---|
| Beef | 100g | 3.6mg | 3.6mg |
| Chicken, lean | 100g | 8.2mg | 8.2mg |
| Cod | 100g | 1.7mg | 1.7mg |

| Source | Average serving | Amount of vitamin per serving | Amount per 100g food |
|---|---|---|---|
| Pork chops | 100g | 5.7mg | 5.7mg |
| Potatoes | 100g | 0.5mg | 0.5mg |
| Wheatgerm | 25g | 1.12mg | 4.5mg |
| White bread | 50g | 0.85mg | 1.7mg |
| Wholemeal bread | 50g | 2mg | 4.1mg |

## Vitamin B6

| Source | Average serving | Amount of vitamin per serving | Amount per 100g food |
|---|---|---|---|
| Baked beans | 200g | 0.28mg | 0.14mg |
| Banana | 100g | 0.29mg | 0.29mg |
| Beef | 100g | 0.3mg | 0.3mg |
| Brussels sprouts | 50g | 0.1mg | 0.19mg |
| Chicken | 100g | 0.26mg | 0.26mg |
| Cod | 100g | 0.38mg | 0.38mg |
| Turkey | 100g | 0.32mg | 0.32mg |
| Oranges | 1 | 0.03mg | 0.10mg |
| Potatoes | 100g | 0.33mg | 0.33mg |
| Wheatgerm | 25g | 0.8mg | 3.3mg |
| White bread | 50g | 0.03mg | 0.07mg |
| Wholemeal bread | 50g | 0.06mg | 0.12mg |
| Yam | 50g | 0.06mg | 0.12mg |

## Vitamin B12

| Source | Average serving | Amount of vitamin per serving | Amount per 100g food |
|---|---|---|---|
| Beef | 100g | 2.0µg | 2.0µg |
| Cereals, fortified | 35g | 0.56µg | 1.7µg |
| Cheese | 25g | 0.27µg | 1.1µg |
| Cod | 100g | 2.0µg | 2.0µg |

| Source | Average serving | Amount of vitamin per serving | Amount per 100g food |
|---|---|---|---|
| Eggs | 1 | 0.83µg | 2.5µg |
| Liver | 50g | 2.0µg | 81.0µg |
| Liver pate | 25g | 1.8µg | 7.2µg |
| Marmite | 10g | 0.05µg | 0.5µg |

## Folic acid

| Source | Average serving | Amount of vitamin per serving | Amount per 100g food |
|---|---|---|---|
| Almonds | 10g | 4.8µg | 48µg |
| Broccoli | 35g | 21µg | 64µg |
| Brussels sprouts | 50g | 55µg | 110µg |
| Cereals, fortified | 35g | 83µg | 250µg |
| Eggs | 1 | 13µg | 39µg |
| Chick peas, cooked | 50g | 27µg | 54µg |
| Legume beans | 50g | 105µg | 210µg |
| Lettuce | 25g | 14µg | 55µg |
| Peanuts | 25g | 28µg | 110µg |
| Peas | 50g | 13µg | 26µg |
| Potatoes | 100g | 26µg | 26µg |
| White bread | 50g | 30µg | 29µg |
| Wholemeal bread | 50g | 20µg | 40µg |

## Vitamin C

Possible signs of insufficiency:

- Low energy
- Poor wound healing
- Frequent infections
- Bleeding gums
- Easy bruising
- Nose bleeds

Good sources:

| Source | Average serving | Amount of vitamin per serving | Amount per 100g food |
|---|---|---|---|
| Branflakes | 35g | 8.3mg | 25mg |
| Beetroot | 25g | 2.5mg | 10mg |
| Blackcurrants | 25g | 32.5mg | 130mg |
| Brussels sprouts | 50g | 30mg | 60mg |
| Cabbage, cooked | 35g | 6.6mg | 20mg |
| Cabbage, raw | 35g | 16.3mg | 49mg |
| Cauliflower, cooked | 35g | 9mg | 27mg |
| Citrus | 80g | 24–44mg | 30–55mg |
| Kiwis | 80g | 48mg | 59mg |
| Liver/kidney | 50g | 5mg | 10mg |
| Mango | 80g | 31mg | 37mg |
| Orange juice | 80g | 32mg | 39mg |
| Peppers, raw | 80g | 96mg | 120mg |
| Potatoes | 100g | 10–25mg | 10–25mg |
| Raspberries | 80g | 25mg | 32mg |
| Strawberries | 80g | 60mg | 77mg |
| Tomatoes | 80g | 14mg | 17mg |
| Watercress | 35g | 20mg | 62mg |

## Fat-soluble Vitamins

### Vitamin A
Possible signs of insufficiency:

- Poor night-time vision
- Frequent infections
- Mouth ulcers
- Acne
- Dry flaky skin
- Dandruff
- Thrush/cystitis
- Diarrhoea

Good sources:

| Source | Average serving | Amount of vitamin per serving | Amount per 100g food |
|---|---|---|---|
| Butter/margarine, fortified | 10g | 83µg | 830µg |
| Cod liver oil | 1 tsp (5ml) | 900µg | N/A |
| Cheddar | 50g | 160µg | 320µg |
| Cream cheese | 30g | 130µg | 433µg |
| Egg | 1 | 110µg | 330µg |
| Herrings | 50g | 50µg | 100µg |
| Liver | 50g | 20,000µg | 40,000µg |
| Milk, whole | ¼ pt/140ml | 75µg | 50µg |
| Yoghurt, whole milk | 150g | 45µg | 30µg |

## Betacarotene

This water-soluble nutrient converts to vitamin A in the body. Possible signs of insufficiency are similar to vitamin A but it also has its own functions as an antioxidant. It is best utilized from foods cooked or processed with a little fat.

Good sources:

| Source | Average serving | Amount of nutrient or betacarotene per serving | Amount per 100g food |
|---|---|---|---|
| Apricots | 80g | 400µg | 500µg |
| Cabbage | 35g | 333µg | 1,000µg |
| Cantaloupe melon | 80g | 1,360µg | 1,700µg |
| Carrots | 80g | 10,400µg | 13,000µg |
| Guava | 50g | 200µg | 400µg |
| Kale | 25g | 750µg | 3,000µg |
| Lettuce, average | 50g | 500µg | 1,000µg |
| Mange tout | 50g | 300µg | 600µg |
| Mangoes | 80g | 560µg | 700µg |

| Source | Average serving | Amount of nutrient or betacarotene per serving | Amount per 100g food |
| --- | --- | --- | --- |
| Passion fruit | 40g | 280µg | 700µg |
| Plums | 80g | 280µg | 350µg |
| Spinach, boiled | 50g | 3,250µg | 6,500µg |
| Spring greens, raw | 50g | 4,000µg | 8,000µg |
| Sweet potato | 50g | 1,950µg | 3,900µg |
| Tomatoes, fried | 50g | 250µg | 500µg |

## Vitamin D

Possible signs of insufficiency:

- Poor balance
- Rheumatism
- Osteoporosis
- Tooth decay
- Joint pain/stiffness
- Muscle cramps

Good sources:

| Source | Average serving | Amount of vitamin per serving | Amount per 100g food |
| --- | --- | --- | --- |
| Milk, evaporated (not reconstituted) | 10g | 0.39µg | 3.9µg |
| Milk, skimmed | ¼ pt/140ml | 0.0µg | 0.0µg |
| Milk, skimmed, fortified | ¼ pt/140ml | 1.4µg | 2.1µg |
| Milk, whole | ¼ pt/140ml | 0.02µg | 0.03µg |
| Butter | 10g | 0.08µg | 0.8µg |
| Cheddar cheese | 25g | 0.07µg | 0.3µg |
| Cornflakes (fortified) | 35g | 0.7µg | 2.1µg |
| Eggs | 1 | 0.5µg | 1.7µg |
| Liver | 50g | 0.25µg | 0.5µg |
| Cod liver oil | 1 tsp/5ml | 10.5µg | N/A |

| Source | Average serving | Amount of vitamin per serving | Amount per 100g food |
|---|---|---|---|
| Herring/kipper | 50g | 12.5µg | 25.0µg |
| Margarine (fortified) | 10g | 0.8µg | 7.9µg |
| Salmon, canned | 100g | 12.5µg | 12.5µg |

Fifteen minutes in a bathing suit in the sunshine (avoid the hottest part of the day due to risk of burning) provides 200µg of vitamin D, 30–45 minutes with just face, arms and hands a day is sufficient (the darker the skin colour the longer needed).

## Vitamin-E

Possible signs of insufficiency:

- Dry skin
- Premature ageing
- Poor fertility
- Easy bruising
- Frequent infections
- Cardiovascular disease

Good sources:

| Source | Average serving | Amount of vitamin per serving | Amount per 100g food |
|---|---|---|---|
| Almonds, shelled | 15g | 4.2mg | 25.4mg |
| Avocado pear | 1/2 | 3.0mg | 3.0mg |
| Chickpeas, cooked | 50g | 1.5mg | 2.9mg |
| Margarine, spread | 10g | 3.2mg | 32.6mg |
| Olive oil | 1 tbsp | 0.9mg | 5.1mg |
| Sunflower seeds | 15g | 12mg | 38mg |
| Tomatoes | 80g | 0.9mg | 1.2mg |

| Source | Average serving | Amount of vitamin per serving | Amount per 100g food |
|---|---|---|---|
| Walnuts, shelled | 15g | 1.2mg | 3.8mg |
| Wheatgerm oil | 1 tbsp | 40mg | 136mg |
| Wholemeal bread | 50g | 0.15mg | 0.3mg |

## Vitamin K

Possible signs of insufficiency:

– Poor blood clotting
– Intestinal upset/antibiotic use
– Osteoporosis

Good sources:

| Source | Average serving | Amount of vitamin per serving | Amount per 100g food |
|---|---|---|---|
| Broccoli, cooked | 35g | 58µg | 175µg |
| Brussels sprouts, cooked | 35g | 33µg | 100µg |
| Cabbage, cooked | 35g | 42µg | 125µg |
| Cauliflower, raw | 35g | 1,200µg | 3,600µg |
| Cheese, hard | 25g | 12µg | 50µg |
| Liver | 50g | 300µg | 600µg |
| Meat, average | 100g | 50µg | 50µg |
| Potatoes, boiled | 100g | 80µg | 80µg |
| Runner beans | 50g | 145µg | 290µg |
| Soya beans, cooked | 50g | 95µg | 190µg |
| Tomatoes | 80g | 320µg | 400µg |

# Essential Fatty Acids

## Omega-3 family

Possible signs of insufficiency:

- Dry skin and lustreless hair
- Arthritis or rheumatism
- Hyperactivity
- Depression
- Mood and behavioural disorders
- Heart disease
- Frequent infections
- Psoriasis
- Allergies

Good sources:

Oily fish provide EPA and DHA fatty acids: 100 grams of oily fish will provide around 2 grams of EPA/DHA fatty acids. High amounts of essential fatty acids are found in herring, mackerel, tuna (fresh), salmon, sardines (fresh or canned), anchovies, pink trout, kippers, mullet, sprats, sturgeon and eel. Cod liver oil supplements are a good source, but provide about half the amount of fatty acids as high EPA/DHA fish oil supplements. Medium amounts are found in halibut, smelt, shark, oyster, swordfish and trout. Low amounts can be obtained from tuna (canned, vegetable oil packed or water packed), bass, bream, cod, coley, prawns, mussels and haddock.

There are few sources of the omega-3 essential fatty acid (alpha-linolenic acid), and these include flax oil (58 per cent), hemp seed oil (25 per cent), pumpkin seed oil (15 per cent), and pumpkin seeds, soya bean oil (9 per cent), canola (rape) oil (7 per cent), walnut oil (5 per cent) and walnuts.

Other sources of Omega-3s are game and free-ranging grass-fed animals. These provide better amounts than intensively reared meats, and organic milk has been shown to have better levels than non-organic milk. In the plant world only algae produce these fatty acids, and these are now being used as DHA (but not EPA) supplements for vegetarians. Omega-3 enriched eggs, bread and orange juice are also now available – three eggs equals one portion of oily fish in terms of omega-3 content.

## Omega-6 family
Possible signs of insufficiency:

- Dry skin and lustreless hair
- Excessive thirst
- Frequent infections
- PMS or breast pain
- Eczema or dry skin
- Neuropathy in diabetes
- Infertility

Good sources:
There is an excess of omega-6 fatty acids in the Western diet, mostly those of low quality from sources such as refined oils, processed foods and margarines. The main nutritional aim is to redress the balance by consuming more omega-3 oils (see above) and to improve the quality, but not the quantity, of omega-6 oils.

High-quality omega-6 fatty acids are found in *cold-pressed* seed and nut oils such as sunflower, safflower, sesame, walnut and grape. It is also found in unsalted nuts, and seeds such as sesame, sunflower, pumpkin and pine nuts. Evening primrose oil is a rich source of the omega-6 essential fatty acid linoleic acid and in GLA (gamma-linolenic acid).

# Appendix I:
# Sugar, Sweeteners and
# Glycaemic Index

A century ago, we each consumed around 1 kilo of sugar each year – now it is 50–60 kilos. On nutrition panels on the side of food packets, sugars are listed as grams per 100 gram of product. So a breakfast cereal that is 35g sugars per 100 grams of cereal is 35 per cent sugar – or slightly more than one-third sugar. Government guidelines say to choose products with around 10 per cent sugar maximum. It is easy to see that this sample product exceeds the recommended amounts. Common sources of excess sugar are breakfast cereals, juices, soft drinks, cordials, yoghurts, novelty desserts, ice-cream sauces, biscuits, sweets and chocolates. Low-fat foods are also often high in sugar. Manufacturers have caught on to the healthy eating fruit message and blazon fruit across all sorts of foods that either contain no fruit (such as yoghurts), or that are so refined that the sugar content is similar to any other confectionery (such as chewy fruit strips). Adding a teaspoon of sugar at table is often a less sugary option than buying foods with high sugar levels.

- *Sweet-tasting fruit*: Using fruit to satisfy a sweet tooth is ideal. Bananas, raisins, dried apricots, prunes, dried berries and other fruit are sweet, but they have the advantage of also adding fibre and antioxidants into the diet. Refined sugar has none of these advantages and gives us empty calories (calories that are devoid of any nutritional merit).
- *Fructose*: This is fruit sugar and it has a low Glycaemic Index ranking of 19 (see page 352). This makes it suitable for use, in moderation, by diabetics and others who want

to control blood sugar. It still contains as many calories as table sugar.

- *Artificial sweeteners*: Artificial sweeteners are aspartame, saccharine and acesulphame K. They have no calories. Aspartame is implicated in headaches and other problems. Artificial sweeteners should not be given in any quantity to children, and not at all to under threes – this is, of course, not what happens, since many products targeted at children include these sweeteners (though they are not supposed to). Even 'normal' products which are not low-sugar use these sweeteners, as they are a much cheaper ingredient than sugar. Any product that says 'No Added Sugar' on the label is likely to have artificial sweeteners in it.

- *Bulk sweeteners*: Bulk sweeteners are sweet tasting but are not metabolized and so do not affect blood sugar. The most common bulk sweetener is sorbitol, which is used in diabetic jams and sweets. Low-carbohydrate products that are now available tend to use another bulk sweetener, maltitol. The side-effect of bulk sweeteners is that they trigger diarrhoea when consumed above the person's tolerance level.

- *FOS*: FOS (fructo-oligosaccharides) is another bulk sweetener, which has the advantage of improving bowel bacteria health (see Chapter 4: Bacterial Balance, page 35).

- *Xylitol*: Yet another bulk sweetener, used in some chewing gums and mouthwashes, is of tremendous use for dental and oral health, as it stops bacteria from adhering.

## Glycaemic Index (GI) Ranking of Carbohydrate Foods

The GI of over 600 carbohydrate-containing foods have been measured. The foods are measured on a scale where 100 represents glucose, which is the sugar found in the blood.

The foods are tested in amounts of 50 grams of carbohydrate in the food (not 50 grams of the food itself). In practice, this means that some foods need to be eliminated. For instance, you would need to eat implausibly large amounts of celery in order to consume 50 grams of carbohydrates from that source. Protein and fat, or foods that contain mainly these two ingredients but little carbohydrate, such as meat, eggs, avocados and nuts, are ranked as 0.

Remember that a scoring system such as this gives averages for foods, so at best this is a guide. If two foods containing an equal amount of carbohydrates are combined, the GI is the average of the two. Fat and protein slow down the absorption of food, thus lowering the GI. Therefore, fatty foods such as crisps and chocolate have lower GIs than you would expect for their carbohydrate content – this does not make them healthy foods, however. Equally, some fruits and vegetables such as watermelon, banana, raisins and parsnips have highish GI rankings as they are quite sugary. Yet as these foods have many other advantages, such as increasing antioxidant and fibre intakes, they remain healthy foods for most people most of the time (it is only in cases of severe blood sugar control problems that they need to be moderated).

Composite dishes are difficult to figure out unless you are cooking from scratch and keep a calculator nearby. In Australia, many packaged foods are now listed with GI ranking, which is starting to be introduced in the UK.

Most alcohols have almost no carbohydrates, wine has a little and beer a bit more but still considerably less than soft drinks. In moderation these will not raise blood sugar, but large volumes of beer will have a significant effect on blood glucose.

The quantity of a food eaten impacts on blood glucose levels. The GI ranking of the food won't change if a double portion is eaten – the GI number on the scale remains the same. It will, however, affect blood glucose levels and affect the glucose impact of the whole meal. If one slice of white bread is eaten with meat and tomato, the ratio is about one-third of each ingredient with the bread (which ranks 70, fairly high on the scale) affecting blood glucose levels. If two slices of bread are eaten with the same amount of meat and tomato (the ranking of white bread remains 70), the balance of carbohydrate foods to other foods changes to about 50 per cent. Therefore, this will have a different effect on blood sugar from the previous meal, where the bread is only one-third of the ingredients.

Low GI foods remain in the digestive system and the feeling of 'being full' triggers the brain to suppress hunger pangs – this reduces the urge to snack too frequently. Conversely, high-GI foods cause blood glucose levels to rise quickly, followed by a fairly fast decline, which stimulates hunger. After the blood sugar rebound, stress hormones – adrenaline and cortisol – are released and these hormones further stimulate appetite. The effect on appetite can be quite dramatic.

For more information on GI ranking of foods and how they affect health, read *The Glucose Revolution* by Dr A. Leeds, Professor J. Brand Miller and colleagues (Hodder Mobius).

## LOW GI FOODS

| GI of 0 | GI of less than 10 | GI of 11–20 | GI of 21–30 |
|---|---|---|---|
| Avocados | Aubergines | Fructose (fruit | All Bran |
| Butter | Broccoli | sugar) | Apricots, dried |
| Cheese | Cabbage | Peanuts | Barley, pearl |
| (hard) | Mushrooms | Rice bran | Cherries |
| Eggs | Onion | Soya beans, | Chocolate, dark, |
| Fish | Peppers | canned | 70% cocoa |
| Meat | Tomatoes | Yoghurt, | solid |
| Nuts | Vegetables, | low-fat, | Grapefruit |
| Olives | green/lettuce | plain | Lentils, green/ |
| | | | brown |

| GI of 0 | GI of less than 10 | GI of 11–20 | GI of 21–30 |
|---------|--------------------|-------------|-------------|
|         |                    |             | Lentils, red |
|         |                    |             | Peas, split |
|         |                    |             | Prunes |
|         |                    |             | Sausages (with rusks/fillers) |

## MEDIUM GI FOODS

| GI of 31–40 | GI of 41–50 | GI of 51–60 |
|-------------|-------------|-------------|
| Apple, fresh | Baked beans, canned | Apricots, fresh |
| Apple juice | Bread, mixed grain | Banana |
| Beans, French/ haricot | Bulgar | Bran muffin |
| Butter beans | Carrots, boiled | Bread, rye flour |
| Carrots, raw | Custard | Bread, pitta, white |
| Milk, full fat/ semi-skimmed/ skimmed | Cake, sponge/pound | Buckwheat |
| | Chickpeas, canned | Buckwheat flour |
| Pear, fresh | Chocolate, milk | Cola drink |
| Pizza, 11–14% fat | Corn chips | Digestive biscuits |
| Plum, fresh | Grapefruit juice | Fruit cocktail |
| Quinoa, cooked (grain) | Grapes | Honey |
| | Lactose (milk sugar) | Jam |
| Ravioli, durum, meat filled | Lentil soup, canned | Kidney beans, canned |
| | Macaroni | |
| Rye cereal | Noodles, instant | Kiwi fruit |
| Spaghetti, white | Orange, fresh | Mango, fresh |
| Spaghetti, wholemeal | Peach, fresh | Mars bar |
| | Pear, canned (not in syrup) | Muesli |
| Split peas, yellow | Peas, green | Muffins, bran |
| Tomato soup, canned | Pineapple juice | Oat bran |
| | Pinto beans, canned | Oatmeal biscuits |
| Vermicelli, Chinese (mung bean) | Porridge | Orange juice |
| | Pumpernickel | Papaya (pawpaw) |
| Yam | Soya milk | Popcorn, plain |
| Yoghurt, full milk | Sushi, salmon | Potato crisps |
| | Sweetcorn | Pastry |
| | Sweet potato | Pea, split, soup, canned |

| GI of 31–40 | GI of 41–50 | GI of 51–60 |
|---|---|---|
| | Yakult | Rich tea biscuits |
| | | Rice, basmati |
| | | Rice, brown |
| | | Special K, cereal |
| | | Sultanas |
| | | Shortbread biscuits |

## HIGHER GI FOODS

| GI of 61–70 | GI of 71–80 | GI of 81–90 | GI of 91–100+ |
|---|---|---|---|
| Apricots, canned in syrup | Bagel, white | Bread, gluten free | Bread, French baguette |
| Beetroot | Bran buds/ flakes | Cupcake | Dates, dried |
| Black bean soup | Bread, black (German) | Potato, instant | Glucose |
| Bread, wheat, white | Broad (fava) beans | Potato (old) baked | Lucozade |
| Bread, wheat, wholemeal | Cheerios cereal | Pretzels | Maltodextrine |
| Cornmeal | Cornflakes cereal | Rice cakes | Maltose |
| Cous-cous | Crackers, wheat | Rice krispies cereal | Pancakes, gluten-free mix |
| Crispbread, rye, high fibre | Doughnut | Rice, instant | Parsnips |
| Croissant | French fries, frozen, microwave | Tapioca, boiled with milk | Potatoes, Desirée, boiled |
| Crumpet | Fruit bars, processed | | Rice, Jasmin/ glutinous |
| Fanta | Jelly beans | | |
| Fig, dried | Millet cereal | | |
| Gnocchi | Puffed wheat cereal | | |
| Grapenuts cereal | Pumpkin | | |
| Hamburger bun | Scones, packet mix | | |
| Ice cream | Shredded wheat cereal | | |
| Macaroni cheese, frozen | | | |

| GI of 61–70 | GI of 71–80 | GI of 81–90 | GI of 91–100+ |
| --- | --- | --- | --- |
| Mars bar | Sultana bran | | |
| Melon |   cereal | | |
| Melba toast | Swede | | |
| Pancakes, | Vanilla wafers | | |
|   packet mix | Waffles | | |
| Pineapple | Water biscuits | | |
| Raisins | Watermelon | | |
| Rice, arborio | | | |
| Rice, long | | | |
|   grain, white | | | |
| Stone wheat | | | |
|   thins | | | |
| Sucrose (table | | | |
|   sugar) | | | |
| Sustain cereal | | | |
| Taco shells | | | |
| Turnip | | | |

# Appendix II:
# Salt – Reducing Intake

The average daily salt intake per adult in the UK and USA is 9–12 grams, in contrast to the recommended maximum of 6 grams, with children consuming similarly high levels. It is a major public and personal health goal to reduce salt intakes to reduce hypertension and heart disease.

Recommended Daily Sodium/Salt Intakes

|  | Sodium | Salt | Maximum salt* |
|---|---|---|---|
| 1–3 years | 0.5g | 1.25g | 2g |
| 4–6 years | 0.7g | 1.75g | 3g |
| 7–10 years | 1.2g | 3.0g | 5g* |
| 11–18 years | 1.6g | 4.0g | 5g |
| Adults (women) | 1.6g | 4.0g | 5g |
| Adults (men) | 1.6g | 4.0g | 7g |

\* *These are the levels proposed by SACN (Scientific Advisory Committee on Nutrition) – some authorities believe the 7–10 year old figure would be better set at 4g.*

In order to find the figure for salt from the sodium levels declared on food packaging, you need to convert the sodium figure per portion or per 100g. To get the salt figure, multiply the sodium figure given by 2.5. Therefore:

| 0.5g sodium | = | 1.25g salt |
|---|---|---|
| 1.0g sodium | = | 2.5g salt |
| 2.0g sodium | = | 5g salt |

It also helps to know that:

5g of salt  =  1 level teaspoon

The above is a slight oversimplification, because some products give the total *added* sodium (ignoring natural sodium) and some give the total sodium content (natural salt present in the food, plus the added sodium). Monosodium glutamate (E621) and bicarbonate (baking soda) may be ignored in the sodium count. MSG can be disguised on the ingredients' listing as: hydrolyzed protein, natural flavouring, seasoning, spices, vegetable bouillon, and plant protein extract.

- Sea salt is made up of sodium chloride, but also contains other minerals such as magnesium, potassium and iodine. This means that the sodium in sea salt is about two-thirds of the equivalent amount of table salt.
- Cutting out salt is not necessarily as straightforward as it appears. For instance, you might think that cutting out crisps would be a good place to start to reduce salt intake. And yet an equivalent amount of corn flakes has a lot more salt than most crisps. Because of the amount we eat, bread can account for a major portion of salt intake (though salt levels in bread have recently been reduced, there is still far too much). Foods such as sausages, cheese and tinned pasta take levels sky-high. Believe it or not, products such as spaghetti hoops that are marketed specifically at children, are often higher in salt than their equivalent products not aimed at children. Take-away and convenience foods, smoked and preserved foods are other familiar sources.
- Processed, packaged and convenience foods contribute about three-quarters of our salt intake. The low levels in the DASH-Sodium trial were largely achieved using low-salt alternatives to staples such as bread and pasta sauce. The

Food Standards Agency says that 0.5g sodium per 100g product is too high, and that less than 0.1g should be considered a good level. The figures below illustrate the difference that cooking using unprocessed ingredients can make to sodium intake. Look at these comparable foods, per 100g:

| | | | |
|---|---|---|---|
| Frozen peas | 0.003g | Canned processed peas | 0.25g |
| Unsalted butter | 0.01g | Salted butter | 0.75g |
| Beef, lean | 0.06g | Beefburger | 0.60g |
| Tomato purée | 0.02g | Ketchup | 1.12g |
| Pork, lean | 0.07g | Sausages | 0.76g |
| Haddock, fresh | 0.07g | Haddock, smoked | 0.99g |
| Pasta, cooked | 0.05g | Pasta shapes, tinned | 0.40g |

Typical Portions of Foods and Amount of Sodium/Salt

| Source | Portion | Sodium | Salt |
|---|---|---|---|
| Bacon | 25g – 2 rashers | 0.37g | 0.92g |
| Baked beans | 200g | 1.06g | 2.65 |
| Bread, 1 medium slice | 35g | 0.18g | 0.45g |
| Burger, take-away kid's meal with bun, small fries/small cola | | 1.32g | 3.3g |
| Butter, salted | 10g (2 tsp, average one slice bread) | 0.07g | 0.18 |
| Cheese, yellow | 50g | 0.35g | 0.87g |
| Chicken nuggets | 50g | 0.5g | 1.25g |
| Convenience lunch box with crackers, ham/cheese | | 1.1g | 2.75g |
| Corn flakes | 35g | 0.33g | 0.82g |
| Crisps | 35g – 1 small pkt | 0.2g | 0.5g |
| Egg | 1 | 0.14g | 0.35g |
| Fish fingers | 3 – 100g | 0.3g | 0.75g |
| Ketchup, 1 level tsp | 5g | 0.06g | 0.15g |
| Marmite/Bovril, 1 level tsp | 5g | 0.25g | 0.62g |

| | | | |
|---|---|---|---|
| Noodle snack | 89g | 1.8g | 4.5g |
| Pasta shapes | 205g tin | 0.8g | 2.0g |
| Pizza, slice | 200g | 1.2g | 3.0g |
| Sausages | 50g | 0.38g | 0.95g |
| Tomato soup | 100g can | 0.45g | 1.12g |

- If recommendations to lower salt were successful, it is estimated that there would be a corresponding fluid intake reduction of 350 mililitres per day per person. One-quarter of fluid intake is from soft-drinks, so this would impact sales by 5 billion pounds per annum in the UK. Yet, not surprisingly, many soft-drink companies also sell high-salt snacks.
- By eating a can of pasta shapes, some sausages and marmite sandwiches, a child easily exceeds the maximum recommended level. The most effective way to cut back is to switch from regular use of packaged foods to making more meals from scratch, where you can control the amount of salt used.
- Don't put salt-cellars on the table and don't add salt when cooking. It is unnecessary to add salt to the cooking water of rice or pasta, which increases sodium levels in cooked foods.
- A taste for salt can be curbed over time by gradually reducing dependency on salt and salty foods. Using chopped herbs and ground spices in your cooking instead of salt is a great way to 'divert' taste interest elsewhere. You could experiment with a sprinkle of lemon, parsley, chives, coriander, cumin, tarragon and others.
- Increasing potassium intakes from fruits and vegetables may partly counteract the negative effects of sodium (this is one strategy to follow if, for instance, a partner refuses to reduce salt intake!). Trials show a blood pressure-lowering effect

in hypertensives when potassium is increased, though the compound effect of raising potassium alongside sodium-reduction is probably most useful. Potatoes, bananas and watermelon are particularly high in potassium.

# Appendix III:
# Fibre – Increasing Intake

Average daily fibre intake in the UK is 9–12 grams, while the recommended intake is 18 grams. In the US, the recommended intake is 25 grams daily. High fibre diets, and those aimed at preventing diseases such as diabetes and some forms of cancer, can suggest 35 grams of fibre. There are two main types of dietary fibre: soluble and insoluble. All foods contain both in different proportions, but some favour more of one than the other. Oats, fruit, vegetables, pulses (beans and lentils) and linseeds are rich in soluble fibre. Wheat and rye are high in insoluble fibre. For digestive and bowel health, it is generally better to increase levels of soluble fibre, as this is more gentle on the digestive system.

Meat, dairy products, eggs, fish, sugar and fat contain no fibre. Fibre is only found in carbohydrate (starchy) foods such as bread, rice, potatoes, beans, vegetables and fruit. Generally speaking, the easier it is to cook a food the less fibre it is likely to contain (so easy-cook rice has less fibre than brown rice) and the more refined or processed a product, the less fibre it contains. Packaged products will generally, but not always, include the amount of fibre in a product. If moving from a low-fibre to a high-fibre diet, it is advisable to increase by increments of 5 grams of fibre daily, each week or so, in order that the digestive tract can learn to adapt to this new level; otherwise bloating, wind, cramp and/or constipation can result. Adding spoonfuls of wheat bran to cereal is generally a bad idea, while increasing food sources of fibre is beneficial. Adding fibre such as ground linseeds, psyllium husks or rice bran to cereals is a better option than wheat fibre.

## Suggested Menu

The following daily menu will provide in excess of 25 grams of fibre:

| | |
|---|---|
| *Breakfast*: | 1 bowl of porridge or muesli |
| | 1 tablespoon of linseeds added to cereal |
| | 1 portion of berries or other fruit |
| *Lunch*: | 2 slices wholemeal or rye bread |
| | 1 serving vegetable |
| | 1 portion of fruit |
| *Evening*: | 1 serving brown rice, or 1 medium jacket potato or 1 serving pasta |
| | 1 serving pulses/legumes |
| | 1 serving vegetables |
| *Snacks*: | 2 servings fruit |

### Foods that are Good Sources of Fibre

| Source | Portion | Grams fibre |
|---|---|---|
| Almonds | 10g | 1.4 |
| Apples | 1 medium | 2.0 |
| Apricots, dried | 15g | 3.6 |
| Apricots, fresh | 2 medium | 1.0 |
| Asparagus | 50g | 0.5 |
| Avocado | 1/2 medium | 2.0 |
| Bananas | 1 medium | 2.0 |
| Barley, cooked | 50g | 1.0 |
| Beans, butter, cooked | 50g | 2.5 |
| Beans, French | 25g | 0.7 |
| Beans, haricot, cooked | 50g | 3.5 |
| Beetroot, raw | 25g | 1.5 |
| Blackberries | 15g | 1.0 |
| Blackcurrants | 15g | 1.5 |
| Bread, white | 25g | 1.0 |
| Bread, wholemeal | 25g | 2.0 |
| Broccoli | 25g | 1.0 |
| Brussels sprouts | 25g | 1.0 |
| Buckwheat (kasha) cooked | 50g | 3.0 |

| Source | Portion | Grams fibre |
|---|---|---|
| Cabbage | 25g | 0.7 |
| Carrots | 25g | 0.7 |
| Cauliflower | 25g | 0.5 |
| Cherries | 25g | 0.5 |
| Chestnuts | 15g | 1.1 |
| Chickpeas, cooked | 50g | 3.0 |
| Coconut, fresh | 15g | 2.3 |
| Corn on the cob | 1 medium | 5.0 |
| Currants | 10g | 0.7 |
| Dates, dried | 15g | 1.5 |
| Figs, dried | 15g | 3.1 |
| Figs, fresh | 25g | 0.7 |
| Flour, rye | 100g | 6.0 |
| Flour, white | 100g | 3.0 |
| Flour, wholemeal | 100g | 9.0 |
| Leeks | 50g | 1.5 |
| Lentils, cooked | 50g | 2.0 |
| Lettuce | 25g | 0.3 |
| Linseeds | 1 tablespoon | 2.0 |
| Melons | 50g | 0.5 |
| Muesli | 25g | 2.0 |
| Mushrooms | 15g | 0.5 |
| Oatmeal, uncooked | 25g | 1.7 |
| Okra | 25g | 0.5 |
| Oranges | 1 medium | 2.0 |
| Parsnips | 50g | 2.0 |
| Peaches | 1 medium | 2.3 |
| Peanuts | 15g | 1.4 |
| Pears | 1 medium | 2.0 |
| Peas | 25g | 1.3 |
| Pineapple | 50g | 0.5 |
| Plantain | 25g | 2.0 |
| Plums | 1 medium | 1.0 |
| Potatoes, whole (with skins) | 100g | 2.0 |
| Prunes, dried | 15g | 2.6 |
| Raisins | 15g | 1.2 |
| Raspberries | 25g | 2.0 |
| Rhubarb | 50g | 1.0 |

| Source | Portion | Grams fibre |
|---|---|---|
| Rice, brown, cooked | 100g | 1.7 |
| Rice, white, cooked | 100g | 1.0 |
| Soya flour | 100g | 11.0 |
| Spaghetti, brown, cooked | 100g | 4.0 |
| Spaghetti, white, cooked | 100g | 2.0 |
| Spinach, cooked | 25g | 1.5 |
| Strawberries | 25g | 0.5 |
| Sunflower seeds | 15g | 1.2 |
| Swedes | 50g | 1.5 |
| Tofu | 100g | 0.4 |
| Tomatoes | 50g | 0.7 |
| Walnuts | 15g | 0.8 |
| Yam | 50g | 2.0 |

# Appendix IV:
# Supplement Safety

One in three adults in the UK take supplements: vitamins, minerals, fatty acids, herbs and other products. Since these can have a pronounced effect on health, mainly positive but sometimes negative, it pays to know something about how and when it is safe to take them and when it is sensible to be cautious or to seek further advice. Patients may not tell their doctors about supplement use, and their doctor may not, likewise, ask about preparations they are taking or planning to take. Doctors may not take into account the effects of drug therapy on nutritional status, or of diet on drug efficacy. Drugs can affect nutrient levels by influencing nutrient absorption, metabolism or excretion.

Some medications have narrow therapeutic margins between efficacy and toxicity (drugs such as Digoxin, Phenytoin, Warfarin and Theophylline) which makes advice and monitoring important. Other drugs have wider margins, which involves less concern; however, multiple and long-term drug therapy are an issue. Many drugs trigger nutritional deficiencies, meaning that taking a multivitamin/mineral may be important in those circumstances. Antibiotics have a strong negative effect on digestive and immune health, if taken long term, via their effects on bowel bacteria.

## Who Should take Nutritional Supplements?

It is true to say that it is often those who need them least who are most likely to take supplements, while those that need them most are least likely to take them. Supplements are not a substitute for a healthy background diet. However, in our 'pill-for-an-ill' world, it is common for people to take supplements in the vague hope that these will counteract a poor diet. This may work to some degree, for a short time, but won't be the whole answer and eventually the diet needs to be addressed. At-risk groups, on the other hand, should probably seriously consider taking a vitamin and mineral supplement that at least gives the RDAs for their age group of the basic micro-nutrients. These groups include children, women planning a pregnancy or who are pregnant or breast-feeding and the elderly. Young adults often do not get the recommended daily intakes of certain nutrients, which is probably related to their intake of convenience foods, a general loss of cooking skills, and possibly time factors created by career and family needs. They are also the group most at risk for behaviour habits that have an anti-nutrient effect, such as excess drinking and smoking. Those in the lower economic group are also at risk. According to the National Diet and Nutrition Surveys in the UK, many young adults are low in vitamin A, riboflavin (vitamin B2), iron and vitamin D. Women tend to be lower in nutrient intakes than men (often due to a lower calorie intake from dieting). Between one-third and one-half don't get enough calcium, and around three-quarters don't get enough magnesium (the most deficient mineral). Fish eating is at an all-time low, which means that omega-3 fatty acids are low in much of the population.

## Are there Any Problems with Taking Nutritional Supplements?

For most people, it is entirely safe to take a multivitamin/multimineral, a fatty acid supplement and bowel bacteria supplement. When taking a combination of supplements, however, it is wise to check for high levels of any one particular nutrient, especially vitamin A ( toxic in very high doses), iron (which should not be overdone, as it promotes oxidation at high levels) and zinc. While zinc would be highly unlikely to cause an overdose, it could lead to an imbalance of other nutrients – more than 45mg of zinc over the long term imbalances copper and causes excretion of magnesium. For instance, you could take a multivitamin that includes vitamin A, cod liver oil, which is high in vitamin A (though fish oil supplements aren't), alongside an antioxidant supplement that also features vitamin A, and end up taking too much of this nutrient. Equally, a person taking zinc lozenges several times daily for cold symptoms could reach 150mg, which in the short term is not a problem, but over the long term could be. Choose good quality products, to be reasonably sure that you are getting the dosage stated on the package. High doses of individual nutrients are best taken only with professional advice from a nutritionist, who will take into account the individual's health history. There are several specific contraindications to taking supplements or foods and some common examples are outlined below.

### Pregnancy and supplements

Only supplements that are specifically formulated for use during pregnancy should be taken. This is to avoid taking vitamin A, which is contraindicated in pregnancy, to ensure adequate intakes of folic acid, and because pregnancy-formulated supplements avoid herbs that are contraindicated (of which there are many).

### What about herbal supplements?

For many years it has been known that drug/drug interactions are a serious consideration. These can particularly affect the elderly, who are often taking a variety of medications. Hot on the heels of this is the realization that herbal medicines, tinctures and teas with potent pharmacological – and thus positive therapeutic – effects can affect the metabolism of drugs. They do this by affecting the rate at which they are processed by the liver or by enhancing or blocking the actions of the drugs. Consequently, it is always best to seek the advice of a qualified herbalist before taking herbs alongside prescribed or over-the-counter drugs. For instance, St John's wort, while having extremely useful antidepressant actions, could easily interfere with the efficacy of the contraceptive Pill (which many women would not consider a drug). Echinacea, which boosts immune health, can interfere with some chemotherapy drugs. The simple guiding principles are:

- Don't use herbs with medicines that have a similar effect. For instance, an anti-anxiety herb such as valerian should not be used with other anti-anxiety substances such as barbiturates, sedatives (sleeping pills), alcohol or anaesthetics
- If taking any prescribed or over-the-counter medicine, speak to your doctor or a medical herbalist for advice regarding potential interactions
- Many herbs are not safe in pregnancy, so unless you know something is safe, don't use it. Many herbs are also contraindicated during breast-feeding, when the substances can pass into the mother's milk
- If any adverse symptoms are experienced, stop taking the herb immediately and seek the advice of a doctor or medical herbalist.

## Food/Nutrient/Drug Interactions and Contraindications

- *Grapefruit juice*: This citrus juice, but not others such as orange or tangerine, affects the rate at which a glycoprotein in the digestive tract and cytochrome P-450 enzymes process some drugs. It can significantly raise drug levels in the blood beyond acceptable limits for up to 12 hours after consumption of just one glass of juice. Most commonly affected drugs are cholesterol-lowering medication, calcium channel blockers used to lower blood pressure, sedatives, immunosuppressive drugs and Cyclosporin (a chemotherapy drug). The Pomelo (another citrus fruit with a grapefuit taste) may have similar actions on some drugs (such as renal drugs).

- *Vitamin K-rich foods and anti-blood clotting drugs*: Blood-thinning medication such as Warfarin acts by inhibiting vitamin K metabolism, and increases in dietary vitamin K can induce Warfarin resistance. Green leafy vegetables, such as cabbage, broccoli, Brussels sprouts and cauliflower (richest source) are particularly high in vitamin K. A constant daily level of 65–80µg vitamin K is best practice. This means that more than 250g to 500g daily of green vegetables is contraindicated (spinach, Brussels sprouts, broccoli, kale, parsley, peas, cabbage, pickled cucumbers). Other sources of vitamin K include lentils, chickpeas, soya beans, soybean oil and liver. Herbs which are antagonistic to Warfarin include alfalfa (high vitamin K), green tea in excess, St John's wort (which potentiates liver P450 enzymes), and foxglove (also called digitalis). Co-enzyme Q10 (popularly called CoQ10) is structurally similar to vitamin K, which may or may not be relevant. In the US, Olestra is enriched with vitamin K because of the fat-blocking effects of the product in offsetting deficiency in fat-soluble vitamins (though this product is not available in the UK).

- *Blood thinning agents*: Many foods and supplements have an effect on blood viscosity and this is an important means by which foods can keep you healthy. However, if you are on blood-thinning medication such as Warfarin, or about to have an operation, care must be exercised. Drugs such as

Warfarin have a narrow therapeutic/toxicity range and it is easy to interfere with their efficacy or increase their toxicity. Eating foods with a blood-thinning effect, such as oily fish and garlic, is likely to be quite safe, though dosages of blood-thinning medication should be accordingly monitored. A daily glass of tomato juice also thins blood significantly. Taking fish oil supplements and garlic supplements may be contraindicated – speak to your doctor. Many herbals have blood-thinning actions and should not be taken unless your doctor is aware and is monitoring medication levels. Blood-thinning herbals with an anticoagulant effect include: bilberry, blue cohosh, bochu, capsicum, chamomile, dandelion, fenugreek, feverfew, fucus, garlic, ginger, ginseng, hawthorn, kelp, p'au darco, red clover and white willow (also called herbal aspirin). Excessively high doses of vitamin E, another blood thinning agent, is also contraindicated, though some research suggests that up to 1200ius is acceptable.

Any blood-thinning supplements should be stopped in the couple of weeks before an operation (or if you are about to give birth) as a precautionary measure against increased blood loss. The same is usually true of aspirin, though your doctor's advice should be sought. Large amounts (more than one litre) of ice cream may interfere with Warfarin, and avocado has also been implicated, though these are not yet substantiated.

- *Alcohol*: This is contraindicated with many types of medication, particularly antihistamines, blood pressure medication and Warfarin. Speak to your doctor about any medication you are taking.
- *Liquorice and other herbs and hypertension*: The herb liquorice root, as well as liquorice sweets, has a strong effect on raising blood pressure and should not be consumed by anyone with elevated blood pressure. Ginger and Ginkgo

biloba should also be avoided when taking blood pressure lowering medication, as they can make the effects of the drugs more pronounced.

- *ACE inhibitors and potassium supplements*: ACE inhibitors may be taken long term if high blood pressure cannot be brought under control by addressing diet. Potassium supplements (though these are rarely taken) should be discontinued, because of the risk of hyperkalaemia (potassium excess), though a potassium-rich diet featuring fruits and vegetables is safe and beneficial. Alcohol can enhance the hypotensive effect of ACE inhibitors. Chronic use of ACE inhibitors can raise blood zinc levels and increase urinary loss.

- *Loop diuretics and magnesium and calcium balance*: Diuretics affect sodium/potassium/magnesium balance. Side effects include low potassium and low magnesium and significant calcium excretion. A good level of fruit and vegetable intake and 300–400 mg of magnesium supplemented daily might be advised with increased dietary calcium.

- *Folic acid and medication*: Several types of medication, such as Phenytoin prescribed for epilepsy and some anti-cancer and chemotherapy drugs such as Methotrexate (also taken for arthritis and psoriasis) work by influencing folic acid metabolism. In these cases, it is wise only to take folic acid with your doctor's advice. It is unlikely that normal supplemented levels (around 200–400µg) will be a problem, but high doses are probably contraindicated. If on such medication long term, it could be wise to check for homocysteine levels, which can be elevated in the case of low folic acid.

- *Phenytoin (anti-epilepsy medication) and Vitamin D, B6. Evening Primrose oil and epilepsy*: This anti-epilepsy drug is usually taken long term. It lowers vitamin-D levels by speeding up metabolism in the liver, which causes increased output of vitamin-D metabolites in bile. Vitamin-D is important for long-term bone health and requirements from supplementation are possibly increased. Vitamin B6 may reduce Phenytoin effectiveness, and the herbs Ginkgo biloba, kava kava and milk thistle can affect Phenytoin metabolism and so should be avoided. Case reports (in other words, not studies) have implicated evening primrose oil in temporal lobe epilepsy. This may or may not be relevant to other sources of GLA, such as borage (starflower) oil and blackcurrant seed oil.

- *MAOIs and foods*: Anyone prescribed monoamine oxidase inhibitors for depression will be given a list of foods high in tyramine to be avoided as these might interfere with the efficacy of the medication. Symptoms from mixing tyramine with these drugs can include palpitations, nosebleeds and headaches. Occasionally more severe problems result from high blood pressure, which can lead to intra-cranial bleeding. Foods and drinks that contain high levels of tyramine are: beer, liqueurs, red wine, sherry, vermouth, processed ripe cheeses, liver, salami, tinned meat, soya sauce, yeast extract, herrings and kippers. Foods to be moderated include bananas, avocados, figs, chocolate, vanilla, cola, coffee and hot chocolate (up to three cups a day is fine).

# Appendix V: Travel Advice

Long distance travel, or travel to countries with different standards of hygiene or common diseases, can raise some health concerns. If you are travelling to another country, it is always wise to check what health advice is in place. Your doctor can advise you on vaccination requirements or, for instance, anti-malaria medication. Use sun protection for hot countries, including sun blocks and cover-up clothing and hats.

- *Long-distance driving*: If you are tired when driving long distances, stop and rest. It is a common idea that sugary snacks will keep a driver going but these are not that effective, as the sugar burns out quickly. More effective is a strong cup of coffee followed immediately by a 20-minute nap. The nap refreshes and gives the coffee time to take effect.
- *Travel sickness*: Ginger is most effective (more so than some travel sickness drugs) as is mint tea and an acupuncture pressure point on the wrist – see Nausea, page 259. Avoid large meals before a journey and drink regular small amounts of water to avoid dehydration.
- *Deep vein thrombosis (DVT)*: Sometimes called Economy Class Syndrome (this is misleading, as it can occur in susceptible people whichever class they are travelling in) is when a clot forms and travels to a section of vein where it can cause a blockage. This can lead to a heart attack or stroke. Your doctor will be able to advise you on the use of aspirin or other blood-thinning medication where appropriate. Moving around the cabin and wearing support socks is also advised. Nutritional steps are to drink plenty

of water and to avoid all alcohol. Omega-3-rich oily fish, or fish oil supplements and garlic or garlic supplements, are as effective as aspirin at thinning blood – take these for a week before departure.

- *Jet lag*: This can be reduced by avoiding alcohol on a flight and drinking plenty of water. Eat light meals, including lots of fruit, and when you get to your destination start eating at local time as soon as possible to help establish a routine.

- *Food poisoning – preparation*: Traveller's tummy is a problem when exposed to bacteria to which you are unused, or to food poisoning bugs. There is good evidence that people who take probiotic supplements (*Bifidobacteria* and *Lactobacillus acidophilus*) for two to four weeks prior to travel have significantly enhanced protection against food poisoning, including *E. coli*. Live yoghurt or a probiotic-enhanced drink are other options, though these may be best taken for a minimum of four weeks before travel. See Food Poisoning, page 206.

- *Avoiding food poisoning*: In countries where food poisoning is most likely, drink bottled water, avoid drinks that may have been diluted with water or with ice cubes, salads that may be washed in contaminated water and peeled fruit (peel it yourself). Make sure meats are thoroughly cooked, avoid dishes that have been left out on countertops without refrigeration and food exposed to flies. You should be cautious about food bought from roadside vendors (though this can be the most delicious traditional food). If you contact food poisoning, seek medical help immediately.

- *Sun damage*: Keep sun exposure to early and late in the day, when the sun is less strong, and be particularly careful if you have red hair or light skin. Eating an antioxidant rich diet, particularly vegetables and fruits rich in betacarotene (carrots, cantaloupe, papaya, mango and spinach) helps to protect the skin against sun damage. Taking the antioxidant betacarotene for eight to 12 weeks prior to sun exposure has been shown in studies to reduce damage to the growth layer of skin exposed to UV light. When used along with vitamin E the results were even better – together they fight lipid peroxidation damage in cell membranes.

# Appendix VI:
# Useful Contacts

**Health & Nutrition**
To find out more about Suzannah Olivier's activities visit
www.healthandnutrition.co.uk

**Allergy UK (previously Allergy Foundation)**
For information on intolerances and allergies
Helpline: 01322 619864
www.allergyuk.org

**British Association for Nutritional Therapy (BANT)**
For a register of nutritional therapists
Tel: 08706 061284
www.bant.org.uk

**British Society for Allergy, Environmental and Nutritional
Medicine (BSAENM)**
Medical doctors who practise nutritional therapy
Tel: 0906 3020010 (premium line)
www.bsaenm.org

**Food Standards Agency**
The Government's voice on food and eating-related issues.
Useful advice on many aspects of healthy eating
www.foodstandards.gov.uk

**General Council and Register of Consultant Herbalists and Homoeopaths**
For a register of qualified herbalists
Tel: 01792 655886
www.irch.org

**National Institute of Medical Herbalists (NIMH)**
For a register of qualified herbalists
Tel: 01392 426022
www.nimh.org.uk

**Soil Association**
Certification body for organic food with lists of local suppliers and box schemes.
Tel: 0117 314 5000
www.soilassociation.org

**York Nutrition Laboratories**
Food allergy and intolerance testing and homocysteine testing
0800 074 6185
www.allergy-testing.com

# Selected References and Resources

## Acne

1. **Cordain L. et al.** Acne vulgaris: a disease of western civilization. *Arch Dermatol.* 138:1584–90, (2002).
2. **Dreno B. et al.** Multicentre randomized comparative double-blind controlled clinical trial of the safety and efficacy of zinc gluconate versus minocycline hydrochloride in the treatment of inflammatory acne vulgaris. *Dermatology.* 203:135–40, (2001).
3. **Logan A.C.** Omega-3 fatty acids and acne. *Arch Dermatol.* 139:941–2, (2003).
4. **Michaelsson G., Edqvist L.E.** Erythrocyte glutathione peroxidase activity in acne vulgaris and the effect of selenium and vitamin E treatment. *Acta Derm Venereol.* 64:9–14, (1984).
5. **Treloar V.** Diet and acne redux. *Arch Dermatol.* 139:941, (2003).

## Acne Rosacea

1. **Baba A. et al.** Pancreatic exocrine function in rosacea. *Dermatologica* 165:601–6, (1982).
2. **Kendall S.N.** Remission of rosacea induced by reduction of gut transit time. *Clin Exp Dermatol.* 29:297–9, (2004).

## Addiction

1. **Brain Bio Centre,** London. Tel: 020 8877 9261.
2. **Buydens-Brancey L. et al.** Polyunsaturated fatty acid status and relapse vulnerability in cocaine addicts. *Psychiatry Res.* 120:29–35, (2003).
3. **Colantuoni C. et al.** Evidence that intermittent, excessive sugar intake causes endogenous opioid dependence. *Obes Res.* 10:478–88, (2002).
4. **Moorhouse M. et al.** Carbohydrate craving by alcohol-dependent men during sobriety: relationship to nutrition and serotonergic function. *Alcohol Clin Exp Res.* 24:635–43, (2000).

# Ageing

1. **Bosy-Westphal A. et al.** The age-related decline in resting energy expenditure in humans is due to the loss of fat-free mass and to alterations in its metabolically active components. *J Nutr.* 133(7):2356–62, (2003).
2. **Ettinger R.L.** Changing dietary patterns with changing dentition: how do people cope? *Spec Care Dentist.* 18(1):33–9, (1998).
3. **Evans W.J.** Reversing sarcopenia: how weight training can build strength and vitality. *Geriatrics.* 51(5):46–7, (1996).
4. **Kleessen B. et al.** Effects of inulin and lactose on fecal microflora, microbial activity, and bowel habit in elderly constipated persons. *Am J Clin Nutr.* 65(5):1397–402, (1997).
5. **McKay D.L.** The effects of a multivitamin/mineral supplement on micronutrient status, antioxidant capacity and cytokine production in healthy older adults consuming a fortified diet. *J Am Coll Nutr.* 19(5):613–21, (2000).
6. **Stewart K.J. et al.** Fitness, fatness and activity as predictors of bone mineral density in older persons. *J Intern Med.* 252(5):381–8, (2002).
7. **Newman A.B. et al.** Strength and muscle quality in a well-functioning cohort of older adults: The Health, Aging and Body Composition Study. *J Am Geriatr Soc.* 51(3):323–330, (2003).
8. **Proeuhealth – Crownalife.** The unknown within us – ageing affects our gut flora. www.crownalife.be (2003).
9. **Saunier K., Doré J.** Gastrointestinal tract and the elderly: functional foods, gut microflora and healthy ageing. *Dig Liver Dis.* 34 (Suppl 2):S19–24, (2002).
10. **Sheiham A. et al.** Prevalence of impacts of dental and oral disorders and their effects on eating among older people; a national survey in Great Britain. *Community Dent Oral Epidemiol.* 29(3):195–203, (2001).
11. **Tiemeier H. et al.** Plasma fatty acid composition and depression are associated in the elderly: the Rotterdam study. *Am J Clin Nutr.* 78:40–6, (2003).

# Alcohol, Excessive Intake

1. **Alcoholics Anonymous.** Helpline: 0845 7697 555. www.aa-uk.org.uk

2. **Dudley R.** Fermenting fruit and the historical ecology of ethanol ingestion: is alcoholism in modern humans an evolutionary hangover? *Addiction.* 97:381–8, (2002).

3. **Stranges S.** Alcoholism. *Clinical and Experimental Research.* 28:949, (2004).

# Allergies

1. **Cullinan P. et al.** Early prescriptions of antibiotics and the risk of allergic disease in adults: a cohort study. *Thorax.* 59:11–5, (2004).

2. **Kaliomaki M., Isolauri E.** Role of intestinal flora in the development of allergy. *Curr Opin Allergy Clin Immunol.* 3:15–20, (2003).

3. **Prescott S.L., Calder P.C.** N-3 polyunsaturated fatty acids and allergic disease. *Curr Opin Clin Nutr Metab Care.* 7:123–9, (2004).

4. **Sheikh A., Strachan D.P.** The hygiene theory: fact or fiction? *Curr Opin Otolaryngol Head Neck Surg.* 12:232–6, (2004).

# Alzheimer's Disease

1. **Baum L., Ng A.** Curcumin interaction with copper and iron suggests one possible mechanism of action in Alzheimer's disease in animal models. *J Alzheimer's Dis.* 6(4):367–377, (Aug 2004).

2. **Christen Y.** Oxidative stress and Alzheimer disease. *Am J Clin Nutr.* 71(Supl):621S–9S, (2000).

3. **Grodstein F. et al.** High-dose antioxidant supplements and cognitive function in community-dwelling elderly women. *Am J Clin Nutr.* 77(4):975–84, (2003).

4. **Nourhashemi F. et al.** Alzheimer disease: protective factors. *Am J Clin Nutr.* 71(Suppl):643S–9S, (2000).

5. **Selhub J. et al.** B-vitamins, homocysteine, and neurocognitive function in the elderly. *Am J Clin Nutr.* 71(Suppl):614S–20S, (2000).

6. **Seshadri S. et al.** Plasma homocysteine as a risk factor for dementia and Alzheimer's disease. *N Engl J Med.* 346(7):476–83, (2002).

7. **OPTIMA** – Oxford Project to Investigate Memory and Ageing. www.pharm.ox.ac.uk/optima.htm (2003).

8. **Puglielli L. et al.** Alzheimer's disease: the cholesterol connection. *Nat Neurosci.* 6(4):345–51, (2003).

9. **Reynish W. et al.** Nutritional factors and Alzheimer's disease. *J Gerontol A Biol Sci.* 56(11):M675–80, (2001).

10. **Snowdon D.A. et al.** Serum folate and the severity of atrophy of the neocortex in Alzheimer disease: findings from the Nun Study. *Am Soc Clin Nutr.* 71:993–8, (2000).

## Anaemia, Iron Deficiency

1. **Hulten L.** Iron absorption from the whole diet. Relation to meal composition, iron requirements and iron stores. *Eur J Clinical Nutr.* 49:794–808, (1995).

2. **Lozoff B. et al.** Poorer behavioural and developmental outcome more than 10 years after treatment for iron deficiency in infancy. *Pediatrics.* 105(4):E51, (2000).

3. **Wynn A.** *The Role of Iron.* British Nutrition Foundation. www.nutrition.org.uk (1999).

## Antibiotic Resistance

1. **MRSA Support Group.** 169 Heath Road, Kings Norton, Birmingham B30 1HE (Send SAE).

## Arthritis

1. **Arthritis Research Council.** www.arc.org.uk

2. **Bengtsson U. et al.** Survey of gastrointestinal reactions to foods in adults in relation to atopy, presence of mucus in the stools, swelling of joints and arthralgia in patients with gastrointestinal reactions to foods. *Clin Exp Allergy.* 26(12):1387–94, (Dec 1996).

3. **Calder P.C., Zurier R.B.** Polyunsaturated fatty acids and rheumatoid arthritis. *Curr Opin Clin Nutr Meth Care.* 4:115–21, (2001).

4. **Darlington G.** *Oils and arthritis – can they help?* Arthritis Research Campaign. www.arc.org.co.uk (2003).

5. **James M.J., Cleland L.G.** Dietary n-3 fatty acids and therapy for rheumatoid arthritis. *Semin Arthritis Rheum.* 27:85–97, (1997).

6. **Rennie K.L. et al.** Nutritional management of rheumatoid arthritis: a review of the evidence. *J Hum Nutr Diet.* 16(2):97–109, (2003).

7. **US General Practitioner Research Group.** Calcium pantothenate in arthritic conditions. *Practitioner.* 224:208–11. In: Bowman B.A., Russell R.M. *Present Knowledge in Nutrition 8th Edition.* ILSI Press, Washington, (1980).

# Asthma

1. **Balatsinou L. et al.** Asthma worsened by benzoate contained in some antiasthma drugs. *Int J Immunopathol Pharmacol.* 17:225–6, (2004).
2. **Bolte G. et al.** Margarine consumption and allergy in children. *Am J Respir Crit Care Med.* 163(1):277–9, (Jan 2001).
3. **Hasselmark L. et al.** Selenium supplementation in intrinsic asthma. *Allergy.* 48:30–6, (1993).
4. **Hodge L. et al.** Effect of dietary intake of omega-3 and omega-6 fatty acids on severity of asthma in children. *Eur Respir J.* 11(2):361–5, (1998).
5. **James J.M.** Respiratory manifestations of food allergy. *Pediatrics.* 2003 Jun;111(6 Pt 3):1625–30, (2003).
6. **Oddy W.H. et al.** Ratio of omega-6 to omega-3 fatty acids and childhood asthma. *J Asthma.* 41:319–26, (2004).
7. **Shaheen S.O. et al.** Dietary antioxidants and asthma in adults. *Am J Respir Crit Care Med.* 164:1823–8, (2001).

# Bad Breath, Halitosis

1. **Henker J. et al.** Successful treatment of gut-caused halitosis with a suspension of living non-pathogenic Escherichia coli bacteria – a case report. *Eur J Pediatr.* 160:592–4, (2001).
2. **Ierardi E. et al.** Halitosis and Helicobacter pylori: a possible relationship. *Dig Dis Sci.* 43:2733–7, (1998).
3. **Takarada K. et al.** A comparison of the antibacterial efficacies of essential oils against oral pathogens. *Oral Microbiol Immunol.* 19:61–4, (2004).

# Balance

1. **Dhesi J.K. et al.** Neuromuscular and psychomotor function in elderly subjects who fall and the relationship with vitamin D status. *J Bone Miner Res.* 17:891–7, (2002).

# Behavioural Disorders

## Autism and Asperger's Syndrome
1. For more on this approach go the website set up at Sunderland University http://osiris.sunderland.ac.uk/autism

## Schizophrenia and Bi-polar Disorder
1. **Peet M., Glen I., Horrobin D.F.** *Phospholipid Spectrum Disorders in Psychiatry and Neurology* 2nd Edition. Marius Press, Lancashire, UK, (2003).
2. **Tokdemir M. et al.** Blood zinc and copper concentrations in criminal and non-criminal schizophrenic men. *Arch Androl.* 49:365–8, (2003).

## Antisocial Behaviour
1. **Buydens-Brancey L. et al.** Polyunsaturated fatty acid status and aggression in cocaine addicts. *Drug Alcohol Depend.* 71:319–23, (2003).
2. **Eves A., Gesch B.** Food provision and the nutritional implications of food choices made by young adult males, in a young offenders' institution. *J Hum Nutr Diet.* 16:167–9, (2003).
3. **Gesch C.B.** Influence of supplementary vitamins, minerals and essential fatty acids on the antisocial behaviour of young adult prisoners. *Brit J Psychiatry.* 181:22–8, (2002).
4. **Hibbeln J.R. et al.** A replication study of violent and non-violent subjects: cerebrospinal fluid metabolites of serotonin and dopamine are predicted by plasma essential fatty acids. *Biol Psychiatry.* 44:243–9, (1998).
5. **Iribarren C. et al.** Dietary intake of n-3, n-6 fatty acids and fish: relationship with hostility in young adults – the CARDIA study. *Eur J Clin Nutr.* 58:24–31, (2004).
6. **Virkkunen M., Huttunen M.O.** Evidence for abnormal glucose tolerance test among violent offenders. *Neuropsychobiology.* 8:30–4, (1982).

# Bloating

1. **Heitkemper M.M. et al.** Relationship of bloating to other GI and menstrual symptoms in women with irritable bowel syndrome. *Dig Dis Sci.* 49:88–95, (2004).
2. **Suarez F.L., Levitt M.D.** An understanding of excessive intestinal gas. *Curr Gastroenterol Rep.* 2:413–9, (2000).

# Blood Pressure, High (hypertension)

1. **Banerjee S.K., Maulik S.K.** Effect of garlic on cardiovascular disorders: a review. *Nutr J.* 1:4. (2002).
2. **Sigurjonsdottir H.A. et al.** Subjects with essential hypertension are more sensitive to the inhibition of 11 beta-HSD by liquorice. *J Hum Hypertens.* 17:125–31, (2003).
3. **Vollmer W.M. et al.** *Annals of Internal Medicine.* Effects of diet and sodium intake on blood pressure: subgroup analysis of the DASH-sodium trial. 135(12):1019–28, (Dec 2001).
4. **Wilburn A.J. et al.** The natural treatment of hypertension. *J Clin Hypertens.* 6:242–8, (2004).

# Bowel Bacteria

1. **Gibson G.R.** Dietary modulation of the human gut microflora using prebiotics. *Br J Nutr.* 80:S209–12, (1998).
2. **Gill H.S., Rutherfurd K.J.** Immune enhancement conferred by oral delivery of Lactobacillus rhamnosus HN001 in different milk-based substrates. *J Dairy Res.* 68(4):611–6, (2001).
3. **Kirjavainen P.V., Gibson G.R.** Healthy gut microflora and allergy: factors influencing development of the microbiota. *Ann Med.* 31(4):288–92, (1999).
4. **Langhendries J.P. et al.** Effect of a fermented infant formula containing viable bifidobacteria on the fecal flora composition and pH of healthy full-term infants. *J Pediatr Gastroenterol Nutr.* 21(2):177–81, (1995).
5. **Marteau P.R.** Probiotics in clinical conditions. *Clin Rev Allergy Immunol.* 22(3):255–73, (2002).
6. **Sanders M.E.** Probiotics: considerations for human health. *Nutr Rev.* 61(3):91–9, (2003).
7. **Sheih Y.H. et al.** Systemic immunity-enhancing effects in healthy subjects following dietary consumption of the lactic acid bacterium Lactobacillus rhamnosus HN001. *J Am Coll Nutr.* 20(2 Suppl):149–56, (2001).
8. **Sullivan A., Nord C.E.** The place of probiotics in human intestinal infections. *Int J Antimicrob Agents.* 20:313–9, (2002).
9. **Rubaltelli F.F. et al.** Intestinal flora in breast- and bottle-fed infants. *J Perinat Med.* 26(3):186–91, (1998).

# Breast Tenderness, Lumpiness

1. **London R.S. et al.** Efficacy of alpha-tocopherol in the treatment of the premenstrual syndrome. *J Reprod Med.* 32:400–4, (1987).
2. **Norlock F.E.** Benign breast pain in women: a practical approach to evaluation and treatment. *J Am Med Women's Assoc.* 57:85–90, (2002).
3. **Tschudin S., Huber R.** Treatment of cyclical mastalgia with a solution containing a Vitex agnus castus extract: Results of a placebo-controlled double-blind study. *Breast;* 8:175–181. *Försch Komplementarmed Klass Naturheilkd.* 7:162–4, (2000).

# Cancer Prevention

1. **Combs G.F. Jr et al.** An analysis of cancer prevention by selenium. *Biofactors.* 14:153–9, (2001).
2. **Food Nutrition and the Prevention of Cancer: A Global Perspective.** World Cancer Research Fund and American Cancer Institute, (1997).
3. **Key R.J. et al.** The effect of diet on risk of cancer. *Lancet.* 360:861–8, (2002).
4. **Lai P.K., Oay J.** Antimicrobial and chemopreventive properties of herbs and spices. *Curr Med Chem.* 11:1451–60, (2004).
5. **Mezencev R. et al.** Antiproliferative and cancer chemopreventive activity of phytoalexins: focus on indole phytoalexins from crucifers. *Neoplasma.* 50:239–45, (2003).
6. **Moorman P.G., Terry P.D.** Consumption of dairy products and the risk of breast cancer: a review of the literature. *Am J Clin Nutr.* 80:5–14, (2004).
7. **Moyers S.B., Kumar B.** Green tea polyphenols and cancer chemoprevention. *Nutr Rev.* 62:204–11, (2004).
8. **Purasiri P. et al.** Modulation of cytokine production in vivo by dietary essential fatty acids in patients with colorectal cancer. *Clin Sci.* 87:711–7, (1994).
9. **Woods M.N. et al.** Low fat, high fibre diet and serum estrone sulphate in premenopausal women. *Am J Clin Nutr.* 49:1179–93, (1989).

# Candida

1. **Cater R.E.** Chronic intestinal candidiasis as a possible etiological factor in the chronic fatigue syndrome. *Med Hypotheses*. 44:507–15, (1995).
2. **Lemar K.M. et al.** Garlic (*Allium sativum*) as an anti-Candida agent: a comparison of the efficacy of fresh garlic and freeze-dried extracts. *J Appl Microbiol*. 93:398–405, (2002).
3. **Ota C. et al.** Antifungal activity of propolis on different species of Candida. *Mycoses*. 44:375–8, (2001).
4. **Ruiz-Sanchez D. et al.** Intestinal candidiasis. A clinical report and comments about this opportunistic pathology. *Mycopathologia*. 156:9–11, (2002).

# Carpal Tunnel Syndrome

1. **Aufiero E. et al.** Pyridoxine hydrochloride treatment of carpal tunnel syndrome: a review. *Nutr Rev*. 62:96–104, (2004).

# Cataracts

1. **Chasan-Taber L. et al.** A prospective study of carotenoid and vitamin A intakes and risk of cataract extraction in US women. *Am J Clin Nutr*. 70:509–16, (1999).
2. **Jacques P.F. et al.** Long-term vitamin C supplement use and prevalence of early age-related lens opacities. *Am J Clin Nutr*. 66:911–6, (1997).
3. **Jacques P.F. et al.** Long-term nutrient intake and early age-related nuclear lens opacities. *Arch Ophthalmol*. 119:1009–19, (2001).
4. **Taylor A. et al.** Long-term intake of vitamins and carotenoids and odds of early age-related cortical and posterior subcapsular lens opacities. *Am J Clin Nutr*. 75:540–9, (2002).

# Cholesterol, High

1. **Gorinstein S. et al.** Fresh Israeli jaffa Sweetie juice consumption improves lipid metabolism and increases antioxidant capacity in hypercholesterolemic patients suffering from coronary artery disease. *J Agric Food Chem*. 52:5215–22, (2004).

2. **James S.L. et al.** Dietary fibre: a roughage guide. *Intern Med J.* 33:291–6, (2003).

3. **Li Z. et al.** Fish consumption shifts lipoprotein subfractions to a less atherogenic pattern in humans. *J Nutr.* 134:1724–8, (2004).

4. **Mayo Clin Women's Healthsource.** Oats and soy may cut cholesterol level. 6:3, (2002).

5. **Mensink R.P.** Effects of dietary fatty acids and carbohydrates on the ratio of serum total to HDL cholesterol and on serum lipids and apolipoproteins: a meta-analysis of 60 controlled trial. *Am J Clin Nutr.* 77:1146–55, (2003).

6. **Morgan J.M. et al.** Effects of walnut consumption as part of a low-fat, low-cholesterol diet on serum cardiovascular risk factors. *Int J Vitam Nutr Res.* 72:341–7, (2002).

7. **Pittaway J.K. et al.** The effect of chickpeas on human serum lipids and lipoproteins. *Asia Pac J Clin Nutr.* 13(Suppl):S70, (2004).

## Coeliac Disease and Gluten Avoidance

1. **Coeliac Support Group**. www.coeliac.co.uk
2. **Storsrud S. et al.** Beneficial effects of oats in the gluten-free diet of adults with special reference to nutrient status, symptoms and subjective experiences. *Br J Nutr.* 90:101–7, (2003).

## Cold Sores

1. **Hovi T. et al.** Topical treatment of recurrent mucocutaneous herpes with ascorbic acid-containing solution. *Antiviral Res.* 27(3):263–70, (June 1995).

2. **Thein D.J., Hurt W.C.** Lysine as a prophylactic agent in the treatment of recurrent herpes simplex labialis. *Oral Surg Oral Med Oral Pathol.* 58(6):659–66, (December 1984).

## Colitis and Crohn's Disease

1. **Ballegaard M. et al.** Self-reported food intolerance in chronic inflammatory bowel disease. *Scand J Gastroenterol.* 32(6):569–71, (June 1997).

2. **Fedorak R.N., Madsen K.L.** Probiotics and the management of inflammatory bowel disease. *Inflamm Bowel Dis.* 10(3):286–99, (May 2004).
3. **National Association for Colitis and Crohn's Disease.** www.nacc.org.uk

## Concentration

1. **Benton D., Parker P.Y.** Breakfast, blood glucose and cognition. *Am J Clin Nutr.* 67(Suppl):772S-8S, (1998).

## Constipation

1. **Borody T.J. et al.** Bacteriotherapy using fecal flora: toying with human motions. *J Clin Gastroenterol.* 38(6):475–83, (July 2004).
2. **Daher S. et al.** Cow's milk protein intolerance and chronic constipation in children. *Pediatr Allergy Immunol.* 12(6):339–42, (Dec 2001).
3. **Koebnick C. et al.** Probiotic beverage containing Lactobacillus casei Shirota improves gastrointestinal symptoms in patients with chronic constipation. *Can J Gastroenterol.* 17(11):655–9, (Nov 2003).

## Convalescence

1. **Kirk H.J., Heys S.D.** Immunonutrition. *Br J Surg.* 90:1459–60, (2003).
2. **Rayes N.** Lactobacilli and fibres – a strong couple against bacterial infections in patients with major abdominal surgery. *Nutrition.* 20:579–80, (2004).

## Cramp

1. **Roffe C. et al.** Randomised, cross-over, placebo controlled trial of magnesium citrate in the treatment of chronic persistent leg cramps. *Med Sci Monit.* 8:CR326–30, (2002).

# Cystic Fibrosis

1. **Cystic Fibrosis Trust.** Tel: 020 8462 7211. www.cftrust.org.uk
2. **Freedman S.D. et al.** Association of cystic fibrosis with abnormalities in fatty acid metabolism. *NEJM*. 350:560–9, (2004).

# Cystitis

1. **Patel N., Daniels I.R.** Botanical perspectives on health: of cystitis and cranberries. *J R Soc Health*. 120(1):52–3, (March 2000).

# Depression

1. **Adams P.B. et al.** Arachidonic acid to eicosapentanoic acid ratio in blood correlates positively with clinical symptoms of depression. *Lipids*. 31:S157–S161, (1996).
2. **Bruinsma K.A., Taren D.L.** Dieting, essential fatty acid intake, and depression. *Nutr Rev*. 58(4):98–108, (2000).
3. **Hibbeln J.R.** Fish consumption and major depression. *The Lancet*. 351(9110):1213, (18 April 1998).
4. **Horrobin D.F.** A new category of psychotropic drugs: neuroactive lipids as exemplified by ethyl eicosapentaenoate (E-E). *Prog Drug Res*. 59:171–99, (2002).
5. **Makrides M. et al.** Docosahexaenoic acid and post-partum depression – is there a link? *Asia Pac J Clin Nutr*. 12 (Suppl):S37, (2003).
6. **MIND.** www.mind.org.uk
7. **Nemets B. et al.** Addition of omega-3 fatty acid to maintenance medication treatment for recurrent unipolar depressive disorder. *Am J Psychiatry*. 159(3):477–9, (2002).
8. **Small M.F.** The happy fat. *New Scientist*. August 24:34–7, (2002).
9. **Su K.P. et al.** Omega-3 fatty acids in major depressive disorder. A preliminary double-blind, placebo-controlled trial. *Eur Neuropsychopharmacol*. 13(4):267–71, (2003).

# Diabetes

1. **Grylls W.K. et al.** Lifestyle factors associated with glycaemic control and body mass index in older adults with diabetes. *Eur J Clin Nutr* 57:1386–93, (2003).
2. **Hohnston K.L. et al.** Coffee acutely modifies gastrointestinal hormone secretion and glucose tolerance in humans: glycemic effect of chlorogenic acid and caffeine. *Am J Clin Nutr.* 78:728–33, (2003).
3. **Horrobin D.F.** Essential fatty acids in the management of impaired nerve function in diabetes. *Diabetes.* 46 (Suppl 2):S90–3, (1997).
4. **Jamal G.A., Carmichael H.** The effect of gamma-linolenic acid on human diabetic peripheral neuropathy: a double-blind placebo-controlled trial. *Diabet Med.* 7(4):319–23, (1990).
5. **Keen H. et al.** Treatment of diabetic neuropathy with gamma-linolenic acid. The gamma-Linolenic Acid Multicenter Trial Group. *Diabetes Care.* 16(1):8–15, (1993).
6. **Lazarus S.A. et al.** Tomato juice and platelet aggregation in type 2 diabetes. *JAMA.* 292(7):805–6, (18 Aug 2004).
7. **Parillo M., Riccardi G.** Diet composition and the risk of type 2 diabetes: epidemiological and clinical evidence. *Br J Nutr.* 92:7–19, (2004).
8. **Tuomilehto J. et al.** Coffee consumption and risk of type 2 diabetes mellitus among middle-aged Finnish men and women. *JAMA.* 291(10):1213–9, (10 March 2004).

# Diarrhoea

1. **Beniwal R.S. et al.** A randomized trial of yogurt for prevention of antibiotic-associated diarrhoea. *Dig Dis Sci.* 48(10):2077–82, (October 2003).
2. **Szajewska H., Mrukowicz J.Z.** Probiotics in the treatment and prevention of acute infectious diarrhoea in infants and children: a systematic review of published randomized, double-blind, placebo-controlled trials. *J Pediatric Gastroenterol Nutr.* 33:S17–5, (2001).

## Digestive and Bowel Health

1. **Huovinen P.** *British Medical Journal.* Bacteriotherapy: The time has come. 323:353–4, (Aug 2001).


## Dyslexia and Dyspraxia

1. **Durham Trials** (investigating dyslexia, dyspraxia and ADHD) www.durhamtrial.org
2. **Food and Behaviour Research** (including information on dyslexia and dyspraxia). www.fabresearch.org
3. **Richardson A.J. et al.** Fatty acid deficiency signs predict the severity of reading and related difficulties in dyslexic children. *Prostaglandins Leukot Essent Fatty Acids.* 63:69–74, (2000).
4. **Richardson A.J.** *Dyslexia, dyspraxia and ADHD – Can Nutrition Help?* Paper presented at Nutrition in Developmental Disorders Conference October 2001.


## Eating Disorders

1. **National Centre for Eating Disorders** Tel: 01372 469 493 www.eating-disorders.org.uk
2. **Anorexia and Bulimia Nervosa Association** Tel: 0811 808 6555.
3. **Overeaters Anonymous** Tel: 01426 984 674.


## Eczema

1. **Al-Waili N.S.** Topical application of natural honey, beeswax and olive oil mixture for atopic dermatitis or psoriasis: partially controlled, single-blinded study. *Complement Ther Med.* 11(4):226–34, (Dec 2003).

2. **Dattner A.M.** From medical herbalism to phytotherapy in dermatology: back to the future. *Dermatol Ther.* 16(2):106–13, (2003).

3. **Ferrazzini G. et al.** Microbiological aspects of diaper dermatitis. *Dermatology.* 206(2):136–41, (2003).

4. **Fiocchi A. et al.** Dietary treatment of childhood atopic eczema/dermatitis syndrome (AEDS). *Allergy.* 59(Suppl 78):78–85, (Aug 2004).

5. **Horrobin D.F.** Essential fatty acid metabolism and its modification in atopic eczema. *Am J Clin Nutr.* 71(1 Suppl):367S–72S, (Jan 2000).

# Endometriosis

1. **Parazzini F. et al.** Selected food intake and risk of endometriosis. *Hum Reprod.* 19(8):1755–9, *Epub* (14 July 2004).

2. **Dhillon P.K., Holt V.L.** Recreational physical activity and endometrioma risk. *Am J Epidemiol.* 158(2):156–64, (15 July 2003).

# Epilepsy

1. **Kossoff E.H.** More fat and fewer seizures: dietary therapies for epilepsy. *Lancet Neurol.* 3(7):415–20, (July, 2004).

2. **Pratesi R. et al.** Celiac disease and epilepsy: favorable outcome in a child with difficult to control seizures. *Acta Neurol Scand.* 108(4):290–3, (Oct 2003).

3. **Vaddadi K.S.** The use of gamma-linolenic acid and linoleic acid to differentiate between temporal lobe epilepsy and schizophrenia. *Prostaglandins Med.* 6(4):375–9, (April 1982).

4. **Zelnik N. et al.** Range of neurologic disorders in patients with celiac disease. *Pediatrics.* 113(6):1672–6, (June 2004).

# Exercise and Sport

1. **Brownlie T. et al.** Tissue iron deficiency without anemia impairs adaptation in endurance capacity after aerobic training in previously untrained women. *Am J Clin Nutr.* 79(3):437–43, (March 2004).

2. **Shafat A. et al.** Effects of dietary supplementation with vitamins C and E on muscle function during and after eccentric contractions in humans. *Eur J Appl Physiol,* (7 Aug 2004). [Epub ahead of print].

# Fertility, Female

1. **Barbieri R.L.** The initial fertility consultation: recommendations concerning cigarette smoking, body mass index, and alcohol and caffeine consumption. *Am J Obstet Gynecol.* 185:1168–73, (2001).
2. **Clark A.M. et al.** Weight loss in obese infertile women results in improvement in reproductive outcome for all forms of fertility treatment. *Hum Reprod.* 13(6):1502–5, (1998).
3. **Fujii K., Demura S.** Relationship between change in BMI with age and delayed menarche in female athletes. *J Physiol Anthropol. Appl Human Sci.* 22(2):97–104, (2003).
4. **Hassan M.A., Killick S.R.** Negative lifestyle is associated with a significant reduction in fecundity. *Fertil Steril.* 81:384–92, (2004).
5. **James D.C.** Eating disorders, fertility, and pregnancy: relationships and complications. *J Perinat Neonatal Nurs.* 15(2):36–48, (2001).
6. **Katz M.G., Vollenhoven B.** The reproductive endocrine consequences of anorexia nervosa. *Br J Obstet Gynaecol.* 107:707–13, (2000).

# Fertility, Male

1. **Gonzalez E.R.** Sperm swim singly after vitamin C therapy. *JAMA.* 249:2747–51, (1983).
2. **Jensen T.K. et al.** Semen quality among members of organic food associations in Zealand, Denmark. *Lancet.* 347:1844, (1996).
3. **Jorgensen N. et al.** Regional differences in semen quality in Europe. *Hum Reprod.* 16:1012–9, (2001).
4. **Nudell D.M. et al.** Common medications and drugs: how they affect male fertility. *Urol Clin North Am.* 29:965–73, (2002).
5. **Scott R., MacPherson A.** Selenium supplementation in sub-fertile human males. *Brit J Urol.* 82:76–80, (1998).
6. **Wong W.Y. et al.** Effects of folic acid and zinc sulfate on male factor subfertility: a double-blind, randomized, placebo-controlled trial. *Fertil Steril.* 77:491–8, (2002).

# Fibroids

1. **Chiaffarino F. et al.** Diet and uterine myomas. *Obstet Gynecol.* 94:395–8, (1999).

# Flatulence

1. **Queiroz K. da S. et al.** Soaking the common bean in a domestic preparation reduced the contents of raffinose-type oligosaccharides but did not interfere with nutritive value. *J Nutr Sci Vitaminol (Tokyo)*. 48:283–9, (2002).
2. **Robb-Nicholson C.** By the way, doctor. The more I eat a health diet—one that's rich in whole grains, fruits, and vegetables—the more trouble I have with flatulence. Is this unusual? Any suggestions? *Harvard Women's Health Watch*. 10:8, (2003).

# Fluid Retention (Oedema)

1. **Christie S. et al.** Flavonoids—a new direction for the treatment of fluid retention? *Phytother Res*. 15:467–75, (2001).
2. **Christie S. et al.** Flavonoid supplement improves leg health and reduces fluid retention in pre-menopausal women in a double-blind, placebo-controlled study. *Phytomedicine*. 11:11–7, (2004).

# Food Allergy

1. **Anaphylaxis Campaign.** Helpline: 01252 542029. www.anaphylaxis.org.uk

# Food Intolerance

1. **Anthony H et al.** *Environmental Medicine in Clinical Practice*. BSAENM Publications, Southampton, UK, (1997).

# Food Poisoning

1. **Food Poisoning Prevention and Information**. www.foodlink.org.uk

# Gall Stones

1.  **Tsai C.J. et al.** Frequent nut consumption and decreased risk of cholecystectomy in women. *Am J Clin Nutr.* 80:76–81, (2004).
2.  **Marzio L. et al.** Gallbladder kinetics in obese patients. Effect of a regular meal and low-calorie meal. *Dig Dis Sci.* 33(1):4–9, (Jan 1988).
3.  **Halpern Z. et al.** Bile and plasma lipid composition in non-obese normolipidemic subjects with and without cholesterol gallstones. *Liver.* 13(5):246–52, (Oct 1993).
4.  **Heaton K.W.** Review article: epidemiology of gall-bladder disease— role of intestinal transit. *Aliment Pharmacol Ther.* 14 (Suppl 2):9–13, (May 2000).

# Gout

1.  **Arthritis Research Council.** www.arc.org.uk
2.  **Jacob R.A. et al.** Consumption of cherries lowers plasma urate in healthy women. *J Nutr.* 133:1826–9, (2003).
3.  **Choi H.K. et al.** Alcohol intake and risk of incident gout in men: a prospective study. 1: *Lancet.* 363(9417):1277–81, (17 April 2004).
4.  **Choi H.K. et al.** Purine-rich foods, dairy and protein intake, and the risk of gout in men. 1: *N Engl J Med.* 350(11):1093–103, (11 March 2004).

# Headaches

1.  **Hering-Hanit R., Gadoth N.** Caffeine-induced headache in children and adolescents. *Cephalalgia.* 23(5):332–5, (June 2003).
2.  **Yang W.H. et al.** The monosodium glutamate symptom complex: assessment in a double-blind, placebo-controlled, randomized study. *J Allergy Clin Immunol.* 99(6 Pt 1):757–62, (June 1997).
3.  **Millichap J.G., Yee M.M.** The diet factor in pediatric and adolescent migraine. *Pediatr Neurol.* 28(1):9–15, (Jan 2003).
4.  **Newman L.C., Lipton R.B.** Migraine MLT-down: an unusual presentation of migraine in patients with aspartame-triggered headaches. *Headache.* 41(9):899–901, (Oct 2001).
5.  **Blau J.N. et al.** Water deprivation headache: a new headache with two variants. *Headache.* 44(1):79–83, (Jan 2004).

6. **Awada A., al Jumah M.** The first-of-Ramadan headache. *Headache.* 39(7):490–3, (July–Aug 1999).

# Heart Disease

1. **Durak I. et al.** Effects of garlic extract consumption on plasma and erythrocyte antioxidant parameters in atherosclerotic patients. *Life Sci.* 75–1959–66 (2004). Effects of garlic extract consumption on blood lipid and oxidant/antioxidant parameters in humans with high blood cholesterol. *J Nutr Biochem.* 15:373–7, (2004).
2. **Marchioli R. et al.** *Circulation.* Early protection against sudden death by n-3 polyunsaturated fatty acids after myocardial infarction: time-course analysis of the results of the Gruppo Italiano per lo Studio della Sopravvivenza nell'Infarto Miocardico (GISSI)-Prevenzione. 105:1897–903, (2002).
3. **O'Keefe J.H. Jr, Cordain L.** Cardiovascular disease resulting from a diet and lifestyle at odds with our Paleolithic genome: how to become a 21st century hunter-gatherer. *Mayo Clin Proc.* 79(1):101–8, (2004).
4. **Griffin B.A.** The effects of n-3 fatty acids on low density lipoprotein subfractions. *Lipids.* 36 (Suppl):S91–7, (2001).
5. **Klevay L.M.** Ischemic heart disease: nutrition or pharmacotherapy? *J Trace Elem Electrolytes Health Dis.* 7(2):63–9, (1993).
6. **Engler M.B. et al.** Flavonoid-rich dark chocolate improves endothelial function and increases plasma epicatechin concentrations in healthy adults. *J Am Coll Nutr.* 23(3):197–204, (June 2004).
7. **Corder R. et al.** The procyanidin-induced pseudo laminar shear stress response: a new concept for the reversal of endothelial dysfunction. *Clin Sci.* [Epub ahead of print] (24 Aug 2004).
8. **De Lorgeril M.** 'The Mediterranean-style diet'. Is it ideal for the modern world? *Asia Pac J Clin Nutr.* 13(Suppl):S18, (2004).
9. **Mohanty I. et al.** Protective effects of Curcuma longa on ischemia-reperfusion induced myocardial injuries and their mechanisms. *Life Sci.* 75(14):1701–11, (20 Aug 2004).
10. **Kiefer I. et al.** Supplementation with mixed fruit and vegetable juice concentrates increased serum antioxidants and folate in healthy adults. *J Am Coll Nutr.* 23(3):205–11, (June 2004).

# HIV and AIDS

1. **Sharpstone D.S. et al.** Energy balance in asymptomatic HIV infection. *AIDS.* 10:1377–84, (1996).
2. **Sharpstone D.S. et al.** The influence of nutrition and metabolic status on progression from asymptomatic HIV infection to AIDS-defining diagnosis. *AIDS.* 13:1221–6, (1999).
3. **Kruzich L.A. et al.** US youths in the early stages of HIV disease have low intakes of some micronutrients important for optimal immune function. *J Am Diet Assoc.* 104(7):1095–101, (July 2004).
4. **Hadigan C.** Dietary habits and their association with metabolic abnormalities in human immunodeficiency virus-related lipodystrophy. *Clin Infect Dis.* 37 (Suppl 2):S101–4, (2003).

# Homocysteine

1. **Rosenquist T.H., Finnell R.H.** Genes, folate and homocysteine in embryonic development *Proc Nutr Soc.* 60(1):53–61, (2001).
2. **Vollset S.E. et al.** Plasma total homocysteine, pregnancy complications and adverse pregnancy outcomes: the Hordaland Homocysteine Study. *Am J Clin Nutr.* 71:962–8, (2000).
3. **Nygard O. et al.** Coffee consumption and plasma total homocysteine: The Hordaland Homocysteine Study. *Am J Clin Nutr.* 65(1): 136–43, (1997).
4. **Waldmann A. et al.** Homocysteine and cobalamin status in German vegans. *Public Health Nutr.* 7(3):467–72, (May 2004).
5. **Vrentzos G.E. et al.** Diet, serum homocysteine levels and ischaemic heart disease in a Mediterranean population. *Br J Nutr.* 91(6):1013–9, (June 2004).
6. **Wald D.S. et al.** The dose-response relation between serum homocysteine and cardiovascular disease: implications for treatment and screening. *Eur J Cardiovasc Prev Rehabil.* 11(3):250–3, (June 2004).

# Hyperactivity (ADD and ADHD)

1. **Hyperactive Children's Support Group.** Tel: 01243 551 313 www.hacsg.org.uk

2. **Stevens L. et al.** EFA supplementation in children with inattention, hyperactivity and other disruptive behaviours. *Lipids.* 38:1007–1021, (2003).

3. **Richardson A.J., Puri B.K.** A randomized double-blind placebo-controlled study of the effects of supplementation with highly unsaturated fatty acids on ADHD-related symptoms in children with specific learning disorders. *Prgo Neuro-Psychopharmacol Biol Psychiatry.* 26:233–9, (2001).

4. **Bateman B. et al.** The effects of a double-blind, placebo-controlled, artificial food colourings and benzoate preservative challenge on hyperactivity in a general population sample of preschool children. *Arch Dis Child.* 89(6):506–11, (June 2004).

# Indigestion

1. **Marakis G. et al.** Artichoke leaf extract reduces mild dyspepsia in an open study. *Phytomedicine.* 9:694–9, (2002).

2. **Bhamarapravati S. et al.** Extracts of spice and food plants from Thai traditional medicine inhibit the growth of the human carcinogen Helicobacter pylori. *In Vivo.* 17(6):541–4, (Nov–Dec 2003).

3. **Feinle-Bisset C. et al.** Diet, food intake, and disturbed physiology in the pathogenesis of symptoms in functional dyspepsia. *Am J Gastroenterol.* 99(1):170–81, (Jan 2004).

# Infections, Frequent

1. **Gill H.S. et al.** Enhancement of immunity in the elderly by dietary supplementation with the probiotic Bifidobacterium lactis HN019. *Am J Clin Nutr.* 74(6):833–9, (2001).

2. **Sheih Y.H. et al.** Systemic immunity-enhancing effects in healthy subjects following dietary consumption of the lactic acid bacterium Lactobacillus rhamnosus HN001. *J Am Coll Nutr.* 20 (2 Suppl):149–56, (2001).

# Inflammation

1. **Calder P.C.** n-3 Polyunsaturated fatty acids and inflammation from molecular biology to the clinic. *Lipids.* 38:343–52.

2. **Simopoulos A.P.** Omega-3 fatty acids in inflammation and autoimmune diseases. *J Am Coll Nutr.* 21(6):495–505, (2002).

3. **Calder P.C.** Polyunsaturated fatty acids, inflammation and immunity. *Lipids.* 36(9):1007–24, (2001).

4. **James M.J. et al.** Dietary polyunsaturated fatty acids and inflammatory mediator production. *Am J Clin Nutr.* 71(Suppl):343S–8S, (2000).

5. **Grimble R.F.** Inflammatory response in the elderly. *Curr Opin Clin Nutr Metab Care.* 6(1):21–9, (2003).

## Insulin Resistance

1. **Hawley J.A.** Exercise as a therapeutic intervention for the prevention and treatment of insulin resistance. *Diabetes Metab Res Rev.* 20(5): 383–93, (Sep–Oct 2004).

2. **Lee W.Y. et al.** C-reactive protein concentrations are related to insulin resistance and metabolic syndrome as defined by the ATP III report. *Int J Cardiol.* 97(1):101–6, (Oct 2004).

3. **Qin B., Nagasaki M. et al.** Cinnamon extract prevents the insulin resistance induced by a high-fructose diet. *Horm Metab Res.* 36(2): 119–25, (Feb 2004).

4. **Guerrero-Romero F. et al.** Oral magnesium supplementation improves insulin sensitivity in non-diabetic subjects with insulin resistance. A double-blind placebo-controlled randomized trial. *Diabetes Metab.* 30(3):253–8, (June 2004).

5. **Liese A.D. et al.** Whole-grain intake and insulin sensitivity: the Insulin Resistance Atherosclerosis Study. *Am J Clin Nutr.* 78(5):965–71, (Nov 2003).

## Kidney Health

1. **Hollingbery P.W., Massey L.K.** Effect of dietary caffeine and sucrose on urinary calcium excretion in adolescents. *Fed Proc* 1986;45:375 (abstr #1280).

2. **Curhan G.C. et al.** A Prospective study of dietary calcium and other nutrients and the risk of symptomatic kidney stones. *N Engl J Med* 1993:833–8.

3. **Robertson W.G. et al.** Prevalence of urinary stone disease in vegetarians. *Eur Urol* 1982:334–9.

4. **Silver J. et al.** Sodium-dependent idiopathic hypercalciuria in renalstone formers. *Lancet* 1983:484–6.

5. **Rodgers A.L., Lewandowski S.** Effects of 5 different diets on urinary risk factors for calcium oxalate kidney stone formation: evidence of different renal handling mechanisms in different race groups. *J Urol.* 2002;168(3):931–6.

6. **Curhan G.C. et al.** Beverage use and risk for kidney stones in women. *Ann Intern Med.* 128(7):534–40.

7. **McHarg T. et al.** Influence of cranberry juice on the urinary risk factors for calcium oxalate kidney stone formation. *BJU Int.* 92(7):765–8, (Nov 2003).

# Libido and Sexual Function

1. The Impotence Association, advice for women and men. www.impotence.org.uk

# Liver Health

1. **Lieber C.S. et al.** Silymarin retards the progression of alcoholinduced hepatic fibrosis. *J Clin Gastroenterol.* 37;336–9, (2003)

2. **Scadding G.K. et al.** Poor sulphoxidation ability in patients with food sensitivity. *BMJ.* 297:105–7, (1988).

3. **Speroni E. et al.** Efficacy of different Cynara scolymus preparations on liver complaints. *J Ethnopharmacol.* 86:203–11, (2003).

# Lung health

1. **Humiczewska M. et al.** The effect of the pollen extracts quercitin and cernitin on the liver, lungs, and stomach. *Folia Biol.* 42:157–66, (1994).

# Lupus (SLE)

1. **Danao-Camara T.C., Shintani T.T.** The dietary treatment of inflammatory arthritis: case reports and review of the literature. *Hawaii Med J.* 58:126–31, (1999).
2. **Kovacic P., Jacintho J.D.** Systemic lupus erythematosus and other autoimmune diseases from endogenous and exogenous agents: unifying theme of oxidative stress. *Mini Rev Med Chem.* 3:568–75, (2003).
3. **Shigemasa C. et al.** Effect of vegetarian diet on systemic lupus erythematosus. *Lancet.* 339:1177, (1992).


# Macular Degeneration, Age Related

1. **Blodi B.A.** Nutritional supplements in the prevention of age-related macular degeneration. *Insight.* 29:15–6, (2004).
2. **Clemons T.E. et al.; AREDS Research Group.** Associations of mortality with ocular disorders and an intervention of high-dose antioxidants and zinc in the Age-Related Eye Disease Study: AREDS Report No. 13. *Arch Ophthalmol.* 122:716–26, (2004).
3. **Mayo Clin Women's Healthsource.** Antioxidant supplements plus zinc may slow age-related macular degeneration. 6:3, (2002).
4. **Mitchell P. et al.** Nutritional factors in the development of age-related eye disease. *Asia Pac J Clin Nutr.* 12 (Suppl):S5, (2003).
5. **Mozaffarieh M. et al.** The role of the carotenoids, lutein and zeaxanthin, in protecting against age-related macular degeneration: A review based on controversial evidence. *Nutr J.* 2:20, (2003).
6. **Seddon J.M. et al.** Association between C-reactive protein and age-related macular degeneration. *JAMA.* 291:704–10, (2004).


# ME (Myalgic Encephalomyelitis)

1. **Lim A., Lubitz L.** Chronic fatigue syndrome: successful outcome of an intensive inpatient programme. *J Paediatr Child Health.* 38:295–9, (2002).
2. **Logan A.C., Wong C.** Chronic fatigue syndrome: oxidative stress and dietary modifications. *Altern Med Rev.* 6:450–9, (2001).

## Menopausal Symptoms

1. **Aldercreutz H. et al.** Dietary phyto-estrogens and the menopause in Japan. *Lancet.* 339:123, (1992).
2. **Murkies A.L. et al.** Postmenopausal hot flushes decreased by dietary flour supplementation: effects of soya and wheat. *Am J Clin Nutr.* 68(Suppl):1533S, (1998).


## Migraine

1. **Bianchi A. et al.** Role of magnesium, coenzyme Q10, riboflavin, and vitamin B12 in migraine prophylaxis. *Vitam Horm.* 69:297–312, (2004).
2. **Diener H.C. et al.** The first placebo-controlled trial of a special butterbur root extract for the prevention of migraine: reanalysis of efficacy criteria. *Eur Neurol.* 51:89–97, (2004).
3. **Rios J., Passe M.M.** Evidence-based use of botanicals, minerals, and vitamins in the prophylactic treatment of migraines. *J Am Acad Nurse Pract.* 16:251–6, (2004).


## Mood Swings

1. **Food and Mood Project.** Tel: 01273 478 108. www.foodandmood.org
2. **Lloyd H.M. et al.** Acute effects on mood and cognitive performance of breakfasts differing in fat and carbohydrate content. *Appetite.* 27:151–64, (1996).


## Multiple Sclerosis (MS)

1. **Munger K.L. et al.** Vitamin D intake and incidence of multiple sclerosis. *Neurology.* 62:60–5, (2004).
2. **Swank R.L.** Multiple sclerosis: fat-oil relationship. *Nutrition.* 7:368–76, (1991).
3. **Swank R.L., Goodwin J.** Review of MS patient survival on a Swank low saturated fat diet. *Nutrition.* 19:161–2, (2003).

# Nausea

1. **Willetts K.E. et al.** Effect of a ginger extract on pregnancy-induced nausea: a randomised controlled trial. *Aust N Z J Obstet Gynaecol.* 43(2):139–44, (April 2003).
2. **Lee A., Done M.** Stimulation of the wrist acupuncture point P6 for preventing postoperative nausea and vomiting. *Cochrane Database Syst Rev.* 3:CD003281, (2004).

# Neuropathy

1. **Koltringer P. et al.** Ginkgo biloba extract and folic acid in the therapy of changes caused by autonomic neuropathy. *Acta Med Austriaca.* 16(2):35–7, (1989).

# Osteoporosis

1. **Campion J.M., Maricic M.J.** Osteoporosis in men. *Am Fam Physician.* 1;67(7):1521–6, (2003).
2. **Chapuy M.C. et al.** Combined calcium and vitamin D3 supplementation in elderly women: confirmation of reversal of secondary hyperparathyroidism and hip fracture risk: the Decalyos II study. *Osteoporos Int.* 13(3):257–64, (2002).
3. **de Wardener H.E., MacGregor F.A.** Harmful effects of dietary salt in addition to hypertension. *J Hum Hypertens.* 16(4):213–23, (2002).
4. **Jugdaohsing et al.** Dietary silicon intake is positively associated with bone mineral density in men and premenopausal women of the Framingham Offspring Cohort. *J Bone Min Res.* 19:297–307, (2004).
5. **Lilliu H. et al.** Calcium-vitamin-D3 supplementation is cost-effective in hip fractures prevention. *Maturitas.* 25;44(4):299–305, (2003).
6. **New S.A.** Intake of fruit and vegetables: implications for bone health. *Proc Nutr Soc.* 62(4):889–99, (Nov 2003).
7. **American Academy of Pediatrics Committee on School Health.** Soft drinks in schools. *Pediatrics.* 113(1 Pt 1):152–4, (Jan 2004).
8. **Whiting S.J. et al.** Factors that affect bone mineral accrual in the adolescent growth spurt. *J Nutr.* 134(3):696S–700S, (March 2004).

## Otitis Media (Glue Ear)

1. **Arroyave C.M.** Recurrent otitis media with effusion and food allergy in pediatric patients. *Rev Alerg Mex.* 48(5):141–4, (Sep–Oct 2001).
2. **Tapiainen T. et al.** Ultrastructure of Streptococcus pneumoniae after exposure to xylitol. *J Antimicrob Chemother.* 54(1):225–8, (July 2004). (Epub 9 Jun 2004).

## Pain Management

1. **Tall J.M. et al.** Tart cherry anthocyanins suppress inflammation-induced pain behaviour in rats. *Behav Brain Res.* 153:181–8, (2004).
2. **Chrubasik S.** Devil's claw extract as an example of the effectiveness of herbal analgesics. 1: *Orthopade.* 33(7):804–8, (July 2004).
3. **Akhtar N.M. et al.** Oral enzyme combination versus diclofenac in the treatment of osteoarthritis of the knee – a double-blind prospective randomized study. *Clin Rheumatol.* (Jul 24 2004, Epub ahead of print).
4. **Walker A.F. et al.** Bromelain reduces mild acute knee pain and improves well-being in a dose-dependent fashion in an open study of otherwise healthy adults. *Phytomedicine.* 9(8):681–6, (Dec 2002).

## Pancreatitis

1. **Kuklinsky B., Schweder R.** Acute pancreatitis, a free radical disease; reducing the lethality with sodium selenite and other antioxidants. *J Nutr Environm Med.* 6:393–4, (1996).
2. **Takabayashi F. et al.** The effects of green tea catechins (Polyphenon) on DL-ethionine-induced acute pancreatitis. *Pancreas.* 11(2):127–31, (Aug 1995).

## Parkinson's Disease

1. **Coimbra C.G., Junqueira V.B.** High doses of riboflavin and the elimination of dietary red meat promote the recovery of some motor functions in Parkinson's disease patients. *Braz J Med Biol Res.* 36:1409–17, (2003).

2. **Swerdlow R.H.** Is NADH effective in the treatment of Parkinson's Disease? *Drugs Aging.* 13:26–8, (1998).
3. **Shults C.W. et al.** Pilot trial of high dosages of coenzyme Q10 in patients with Parkinson's disease. *Exp Neurol.* 188(2):491–4, (Aug 2004).
4. **Barnham K.L. et al.** Neurodegenerative diseases and oxidative stress. *Nat Rev Drug Discov.* 3(3):205–14, (March 2004).

## PCOS (Polycystic Ovarian Syndrome)

1. **Thys-Jacobs S. et al.** Vitamin D and calcium dysregulation in the polycystic ovarian syndrome. *Steroids.* 64:430–5, (1999).
2. **Guzick D.S. et al.** Endocrine consequences of weight loss in obese, hyperandrogenic, anovulatory women. *Fertil Steril.* 61(4):598–604, (1994).
3. **Norman R.J. et al.** The role of lifestyle modification in polycystic ovary syndrome. *Trends Endocrinol Metab.* 13:251–7, (2002).

## Pre-conceptual Care

1. **Wynn M., Wynn A.** *The case for preconception care of men and women.* AB Academic Publishers, Oxon, UK. pp. 46–8, 78, 136, (1991).

## Pregnancy

1. **Royal College of Obstetrics and Gynaecology.** *Periconceptual folic acid and food fortification in the prevention of neural tube defects.* Scientific Advisory Committee – Opinion Paper 4. www.rcog.org.uk (April 2003).
2. **Doyle W. et al.** The association between maternal diet and birth dimensions. *J Nutr Health.* 1:9–17, (1990).
3. **Wong W.Y. et al.** Nonsyndromic orofacial clefts: association with maternal hyperhomocysteinemia. *Teratology.* 60(5):253–7, (1999).
4. **Vollset S.E. et al.** Plasma total homocysteine, pregnancy complications and adverse pregnancy outcomes: the Hordaland Homocysteine Study. *Am J Clin Nutr.* 71:962–8, (2000).
5. **Poston L. Chappell L.C.** Is oxidative stress involved in the aetiology of pre-eclampsia? *Acta Paediatr Suppl.* 436:3–5, (2001).
6. **Rayman M.P. et al.** Comparison of selenium levels in pre-eclampsic and normal pregnancies. *Biol Trace Element Res.* 55:9–20, (1996).

7. **Rayman M.P. et al.** Low Selenium status is associated with the occurrence of the pregnancy disease pre-eclampsia in women from the United Kingdom. *Am J Obstet Gynecol.* 189(5): 1343–9, (2003).

8. **Clausen T. et al.** High intake of energy, sucrose, and polyunsaturated fatty acids is associated with increased risk of preeclampsia. *Am J Obstet Gynecol.* 185(2):451–8, (2001).

9. **Chappell L.C. et al.** Effects of antioxidants on the occurrence of pre-eclampsia in women at increased risk: a randomised trial. *Lancet.* 354(9181):810–6, (1999).

# Pre-menstrual Symptoms

1. **de Souza M., Walker A.F.** Premenstrual syndrome: Nutritional aspects and management. *Encyclopedia of Human Nutrition,* Vol 3. Academic Press, (1999).

2. **London R.S. et al.** Effect of a nutritional supplement on premenstrual symptomatology in women with premenstrual syndrome: a double-blind longitudinal study. *J Am Coll Nutr.* 10:494–9, (1991).

3. **Schellenberg R.** Treatment for the premenstrual syndrome with agnus castus fruit extract: prospective, randomised, placebo controlled study. *BMJ.* 322:134–7, (2001).

4. **Thys-Jacobs S.** Micronutrients and the premenstrual syndrome: the case for calcium. *J Am Coll Nutr.* 19:220–7, (2000).

5. **Wyatt K M, et al.** Efficacy of vitamin B-6 in the treatment of premenstrual syndrome: systematic review. *BMJ.* 318:1375–81, (1999).

# Prostate Health

1. **Klein E.A., Thompson I.M**. Update on chemoprevention of prostate cancer. *Curr Opin Urol.* 14:143–9, (2004).

2. **Leitzmann M.F. et al.** Dietary intake of n-3 and n-6 fatty acids and the risk of prostate cancer. *Am J Clin Nutr.* 80(1):204–16, (July 2004).

3. **Wilt T. et al.** Serenoa repens for benign prostatic hyperplasia. *Cochrane Database Syst Rev.* (3):CD001423, (2002).

# Psoriasis

1. **Mayser P. et al.** n-3 fatty acids in psoriasis. *Br J Nutr.* 2002 1987 Suppl 1:S77–82, (2002).
2. **Michaelsson G. et al.** Gluten-free diet in psoriasis patients with antibodies to gliadin results in decreased expression of tissue transglutaminase and fewer Ki67+ cells in the dermis. *Acta Derm Venereol.* 83(6):425–9, (2003).

# Raynaud's Syndrome

1. **DiGiacomo R.A. et al.** Fish-oil dietary supplementation in patients with Raynaud's phenomenon: a double-blind, controlled, prospective study. *Am J Med.* 86(2):158–64, (Feb 1989).
2. **Muir A.H. et al.** The use of Ginkgo biloba in Raynaud's disease: a double-blind placebo-controlled trial. *Vasc Med.* 7(4):265–7, (2002).
3. **Leppert J. et al.** The concentration of magnesium in erythrocytes in female patients with primary Raynaud's phenomenon; fluctuation with the time of year. *Angiology.* 45(4):283–8, (April 1994).

# Seasonal Affective Disorder (SAD)

1. **Cott J., Hibbeln J.R.** Lack of seasonal mood change in Icelanders. *Am J Psychiatry.* 158:328, (2001).
2. **Christensen L.** The effect of carbohydrates on affect. *Nutrition.* 13(6):503–14, (June 1997).
3. **Partonen T.** Possible pathophysiological mechanisms regulating food intake in seasonal affective disorder. *Med Hypotheses.* 47(3):215–6, (Sept 1996).
4. **Levitan R.D. et al.** Characterization of the 'seasonal' bulimic patient. *Int J Eat Disord.* 19(2):187–92, (March 1996).

# Stroke

1. **Keli S.O. et al.** Dietary flavonoids, antioxidant vitamins and incidence of stroke: the Zutphen study. *Arch Intern Med.* 156:637–42, (1996).

2. **Gariballa S.E.** Nutritional factors in stroke. *Br J Nutr.* 84(1):5–17, (July 2000).

3. **He K. et al.** Folate, vitamin B6, and B12 intakes in relation to risk of stroke among men. *Stroke.* 35(1):169–74, (Jan 2004), (Epub 11 Dec 2003).

4. **Jeerakathil T.J., Wolf P.A.** Prevention of strokes. *Curr Atheroscler Rep.* 3(4):321–7, (July 2001).

# Thyroid, Overactive

1. **Vrca V.B. et al.** Supplementation with antioxidants in the treatment of Graves' disease; the effect on glutathione peroxidase activity and concentration of selenium. *Clin Chim Acta.* 341(1–2):55–63, (March 2004).

# Thyroid, Underactive

1. **Chanoine J.P.** Selenium and thyroid function in infants, children and adolescents. *Biofactors.* 19(3–4):137–43, (2003).

2. **Lee K. et al.** Too much versus too little: the implications of current iodine intake in the United States. *Nutr Rev.* 57(6):177–81, (1999).

3. **Cikim A.S. et al.** Evaluation of endothelial function in subclinical hypothyroidism and subclinical hyperthyroidism. *Thyroid.* 14(8):605–9, (Aug 2004).

# Ulcers – Leg

1. **Lusby P.E. et al.** Honey: a potent agent for wound healing? *J Wound Ostomy Coninence Nurs.* 29:295–300. *Crit Rev Food Sci Nutr.* 42(3 Suppl):279–84, (2002). Inhibition of Helicobacter pylori adhesion to human gastric mucus by a high-molecular-weight constituent of cranberry juice. Burger O., Weiss E., Sharon N., Tabak M., Neeman I., Ofek I.

2. **Stotts N.A, Hopf H.W.** The link between tissue oxygen and hydration in nursing home residents with pressure ulcers: preliminary data. *J Wound Ostomy Continence Nurs.* 30(4):184–90, (July 2003).

3. **Schmidt T.** Pressure ulcers. Nutrition strategies that make a difference. *Caring*, 21(6):18–24, (June 2002).

## Ulcers – Oral, Gastric and Duodenal

1. **al Somal N. et al.** Susceptibility of Helicobacter pylori to the antibacterial activity of manuka honey. *J R Soc Med*. 87:9–12, (1994).
2. **Pantoflickova D. et al.** Favourable effect of regular intake of fermented milk containing Lactobacillus johnsonii on Helicobacter pylori associated gastritis. *Aliment Pharmacol Ther*. 18:805–13, (2003).
3. **Segawa K., Nakazawa S., Tsukamoto Y., Kurita Y., Goto H., Fukui A., Takano K.** Peptic ulcer is prevalent among shift workers. *Dig Dis Sci*. 32(5):449–53, (May 1987).
4. **Avijgan M.** Phytotherapy: an alternative treatment for non-healing ulcers, *J Wound Care*. 13(4):157–8, (April 2004).
5. **Morton C.A. et al.** Contact sensitivity to menthol and peppermint in patients with intra-oral symptoms. *Contact Dermatitis*. 32(5):281–4, (May 1995).

## Varicose Veins

1. **Iannuzzi A., et al.** Varicose veins of the lower limbs and venous capacitance in postmenopausal women: relationship with obesity. *J Vasc Surg*. 36(5):965–8, (Nov 2002).
2. **MacKay D.** Haemorrhoids and varicose veins: a review of treatment options. 1: *Altern Med Rev*. 6(2):126–40, (April 2001).

## Vegetarianism and Veganism

1. **Donovan U.M., Gibson R.S.** Dietary intakes of adolescent females consuming vegetarian, semi-vegetarian, and omnivorous diets. *J Adolesc Health*. 18(4):292–300, (1996).
2. **Neumark-Sztainer D. et al.** Adolescent vegetarians. A behavioural profile of a school-based population in Minnesota. *Arch Pediatr Adolesc Med*. 151(8):833–8, (1997).

3.  **Millward D.J.** The nutritional value of plant-based diets in relation to human amino acid and protein requirements. *Proc Nutr Soc.* 58(2): 249–60, (1999).

4.  **Millward D.J.** Meat or wheat for the next millennium? *Proc Nutr Soc.* 58(2):209–10, (1999).

5.  **Sanders T.A.** The nutritional adequacy of plant-based diets. *Proc Nutr Soc.* 58(2):265–9, (1999).

6.  **Mangels A.R., Messina V.** Considerations in planning vegan diets: infants. *J Am Diet Assoc.* 101(6):670–7, (2001).

7.  **Harvard Health Letter.** Vegetarianism: addition by subtraction. An increasing number of studies are finding health benefits from a low- or no-meat diet. 29(4):6, (2004).

# Weight-Loss Diets

1.  **Hays N.P. et al.** Effects of ad-libitum low-fat, high carbohydrate diet on body weight, body composition and fat distribution in older men and women. *Arch Int Med.* 164:210–7, (2004).

2.  **Prentice A.M., Jebb S.A.** Trends in diet and activity in relation to obesity in Britain. *BMJ.* 311:437–9, (1995).

3.  **Prentice A.M., Jebb S.A.** Beyond body mass index. *Obesity Rev.* 2:141–7, (2001).

4.  **Slentz C.A. et al.** Effects of the amount of exercise on body weight, body composition and measures of central obesity. *Arch Int Med.* 164:31–9, (2004).

5.  **Stern L. et al.** The effects of low-carbohydrate versus conventional weight loss diet in severely obese adults: one year follow-up of a randomized trial. *Ann Int Med.* 140:778–85, (2004).

6.  **Stubbs R.J. et al.** Carbohydrate, appetite and feeding behaviour in humans. Symposium: Carbohydrates – Friend or Foe? American Society for Nutritional Sciences. *J Nutr.* 131:2775S–2781S, (2001).

7.  **Treuth M.S. et al.** Metabolic adaptation to high-fat and high-carbohydrate diets in children and adolescents. *Am J Clin Nutr.* 77(2):479–89, (2003).

8.  **Yancy W.S. et al.** A low-carbohydrate, ketogenic diet versus a low-fat diet to treat obesity and hyperlipidemia. *Ann Int Med.* 140:769–777, (2004).

## Appendix II: Salt – Reducing Intake

**CASH (Consensus on Salt and Health).** Tel: 020 8725 2409
www.hyp.ac.uk/cash
**Government website:** www.salt.gov.uk

## Appendix IV: Supplement Safety

1. **Awang D.V., Fugh-Berman A.** Herbal interactions with cardio-vascular drugs. *J Cardiovasc Nurs.* 16:64–70, (2002).
2. **Booth S.L., Centurelli M.A.** *Nutrition Reviews.* Vitamin K: a practical guide to the dietary management of patients on Warfarin. 57(9Pt1):288–96, (Sept 1999).
3. **Couris R.R. et al.** *Journal of the American College of Nutrition.* Assessment of healthcare professionals' knowledge about Warfarin-vitamin K drug-nutrient interactions. 19(4):439–45, (Aug 2000).
4. **Dahan A., Altman H.** Food-drug interactions: grapefruit juice augments drug bioavailability – mechanisms, extent and relevance. *Eur J Clin Nutr.* 58:1–9, (2004).
5. **EVM** 2002 – *Food Standards Agency, Draft Report of the Expert Group on Vitamins and Minerals* (EVM) www.foodstandards.gov.uk/science/ouradvisors/vitandmin/evmreport
6. **Harris J.E.** *Journal of the American Dietetic Association.* Interaction of dietary factors with oral anticoagulants: reviews and applications. 95(5):580–4, (May 1995).
7. **Kim J.M., White R.H.** *American Journal of Cardiology.* Effect of vitamin E on the anticoagulant response to Warfarin. 77:545–46, (1996).
8. **Lininger S.W.** (Editor in Chief). *A-Z guide to drug-herb-vitamin interactions.* Roseville, California, USA: Prima Health, (1999).
9. **Maka D.A., Murphy L.K.** *AACN Clinical Issues.* Drug-Nutrient Interactions: A review. 11(4):580–9, (Nov 2000).
10. **Roe D.A.** *Diet and drug interactions.* New York: Van Nostrand Reinhold, (1989).
11. **Thomas J.A., Burns R.A.** *Clinical Pharmacology.* Important drug-nutrient interactions in the elderly. 13(3):199–209, (Sept 1998).
12. **Welling P.G.** *Annual Review of Nutrition.* Effects of food on drug absorption. 16:383–415, (1996).

# Appendix V: Travel Advice

1. **O'Keeffe D.J., Baglin T.P.** Travellers' thrombosis and economy class syndrome: incidence, aetiology and prevention. *Clin Lab Haematol.* 25(5):277–81, (Oct 2003).

2. **Marteau P.R., de Vrese M., Cellir C.J., Schrezenmeir J.** Protection from gastrointestinal diseases with the use of probiotics. *Am J Clin Nutr.* 73(2 Suppl):430S–436S, (Feb 2001).

3. **Scarpignato C., Rampal P.** Prevention and treatment of traveler's diarrhea: a clinical pharmacological approach. *Chemotherapy.* 41 (Suppl) 1:48–81, (1995).

4. **Cesarini J.P., Michel L., Maurette J.M., Adhoute H., Bejot M.** Immediate effects of UV radiation on the skin: modification by an antioxidant complex containing carotenoids. *Photodermatol Photoimmunol Photomed.* 19(4):182–9, (Aug 2003).

5. **Danel T., Libersa C., Touitou Y.** The effect of alcohol consumption on the circadian control of human core body temperature is time dependent. *Am J Physiol Regul Integr Comp Physiol.* 281(1):R52–5, (July 2001).

6. **De Valck E., De Groot E., Cluydts R.** Effects of slow-release caffeine and a nap on driving simulator performance after partial sleep deprivation. *Percept Mot Skills.* 96(1):67–78, (Feb 2003).

# Index